The Boss Binder Table of Contents

My name is Eli Marini RN-BC,TNCC,CVC and I am the assembler of the Boss Binder. Prior to rising to the top of my nursing class with a 4.0 gpa and becoming a double board certified trauma and cardiovascular care nurse; I had previously dropped out of college 5 times. I knew that nursing school would be the hardest thing that I would probably ever do in my life. I knew that it was time to buckle down and take care of business. So many of my classmates would come to me and say “what do you do to study, I want to get the kind of scores you get”. The Boss Binder is a comprehensive compilation of study guides that encompasses the key points you need to know during nursing school. Unlike a traditional textbook it is a quick easy read that will not give you a headache. I have put everything I can into this study guide and I truly hope it changes your life in nursing school the way that it has changed mine. Don't get discouraged, don't ever give up, and don't ever let anyone tell you that your dreams of becoming a nurse will not happen. I hope that everything works out for you and that this study guide helps you .

THE B.U.R.P.S LIST

I. Roots

R/T Body Parts

Root	Meaning	Example(s)
Angi(o), Vas(o)	Blood vessel	Angioplasty, vasoconstriction
Brachi(o)	Arm	Brachial
Bucc(o)	Cheek	Buccal
Cardi(o)	Heart	Cardiopathy
Carp(o)	Wrist	Carpal tunnel syndrome
Cephal(o)	Head	Cephalic
Colp(o)	Vagina	Colposcopy
Crani(o)	Skull	Craniotomy
Cyst(o)	Bladder	Cystoscopy, cystitis
Cyto	Cell	Cytology, cytomegaly
Dactyl(o)	Finger, toe	Polydactyly
Encephal(o)	Brain	Encephalitis
Enter(o)	Intestine	Enteritis
Gloss(o)	Tongue	Glossitis, glossopharyngeal
Hemo, sanguin(o)	Blood	Hemolytic, serosanguinous
Hyster(o)	Womb, uterus	Hysterectomy
Mast(o), mamm(o)	Breast	Mastitis, mammography
Men(o)	Month, r/t menses	Menopause, menarche, dysmenorrheal
Nephr(o), Ren(o)	Kidney	Nephrectomy, renal
Oophor(o)	Ovary	Oopherectomy
Ophthalm, Ocul(o)	Eye	Ophthalmoscope, ocular
Ot(o), Auri, Aud	Ear	Otitis, auricle, audiometer
Phleb(o), Ven(o)	Vein	Phlebitis, venous
Pod	Foot	Podiatrist
Rhin(o)	Nose	Rhinoplasty, rhinorrhea
Salping(o)	Fallopian tube	Salpingectomy, salpingitis
Thorac(o)	Chest	Thoracotomy, thoracic
Thromb(o)	Clot	Thrombosis, thrombolytic

Other Roots

Root	Meaning	Example(s)
Gluc(o)	Sweet, sugar	Glucose, glucometer
Hydr(o)	Water	Hydrocephalus, hydrophobia
Lact(o)	Milk	Lactosuria, lactating
Lip(o), adip(o)	Fat	Lipoma, adipose
Therm	Heat	Hyperthermia

II. Prefixes

R/T Colors

Prefix	Meaning	Example(s)
Erythr(o)	Red	Erythema, erythrocyte
Leuk(o), leuc(o)	White	Leukocytes, leukemia
Cyan(o)	Blue	Cyanosis
Melan(o)	Black	Melanin
Cirrh(o)	Yellow	Cirrhosis

R/T Descriptions

Prefix	Meaning	Example(s)
Ankyl(o)	Stiff, fixed, crooked	Ankylosis
Sten(o), Stric	Narrow	Stenosis, stricture
Ortho	Straight position	Orthopnea, orthopedic
Kypho	Bent, crooked	Kyphoscoliosis, kyphosis
Pseudo	False	Pseudostrabismus, pseudoaneurysm

R/T Measurements

Prefix	Meaning	Example(s)
Macro	Large	Macrophage, macrocephaly
Micro	Small	Microscopic, microorganism
Poly, Hyper, Multi	Many, much	Polydypsia, hyperthyroidism, multiple
Brady	Slow	Bradypnea
Tachy	Fast	Tachycardia
Oligo, Hypo	Few	Oliguria, hypothermia
Iso	Equal	Isometric, isotonic
Diplo, Ambi	Both, double	Diplopia, ambidextrous
Hemi	Half	Hemiplegia, hemisphere
Pan	All	Pansystolic, pancytopenia

R/T Positions

Prefix	Meaning	Example(s)
Pro, Ante, Pre	Before	Prodromal, antepartum, precapillary
Post	After	Postnatal, posterior
Super, supra	Above	Superior, supraclavicular
Sub	Below	Submandibular, subcutaneous
Dors(o)	Back	Dorsoflexion, dorsal
Retro	Backwards	Retrograde, retrosternal
Para	Beside	Paramedic, paranasal
Re	Again	Rehydrate, recuperate
Later(o)	Side	Lateral
Medi(o)	Middle	Medial, mediastinum
Schizo	Split	Schizophrenia
Inter	Between	Intercostals, interdigital
Heter(o)	Different	Heterogeneous
Hom(o)	Same	Homozygous
Ad(o)	Towards	Adduction, adhesion, adrenal
Ab(o)	Away from	Abduction, abnormal
Anti, Contra	Against	Antigen, contraception
Endo, In, Intra	In, within, inside	Endocarditis, inhale, intrapartum
Ex(o), Ec(to)	Out	Exhale, ectopic
Epi	Upon, above	Epidermis, epigastric, epiglottis
Dia, Trans	Through	Diameter, transfusion
Peri, Circum	Around	Perinatal, circumcision
Sinister(a)	Left	OS (oculus sinister – left eye)
Dextr(o)	Right	OD (oculus dexter – right eye)

R/T the Body

Prefix	Meaning	Example(s)
Aden(o)	Gland	Adenoma, adenoids
Arthr(o)	Joint	Arthritis, arthroscopy
Cervic(o)	Neck	Cervical, cervicitis
Costo	Rib	Costochondritis, costovertebral
Cyto	Cell	Cytology, cytomegaly
Derm	Skin	Dermatitis, dermatological
Gastr(o)	Stomach	Gastritis, gastrointestinal
Glosso	Tongue	Glossopharyngeal, glossitis
Heme	Blood	Hematuria, hematemesis, hemangioma
Hepat(o)	Liver	Hepatitis, hepatocellular
Lingu	Tongue	Lingual, linguistic
Litho	Stone	Lithotomy, lithotripsy
My	Muscle	Myoma, myalgia
Myo, myel	Marrow	Myelitis
Neuro	Nerve	Neuromyalgia
Oto	Ear	Otitis, otolaryngology
Opti, Ocu	Eye	Optician, ocular
Osteo	Bone	Osteoarthritis, osteopenia
Pneum(o), Pulm	Lung	Pneumothorax, pulmonary
Psycho	Mind	Psychology, psychopath, psychosomatic
Rhino	Nose	Rhinorrhea, rhinitis
Thor(a)	Chest	Thoracic, thoracentesis
Vasc	Vessel	Vasculitis

Other Prefixes

Prefix	Meaning	Example(s)
A(n)	Without	Anemia, avascular
Auto	Self	Autoimmune
Dys	Difficult, painful	Dyspnea, dysuria
Gravida	Pregnant, heavy	Gravidity
Neo	New	Neonatal, neoplasm

III. Suffixes

R/T Surgery

Suffix	Meaning	Example(s)
Centesis	Tap, puncture	Thoracentesis
Ectomy	Removal	Mastectomy, appendectomy
Lysis	Separate, destroy	Hemolysis
Ostomy	Form an opening	Colostomy
Otomy	Cut into	Tracheotomy, craniotomy
Plasty	Repair	Rhinoplasty

R/T Diseases

Suffix	Meaning	Example(s)
Algia	Pain	Arthralgia, myalgia
Cele	Hernia, swelling	Hydrocele, cystocele
Emia	Blood	Leukemia, anemia
Gen	Producing	Carcinogen, allergen
Itis	Inflammation	Appendicitis, hepatitis

Megaly	Enlargement	Splenomegaly, hepatomegaly
Oid	Resemble	Fibroid, keloid
Oma	Tumor	Adenoma, myoma
Osis	Abnormal condition	Dermatosis
Pathy	Disease	Neuropathy, psychopathology
Penia	Deficiency	Cytopenia, thrombocytopenia
Phagia	Eating	Dysphagia
Phasia	Speech	Aphasia, dysphasia
Plegia	Paralysis	Paraplegia, quadriplegia
Phobia	Fear	Acrophobia, agoraphobia
Pnea	Air, breathing	Apnea, dyspnea, orthopnea
Rrhage	Burst forth	Hemorrhage
Rrhea	Flow, discharge	Diarrhea
Sclerosis	Hardening	Atherosclerosis
Spasm	Contraction	Bronchospasm
Troph(o)	Nourishment	Atrophy, hypertrophy
Uri(a)	Urine	Nocturia, dysuria

Other Suffixes

Suffix	Meaning	Example(s)
Gram	Picture, record	Electrocardiogram
Ology	Study of	Pathology, dermatology
Phon(o)	Sound	Egophony, bronchophony
Scope	Inspect	Microscope, laproscopic

TALK LIKE A NURSE

A-P	anterior-posterior	**BUN**	blood urea nitrogen
ASA	acetylsalicylic acid (aspirin)	**BX**	biopsy
A&W	alive & well	**c̄**	with (cum)
bid	2x/day (bis in dies)	**CA**	cancer
BKA	below-the-knee amputation (AKA-above)	**CABG**	coronary artery bypass graft
BM	bowel movement	**CAD**	coronary artery disease
BMI	body mass index	**CAGE**	cut down, annoyed, guilty, eye opener
BMR	basal metabolic rate	**CAM**	complementary alternative medicine
BPH	benign prostatic hypertrophy	**CBC**	complete blood count
BR	bed rest	**CBE**	clinical breast exam
BRP	bathroom privileges	**CC**	chief complaint
BS	bowel sounds	**cc**	cubic centimeter
BSE	breast self-examination	**CHF**	congestive heart failure
BSO	bilateral salpingo-oophorectomy	**cm**	centimeter

CN	cranial nerve
CNS	central nervous system
C/O	complains of
Copd	chronic obstructive Pulmonary Disease
C&S	culture & sensitivity
Csf	cerebrospinal fluid
Ct	computed(computerized) tomography
Cta	clear to auscultation
Cts	carpal tunnel syndrome
Cva	cerebrovascular accident (stroke)
Cxr	chest x-ray
D/C	Discharge, Discontinue
D & C	dilatation and curettage
DFA	difficulty falling asleep
DJD	degenerative joint disease
DM	diabetes mellitus
DNR	do not resuscitate
DOA	dead on arrival
DOB	date of birth
DOE	dyspnea on exertion
DPT	diphtheria-pertussis-tetanus (vaccine)
DSM	diagnostic & statistical manual
DTR	deep tendon reflexes
DVT	deep vein thrombosis
Dx	diagnosis
ECG	electrocardiogram (or EKG)
ED	emergency department
EEG	electroencephalogram-gram
EMA	early morning awakening
ENT	ears, nose, and throat
EOM	extraocular muscles or movement
ERT	estrogen replacement therapy
ESR	erythrocyte sedimentation rate
ESRD	end-stage renal disease
ETOH	ethanol (alcohol)
FB	foreign body
FBS	fasting blood sugar
FUO	fever of unknown origin
FX	fracture
GERD	gastroesophageal reflux disease
GI	gastrointestinal
GU	genitourinary
H&P	history and physical
HA	headache
HBP	high blood pressure
Hct	hematocrit
HEENT	head, eyes, ears, nose, throat
hgb	hemoglobin
Hib	hemophilus influenza B
h/o	history of (or Hx)
HOB	head of bed
HPI	history of present illness
HRT	hormone replacement therapy
hs	hour of sleep, bedtime
HTN	hypertension
I & D	incision and drainage
IM	intramuscular
I & O	intake and output
IV	intravenous
IVP	intravenous pyelogram
JCAHO	Joint Commission on Accreditation of Healthcare Organizations
JVD	jugular venous distention
KUB	kidney, ureter and bladder (x-ray)
KVO	keep vein open
LE	lower extremities
LFTs	liver function tests
LMP	last menstrual period
LNMP	last normal menstrual period

LOC	loss or level of consciousness
LP	lumbar puncture
MI	myocardial infarction (heart attack)
MMR	measles, mumps, and rubella (vaccine)
MMSE	mini mental state exam
MRI	magnetic resonance imaging
MS	mental status or multiple sclerosis
NAD	no acute or apparent distress
NGT	nasogastric tube
NKA	no known allergies
NKDA	no known drug allergies
NPO	nothing by mouth (non peros)
NSAID	nonsteroidal anti-inflammatory drug
NSR	normal sinus rhythm
NSS	normal saline solution
NV	nausea/vomiting
NVD	nausea, vomiting, diarrhea
NWB	non-weight bearing
OA	osteoarthritis
OC	oral contraceptives
od	right eye (ocular dexter)
OOB	out of bed
os	left eye (ocular sinister)
OT	occupational therapy
OTC	over-the-counter
ou	both eyes
$\bar{p}$	after
p.c.	after meals
PCN	penicillin
PE	physical examination or pulmonary embolism
PERRLA	pupils equal, round, reactive to light and accommodation
PID	pelvic inflammatory disease
PMH	past medical history
PMI	point of maximal impulse (apical pulse)
S/P	status post (after)
PND	paroxysmal nocturnal dyspnea or post nasal drip
PNS	peripheral nervous system
PPD	purified protein derivative (TB skin test)
pr	per rectum
PRN	as needed (pro re nata)
PROM	passive range of motion or premature rupture of membranes
PSA	prostate specific antigen (test)
PT	physical therapy
PTA	prior to admission
PUD	peptic ulcer disease
PVD	peripheral vascular disease
q4h	every 4 hours
q6h	every 6 hours
qam	every morning
qd	every day**
qh	every hour
qhs	every night
qid	4x/day
qod	every other day**
RA	rheumatoid arthritis or right atrium
RBC	red blood cell
REM	rapid eye movements
RLQ	right lower quadrant (RUQ, LLQ, LUQ)
R/O	rule out
ROM	range of motion or rupture of membranes
ROS	review of systems
RRR	regular rate & rhythm
R/T	related to
$\bar{s}$	without (sans)
SBE	subacute bacterial endocarditis
SC	subcutaneous
Sig	label
SL	sublingual
SOB	shortness of breath

sp.gr.	specific gravity
S.Q.	subcutaneous(ly)
S/S	signs and symptoms
STAT	immediately
STS	serological test for syphilis
Sx	symptoms
TCDB	turn, cough, deep breathe
TIA	transient ischemial attack (mini stroke)
tid	3x/day
TM	tympanic membrane
TMJ	temporomand-ibular joint
TNTC	too numerous to count
TPN	total parenteral nutrition
TURP	transurethral resection of prostate
TSE	testicular self- examination
UA	urinalysis

UE	upper extremities
URI	upper respiratory infection
UTI	urinary tract infection
VS	vital signs
VSS	vital signs stable
WBC	white blood cell
WD/WN	well developed, well nourished
WF/BF	white female/black female
WM/BM	white male/black male
WNL	within normal limits
y/o	years old
△	change

**** appear on the JCAHO "Do Not Use" list – should write out "daily" or "every other day"**

Caution against using: < or >

Head-to-Toe Nursing Assessment

The sequence for performing a head-to-toe assessment is:

- **Inspection**
- **Palpation**
- **Percussion**
- **Auscultation**

However, with ***the abdomen it is changed*** where auscultation is performed second instead of last. The order for the abdomen would be:

- **Inspection**
- **Auscultation**
- **Percussion**
- **Palpation (palpation and percussion are done last to prevent from altering bowel sounds)**

Provide privacy, perform hand hygiene, introduce yourself to the patient, and explain to the patient that you need to conduct a head-to-toe assessment

Ask the patient to confirm their name and date of birth by looking at the patient's wrist band (this helps assess orientation to person and confirms you have the right patient). In addition, ask the patient where they are, the current date, and current events (who is the president and vice president) etc.

Collect vital signs: heart rate, blood pressure, temperature, oxygen saturation, respiratory rate, pain level

NOTE: Before even assessing a body system, you are already collecting important information about the patient. For example, you should already be collecting the following information :

- Looking at the overall appearance of your patient: do they look their age, are they alert and able to answer your questions promptly or is there a delay?
- Does their skin color match their ethnicity; does the skin appear dry or sweaty?
- Is their speech clear (not slurred)?

- Do they easily get out of breath while talking to you (coughing etc.)?
- Any noted abnormalities?
- How is their emotion status (calm, agitated, stressed, crying, flat affect, drowsy)?
- Can they hear you well (or do you have to repeat questions a lot)?
- Normal posture?
- Abnormal smells?
- How is their hygiene?

Assess height and weight and calculate the patient's BMI (body mass index).

Below 18.5 = Underweight

18.5-24.9 = Normal weight

25.0-29.9 = Overweight

30.0 or Higher = Obese

Source: https://www.cdc.gov/healthyweight/assessing/bmi/adult_bmi/index.html

Then start with the hair and move down to the toes:

Head:

Inspect the face and hair:

- Inspect the overall appearance of the face (are the eyes and ears at the same level)?
- Is the head an appropriate size for the body?
- Is the face symmetrical.... no drooping of the face on one side (eyes or lips). This can happen in Bell's palsy or stroke.

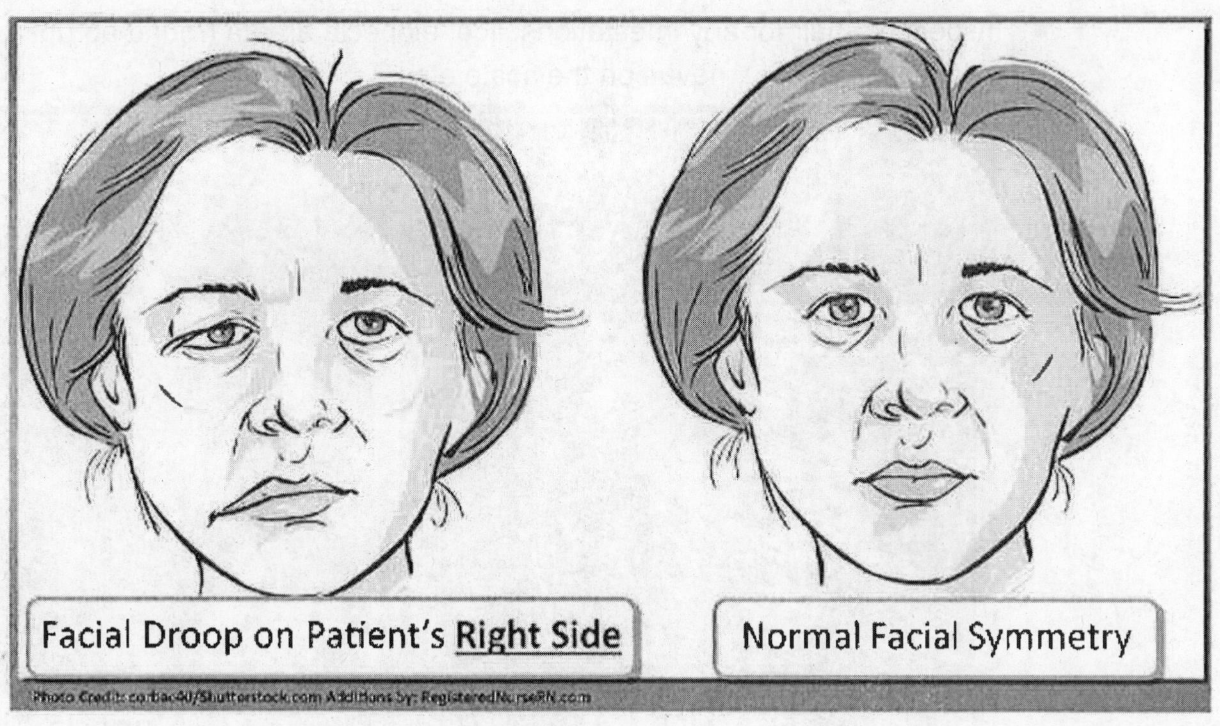

- Are the facial expressions symmetrical (no involuntary movements)?
- Any lesions?
- ***Test cranial nerve VII…facial nerve:*** have the patient close their eyes tightly, smile, frown, puff out cheek. Can they do this will ease?

Palpate the cranium and inspect the hair for infestations, hair loss, skin breakdown or abnormalities:

- Palpate for any masses or indentations
- Skin breakdown (especially on the back of the head in immobile patients)?

- Inspect the hair for any infestations: lice, alopecia areata (round abrupt balding in patches), nevus on the scalp etc.

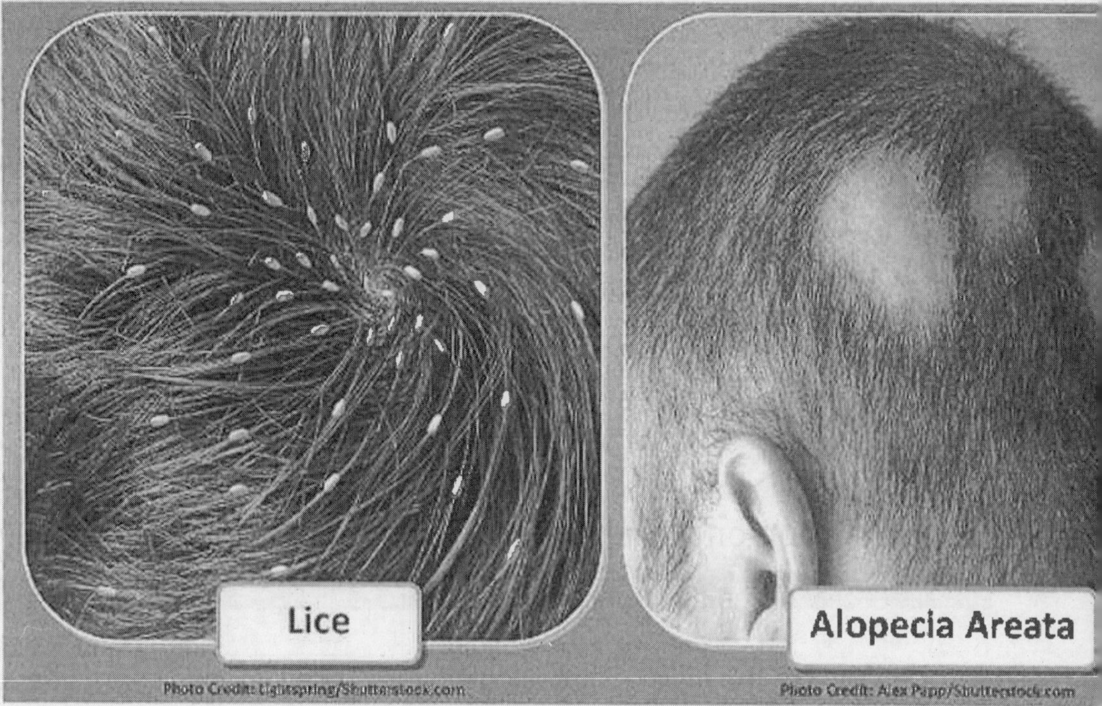

Palpate the temporal artery bilaterally

Test Cranial Nerve V.....trigeminal nerve: This nerve is responsible for many functions and mastication is one of them.

- Have the patient bite down and feel the masseter muscle and temporal muscle
- Then have the patient try to open the mouth against resistance

Palpate the temporomandibular joint for grating or clicking: Have the patient open and close the mouth and feel for any grating sensation or clicking.

Palpate the frontal and maxillary sinuses for tenderness: *patient will* pressure but should not feel pain

Eyes:

Inspect the eyes, eye lids, pupils, sclera, and conjunctiva

- Is there swelling of the eye lids?
- Is the sclera white and shiny?…not yellow as in jaundice

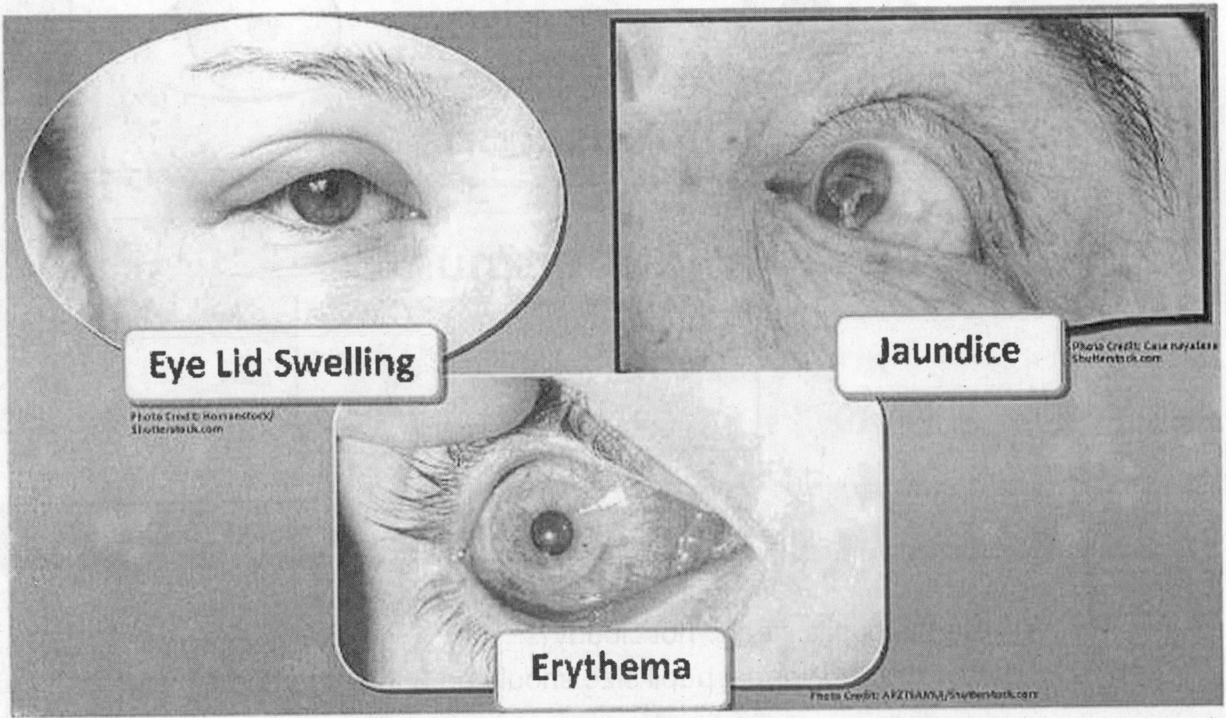

- Is the conjunctiva pink NOT red and swollen?
- Look for Strabismus and Aniscoria:
    - ***Strabismus***: Do the eyes line up with another?
    - ***Aniscoria***: Are the pupils equal in size…or is one pupil larger than the other?

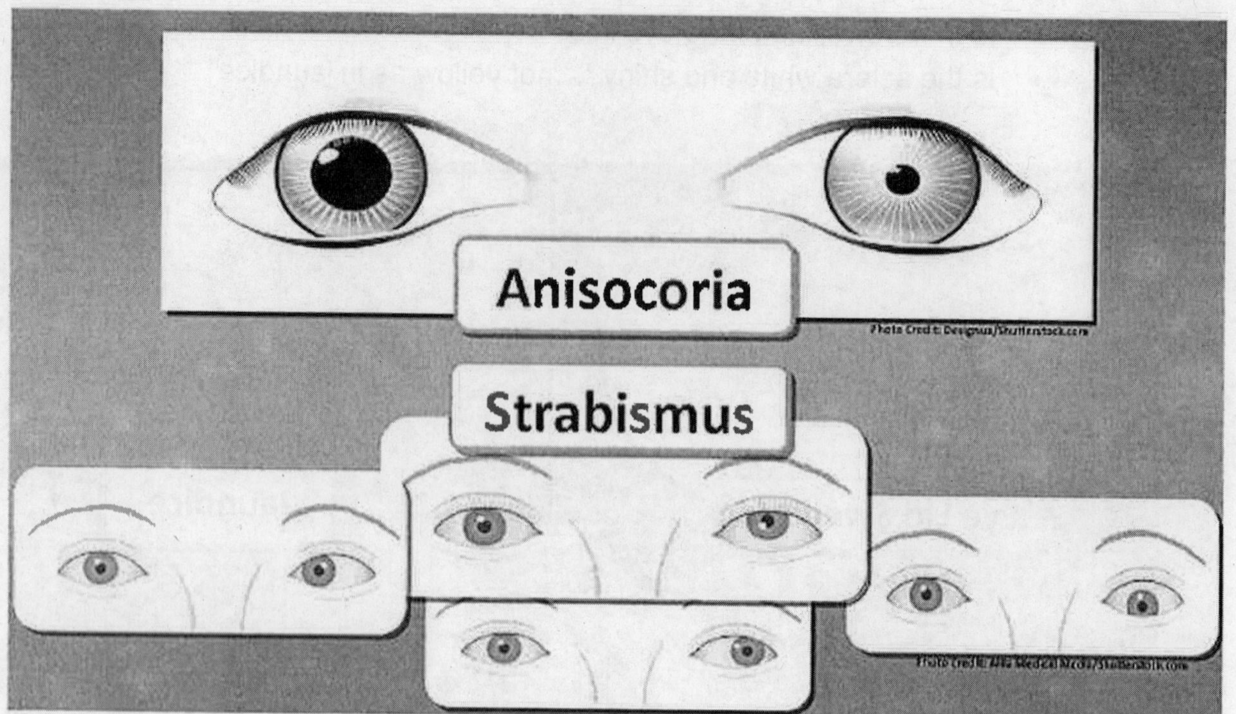

- Are the pupils clear…not cloudy?
    - Normal pupil size should be 3 to 5 mm and equal

Test cranial nerves III (oculomotor), IV (trochlear), VI (abducens)

- Have the patient follow your pen light by moving it 12-14 inches from the patient's face in the six cardinal fields of gaze (start in the midline)
    - Watch for any ***nystagmus*** (involuntary movements of the eye)
- **Reactive to light**?
    - Dim the lights and have the patient look at a distant object (this dilates the pupils)
    - Shine the light in from the side in each eye.
        - Note the pupil response: The eye with the light shining in it should constrict (note the dilatation size and response size (ex: pupil size goes from 3 to 1 mm) and the other side should constrict as well.
    - **Accommodation?**
        - Make the lights normal and have patient look at a distant object to dilate pupils, and then have

patient stare at pen light and slowly move it closer to the patient's nose.

- Watch the pupil response: The pupils should ***constrict and equally move to cross.***

If all these findings are normal you can document **PERRLA.**

Ears:

***Inspect the ears* for:**

- Drainage (ear wax) or abnormalities

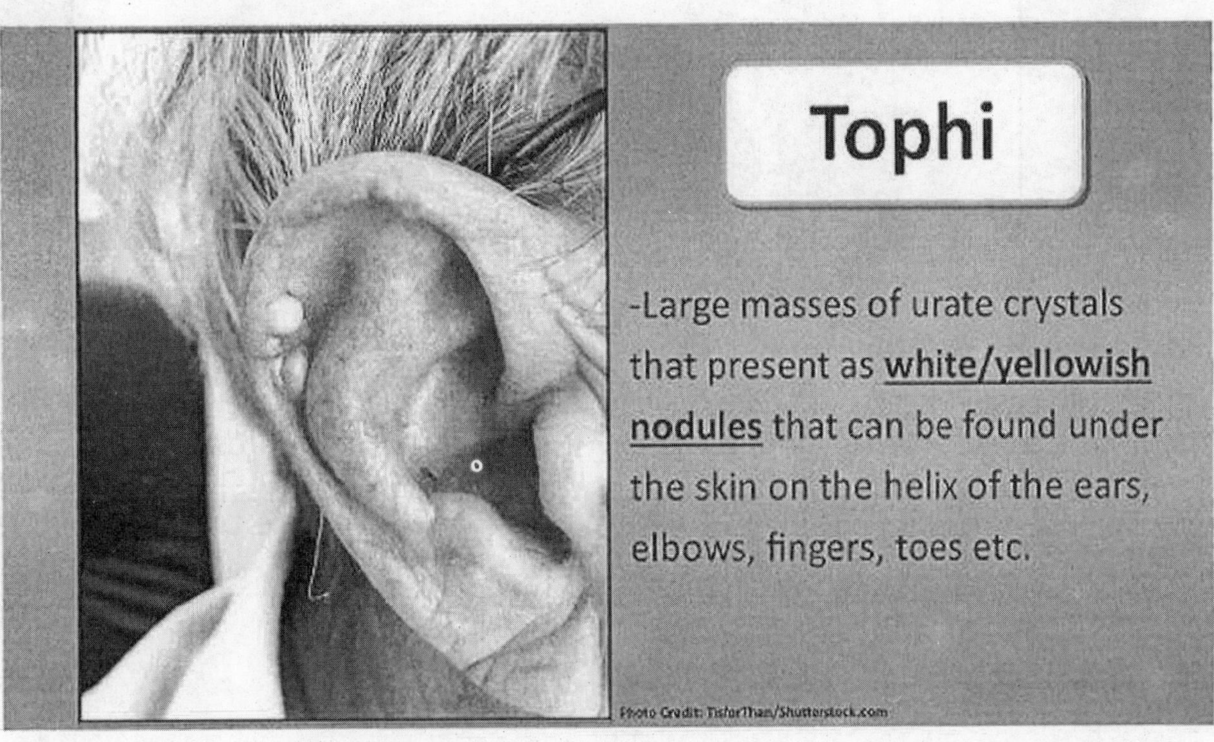

Tophi
-Large masses of urate crystals that present as white/yellowish nodules that can be found under the skin on the helix of the ears, elbows, fingers, toes etc.
Photo Credit: TisforThan/Shutterstock.com

- Ask the patient if they are experiencing any tenderness and palpate the pinna and targus.
- Palpate the mastoid process for swelling or tenderness.

Tests cranial nerve 8 VIII…vestibulocochlear nerve:

- Test the hearing by occluding one ear and whispering two words and have the patient repeat them back. Repeat this for the other ear.

Inspect the tympanic membrane:

- Use an otoscope to look at the tympanic membrane. It should appear as a pearly gray, translucent color and be shiny. Remember for an adult: pull up and back **and** for a child down and back on the pinna.
- Also, the cone of light should be at the 5:00 position in the right ear and 7:00 position in the left ear.

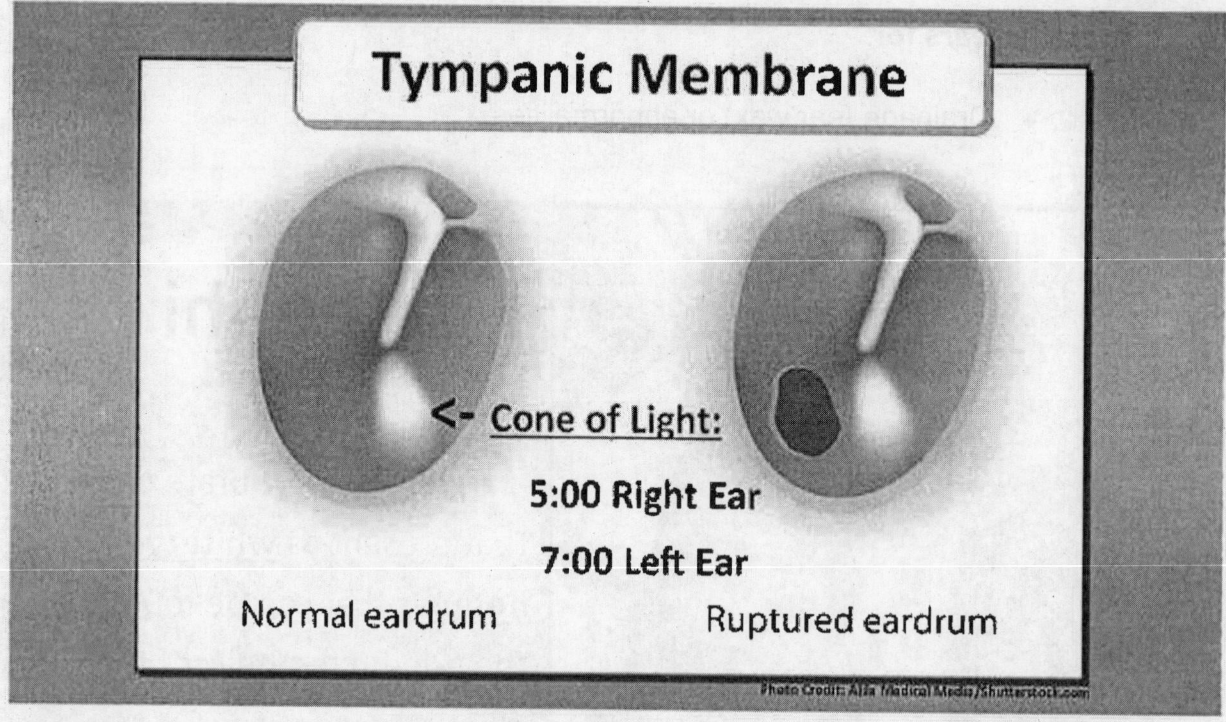

Nose:

Inspect nose

- Symmetrical (midline, look at septum for any deviation)
- Drainage (ask patient if they are having any discharge)
- Use a penlight to shine inside the nose and look for any lesions, redness, or polyps

- Then have the patient close one nostril and have the patient breathe out of it and do the same for the other…**are they patent?**

Test cranial nerve I……olfactory nerve: Have the patient close their eyes and place something with a pleasant smell under the nose and have them identify it.

Mouth:

Inspect lips (lip should be pink NOT dusky or blue/cyanotic or cracked, and free from lesions)

Inspect the inside of the mouth:

- Color of mucous membranes and gums should be pink and shiny. The teeth should be white and free from cavities. Note: any broken or loose teeth too.

Inspect tongue:

- Should be moist and pink (NOT dry or cracked or beefy red (pernicious anemia)
- Underneath the tongue should be no lesions or sores

Inspect hard and soft palate and tonsils (no exudate on tonsils) and uvula should be midline

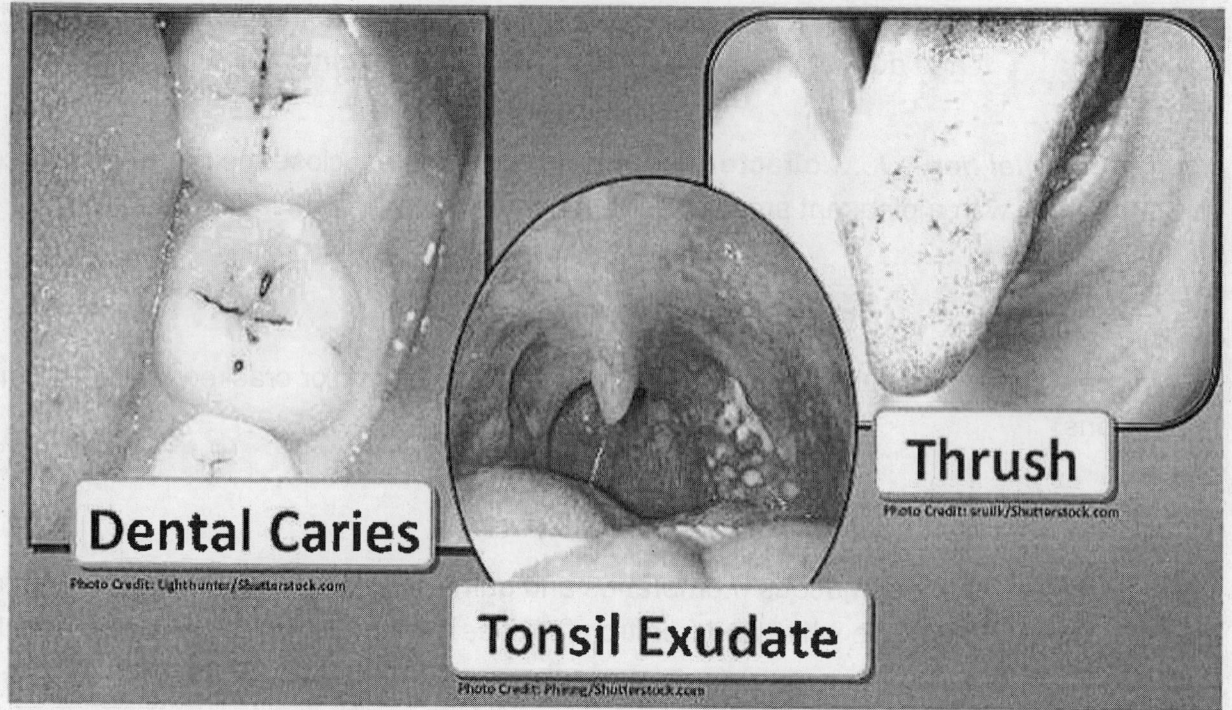

Test cranial nerve XII....hypoglossal: have patient stick tongue out and move it side to side

Test cranial nerve IX (glossopharyngeal) and X (vagus) have patient say "ah"...the uvula will move up (**cranial nerve IX intact**) and if the patient can swallow with ease and has no hoarseness when talking, **cranial nerve X is intact.**

<u>Neck:</u>

Inspect the trachea

- Is it midline, are there any lesions, lumps (goiter), or enlarged lymph nodes (have patient extend the neck up so you can access it better)?

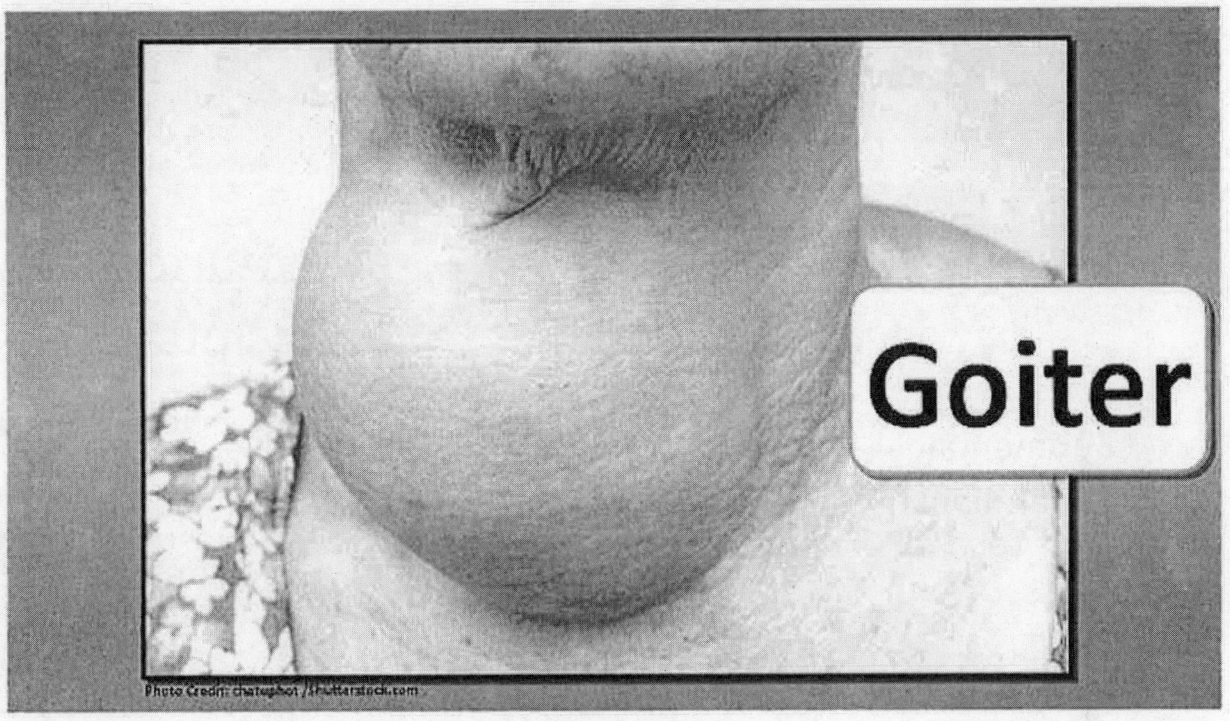

Test cranial nerve XI....accessory nerve: Have the patient move head from side to side and up and down and shrug shoulders against resistance.

Inspect for jugular vein distention

- Place the patient in supine positon at 45 degree angle and have them turn the head to the side and note any enlargement of the jugular vein.

Palpate the lymph nodes with the pads of fingers and feel for lumps, hard nodules, or tenderness:

- *Preauricular, postauricular, occipital, parotid, jugulodiagastric (tonsillar), submandibular, submental, superficial cervical, deep cervical chain, posterior cervical, supravclavicular*

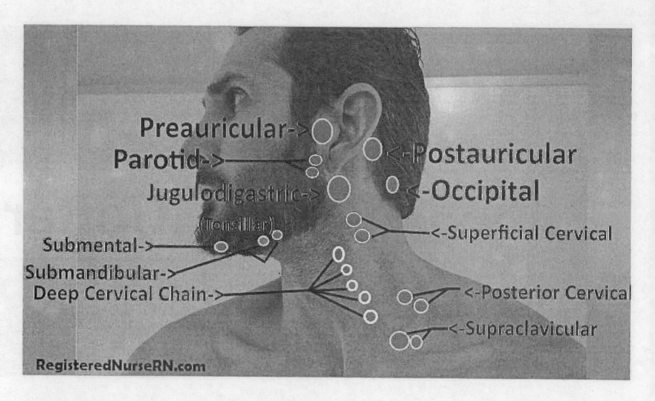

Palpate the trachea and confirm it is midline

Palpate thyroid gland from the back: note for nodules, tenderness or enlargement…normally can't palpate it.

Palpate the carotid artery (one side at a time) and grade it (0 to 4+….2+ is normal)

Auscultate for bruits at the carotid artery with BELL of stethoscope (listen for a swooshing sound which is a bruit)…have patient breathe in and out and hold it while listening.

Upper extremities:

Inspect arms and hands

- Deformities? (Heberden or Bouchard nodes as in osteoarthritis on fingers)

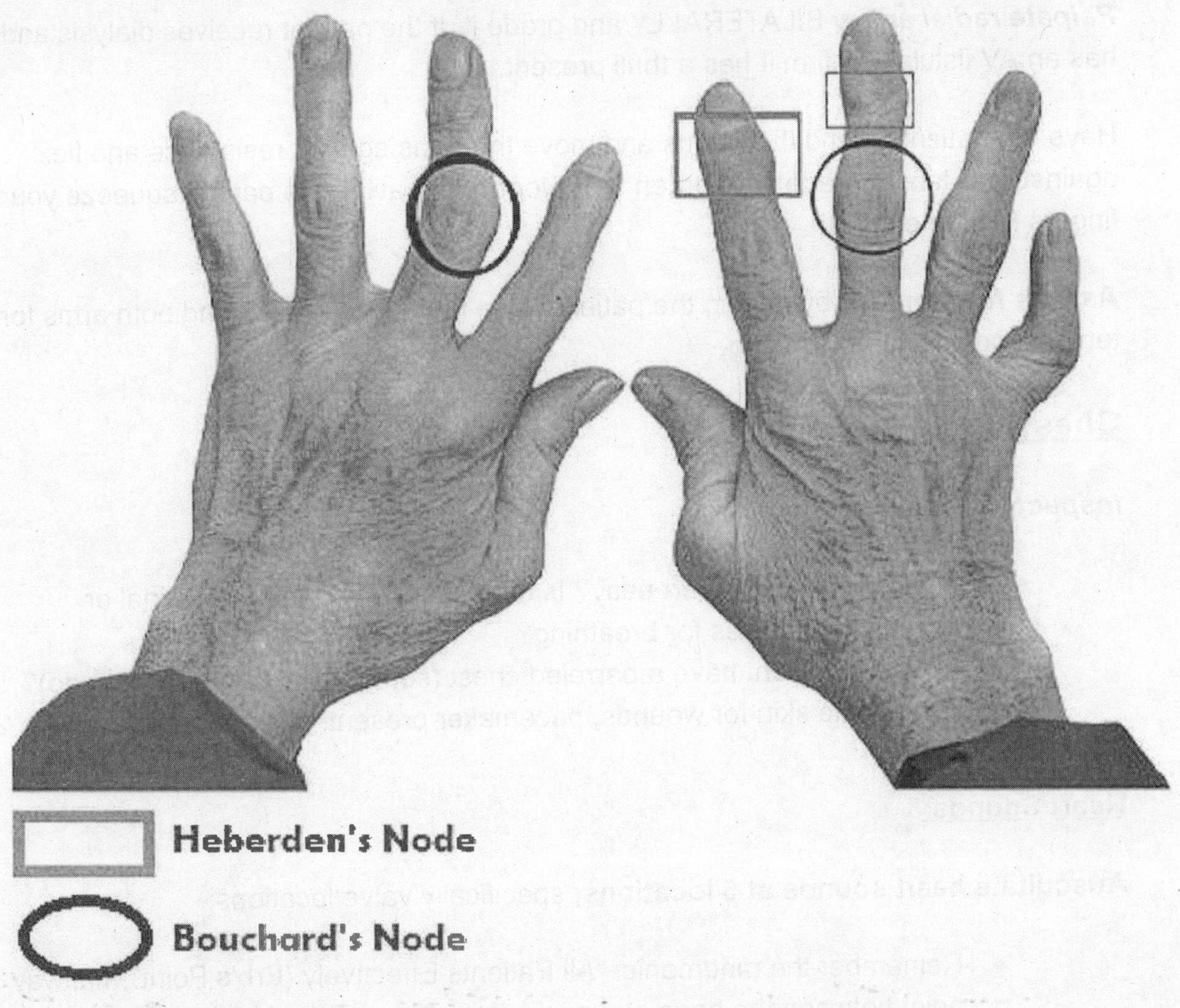

- Any wounds or IVs or central lines? (Assess for redness or drainage, expiration date etc.),
- Hand and fingernails for color: they should be pink and capillary refill should be less than 2 seconds
- Inspect joints for swelling or redness (rheumatoid arthritis or gout)
- Skin turgor (tenting)

Palpate joints (elbows, wrist, and hands) for redness and move the joints (note any decreased range of motion or crepitus)

Palpate skin temperature

Palpate radial artery BILATERALLY and grade it. If the patient receives dialysis and has an AV fistula, confirm it has a thrill present.

Have the patient extend their arms and move the arms against resistance and flex against resistance (grade strengthen 0-5) along with having the patient squeeze your fingers (note the grip).

Assess for arm drift by having the patient close their eyes and extend both arms for ten seconds. Note any drifting.

Chest:

Inspect the chest

- Is the respiratory effort easy? Is the patient using the abdominal or accessory muscles for breathing?
- Does the patient have a barreled chest (some patients with COPD do)?
- Assess the skin for wounds, pacemaker present, subcutaneous port etc.?

Heart Sounds:

Auscultate heart sounds at 5 locations, specifically valve locations:

- Remember the mnemonic: "All Patients Effectively (Erb's Point…halfway point between the base and apex of the heart) Take Medicine"
    - All: **A**ortic
    - Patients: **P**ulmonic
    - Effectively: **E**rb's Point (no valve at this location)
    - Take: **T**ricuspid
    - Medicine: **M**itral

Pulmonic: found left of the sternal border in the 2nd intercostal space REPRESENTS S2 "dub" which is the loudest.

Erb's Point: found left of the sternal border in the 3rd intercostal space…no valve here just the halfway point.

Tricuspid: found left of the sternal border in the 4th intercostal space REPRESENTS S1 "lub".

Mitral: found midclavicular in the 5th intercostal space REPRESENTS S1 "lub" (also the site of point of maximal impulse) APICAL PULSE….count pulse for 1 full minute.

Then listen with the ***BELL of the stethoscope*** at the same locations: for a blowing or swooshing noise…heart murmur.

Lung Sounds:

If you would like to hear some abnormal lung sounds, please watch our video called "abnormal lung sounds".

Auscultate anteriorly:

- Start at: the apex of the lung which is right above the clavicle
- Then move to the 2nd intercostal space to assess ***the right and left upper lobes.***
- Move to the 4th intercostal space, you will be assessing ***the right middle lobe and the left upper lobe.***
- Lastly move to the mid-axillary are at the 6th intercostal space and you will be assessing ***the right and left lower lobes.***

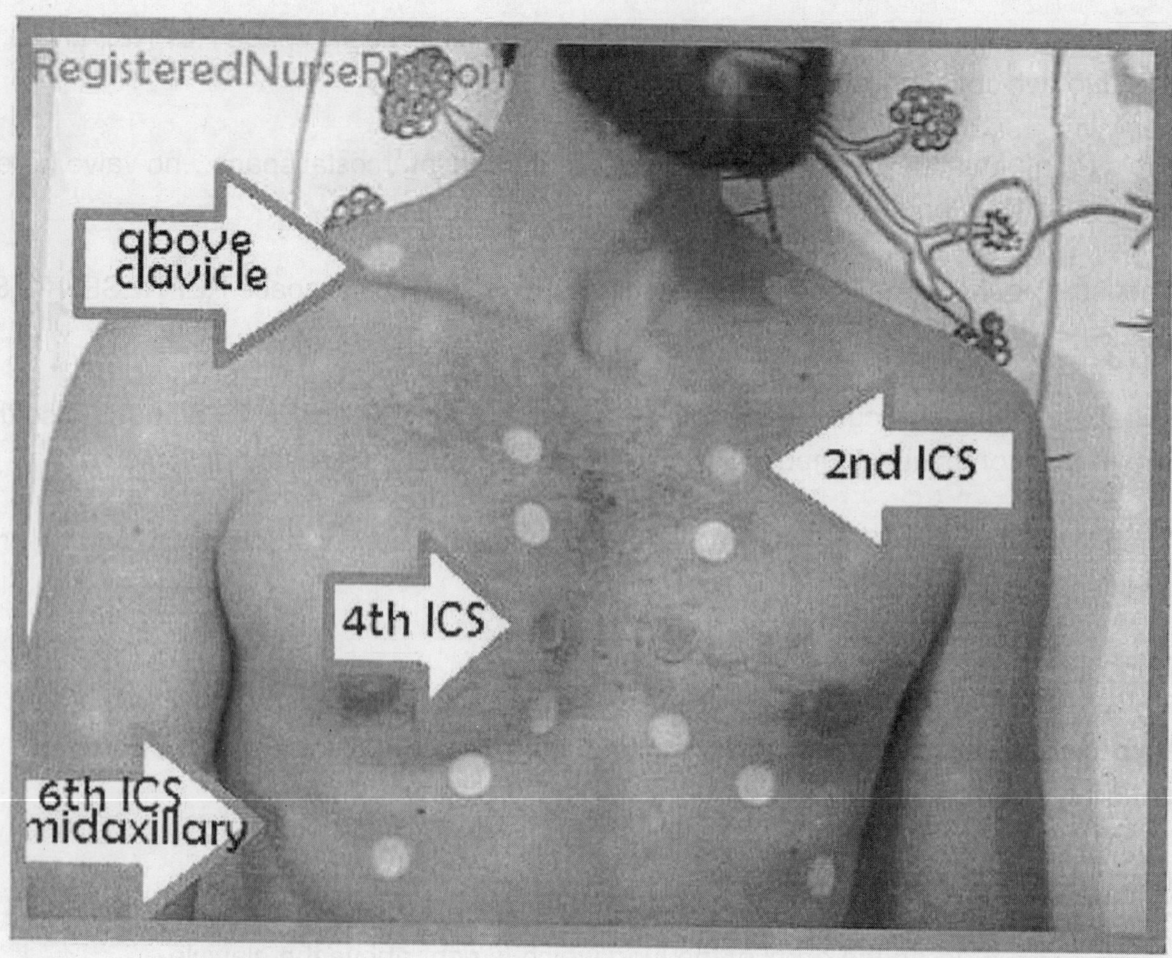

Auscultate posteriorly:

- Start right above the scapulae to listen to the apex of the lungs.
- Then find C7 (which is the vertebral prominence) and go to T3…in between the shoulder blades and spine. This will assess the right and left upper lobes.
- Then from T3 to T10 you will be able to assess the right and left lower lobes.

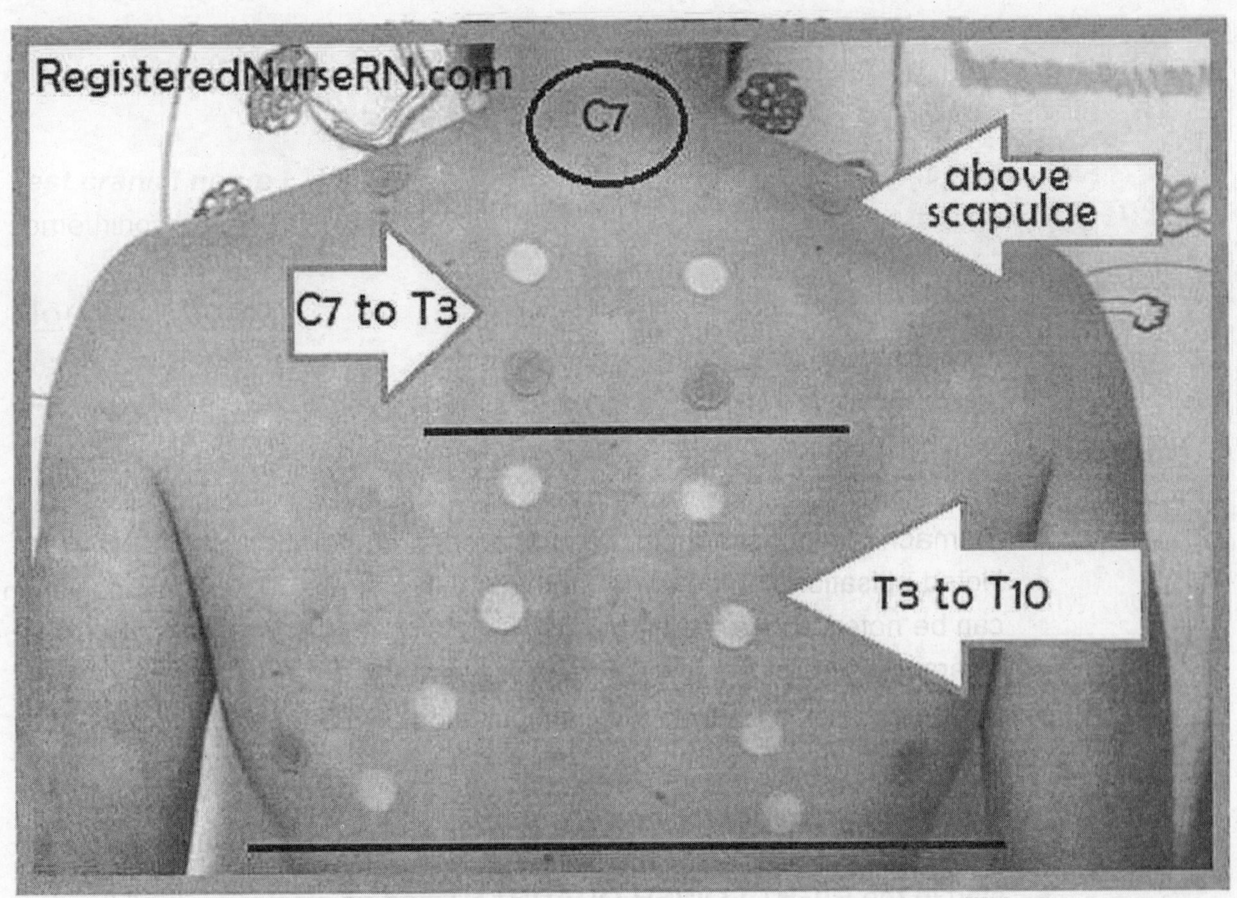

Abdomen:

Switching to Inspection, *Auscultation*, Percussion, and Palpation

- Have patient lay supine
- Ask patient about their last about bowel movement and if they have any problems with urination. If a female patient, ask when their last menstrual period was.
  - If an ostomy is present note the type of ostomy, stoma color (should be pink and shiny), consistency and color of stool?

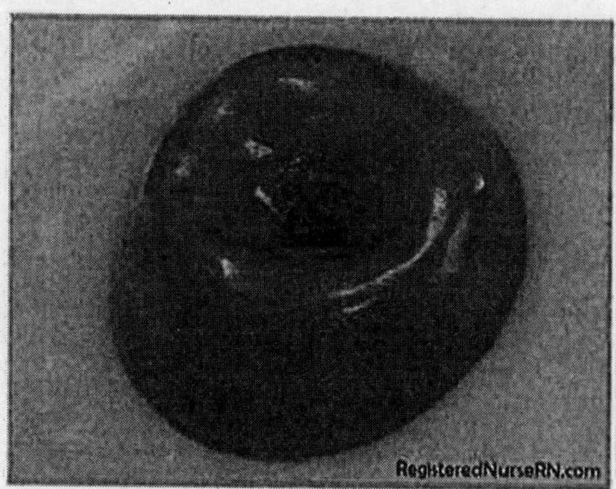

Inspect:

- Stomach contour scaphoid, flat, rounded, protuberant?
- Noted pulsations at the aorta (noted in thin patients): The aortic pulsation can be noted above the umbilicus.
- Characteristics of the navel (invert or everted)
- Masses (check for hernia after auscultation), PEG tube?

Auscultate with the diaphragm for bowel sounds:

- start in the **RIGHT LOWER QUADRANT** and go clockwise in all the 4 quadrants
    - should hear 5 to 30 sounds per minute…if no, bowel sounds are noted listen for 5 full minutes
    - Documents as: normal, hyperactive, or hypoactive

Auscultate for bruits (vascular sounds) at the following locations using the BELL of the stethoscope:

- Aorta: slightly below the xiphoid process midline with the umbilicus
- Renal Arteries: go slightly down to the right and left at the aortic site
- Iliac arteries: go few a inches down from the belly button at the right and left sides to listen
- Femoral arteries: found in the right and left groin.

Check for hernia: have patient raise up a bit and look for hernia (at stomach area or navel area)

Palpation of the abdomen:

- Light palpation (2 cm): should feel soft with no pain or rigidity
- Deep palpation (4-5 cm): feel for any masses, lumps, tenderness

Lower extremities:

Inspect:

- color from legs to toes?
- normal hair growth? (peripheral vascular disease: leg may be hairless, shiny, thin)
- warm (good blood flow)?
- swelling (press down firmly over the tibia…does it pit?)
- any redness, swelling DVT (deep vein thrombosis)?
- capillary refill less than 2 seconds in toes?
- How do the toe nails look (fungal or normal)?
- Sores on the feet (Note: with diabetics, foot care is important. They don't have good sensation on their feet. Therefore, inspect the feet for damage because they may not be aware of it.)
- Is there any breakdown on the heels?
- Assess joints of the toes and knees (any crepitus, redness, swelling, pain)

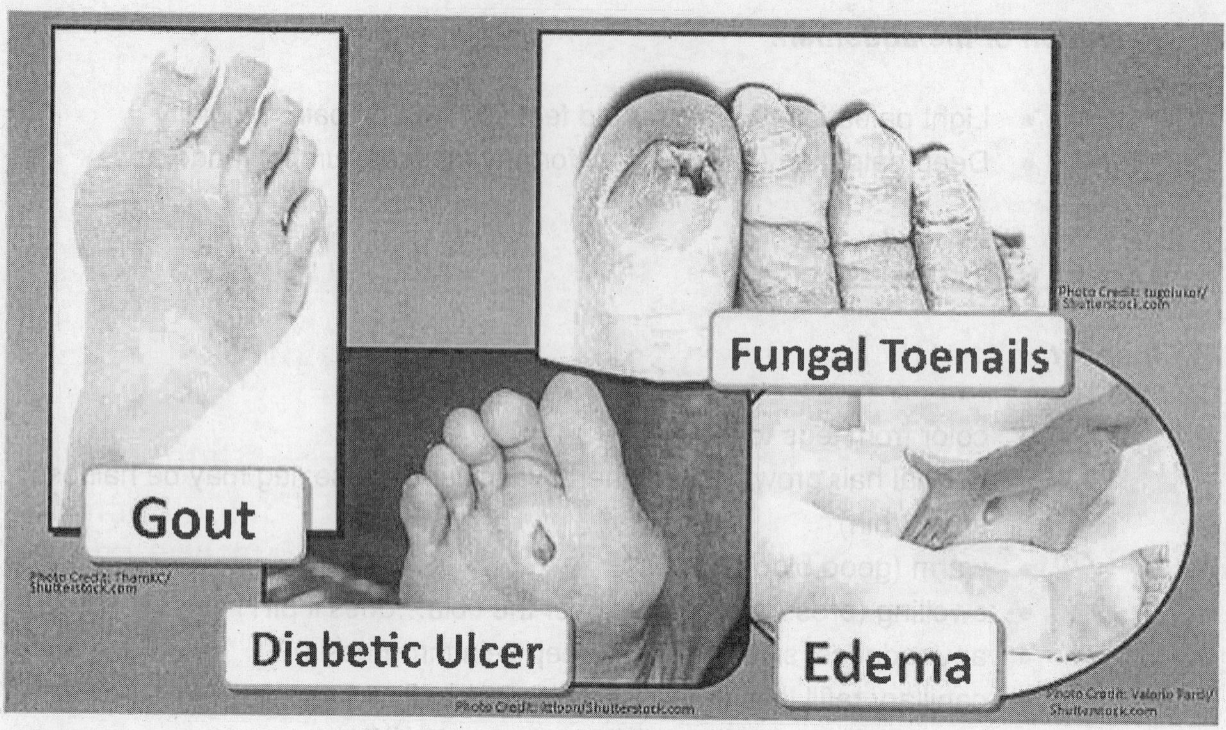

Palpate pulses bilaterally: popliteal (behind the knee), dorsalis pedis (top of foot), posterior tibial (at the ankle) and grade them

Palpate muscle strength: have patient push against resistance with feet and lift legs

Prefix/ Suffix	Class	Examples
Cef-	Cephalosporins (antibiotics)	Cefadroxil, Cefaclor, Cefixime, Ceftibuten
Ceph-	Cephalosporins (antibiotics)	Cephalexin, Cephapirin, Cephradine
Cort-	Corticosteroids (anti-inflammatory)	Cortisone
Rifa-	Antituberculars	Rifamate, Rifampin, Rifapentine, Rifater
Sulf-	Sulfanilamides (antibiotics)	Sulfadiazine, Sulfamethoxazole, Sulfasoxazole
-actone	Potassium-sparing diuretics	Aldactone, Spironolactone
-ane	General Anesthetics	Cyclohexane, Ethane, Fluorane
-ase	Thrombolytics (clot-busters)	Eminase, Retavase, Streptokinase
-azole	Antifungals	Butoconazole, Econazole, Fluconazole
-azosin	Alpha blockers (adrenergic antagonists)	Doxazosin, Prazosin, Terazosin
-barbital	Barbiturates (sedative-hypnotics)	Amobarbital, Phentobarbital, Secobarbital
-caine	Local Anesthetics	Bupivacaine, Cocaine, Lidocaine, Xylocaine
-calci-	Calcium & Vitamin D supplements	Calciferol, Calcitriol, Ergocalciferol
-cillin	Penicillins	Ampicillin, Penicillin
-ciclovir	Antivirals	Famiciclovir, Ganciclovir
-dazole	Nitroimidazole Antimicrobial	Metronidazole
-dipine	Calcium Channel Blockers	Amlodipine, Felodipine, Isradipine, Nifedipine
-dronate	Biphosphonates	Alendronate, Etidronate, Pamidronate, Risedronate
-ergot-	Ergotamines (anti-migraine)	Erogotamine, Dihydroergotamine
-floxacin	Fluoroquinolones (antibiotics)	Ciprofloxacin, Gatifloxacin, Levofloxacin

-ine	Stimulants	Amphetamine, Caffine, Terbutaline, Theophylline
-lam	Benzodiazepines (anxiolytics)	Alprazolam, Midazolam
-lol	Beta Blockers (adrenergic antagonists)	Atenolol, Propanolol, Sotalol
-lone	Corticosteroids (anti-inflammatory)	Methylprednisolone, Prednisolone, Triamcinolone
-micin	Aminoglycosides (antibiotics)	Gentamicin
-mycin	Aminoglycosides/ Macrolides (antibiotics)	Erythromycin, Tobramycin, Vancomycin
-navir	HIV/ AIDS antivirals	Amprenavir, Indinavir, Nelfinavir, Ritonavir
-pam	Benzodiazepines (anxiolytics)	Diazepam, Lorazepam
-parin	Anticoagulant	Enoxaparin
-prazole	Proton Pump Inhibitors (anti-ulcer)	Lansoprazole, Omeprazole, Pantoprazole
-pril	ACE inhibitors (antihypertensives)	Captopril, Moexipril, Quinapril
-profen	NSAIDS (anti-inflammatory)	Fenoprofen, Ibuprofen, Ketoprofen
-quine	Antiparasitics	Chloroquine, Hydroxychloroquine, Mefloquine
-sartan	Angiotensin-II receptor antagonists	Candesartan, Losartan, Telmisartan, Valsartan
-semide	Loop Diuretic	Furosemide
-setron	5-HT3 receptor antagonists (antiemetics)	Dolasetron, Granisetron, Ondansetron
-sone	Corticosteroids (anti-inflammatory)	Cortisone, Dexamethasone, Prednisone
-statin	HMG-CoA Reductase Inhibitor	Rosuvastatin, Atorvastatin, Simvastatin
-stigmine	Cholinergics	Neostigmine, Physostigmine, Pyridostigmine
-stine	Antieoplastics (anti-tumor)	Carmustine, Lomustine, Vinblastine, Vincristine
-terol	Bronchodilators	Albuterol, Bitolterol, Levalbuterol, Pirbuterol

-thiazide	Thiazides Diuretics	Benzthiazide, Hydrochlorothiazide
-tidine	H2 receptor antagonists (anti-ulcer)	Cimetidine, Famotidine, Nizatidine, Ranitidine
-triptan	Anti-migraines	Naratriptan, Rizatriptan
-triptyline	Tricyclics (antidepressants)	Amitriptyline, Nortriptyline, Protriptyline
-vir	Antivirals	Abacivir, Zanamivir
-vudine	HIV/ AIDS antivirals	Lamivudine, Stavudine, Zidovudine
-zolam	Benzodiazepines (anxiolytics)	Alprazolam, Midazolam
-zine	Phenothiazines (antipsychotics, antiemetics)	Chlopromazine, Perphenazine, Prochlorperazine
-zoline	Nasal decongestants	Oxymetazoline, Xylometazoline

Acetaminophen (Tylenol)
Generic Name: Acetaminophen
Trade Name: Tylenol
Indications: Pain, Fever
Actions: Inhibit the synthesis of prostaglandins which play a role in transmission of pain signals and fever response.
Therapeutic Class: Antipyretic, Non-opioid analgesic

Acyclovir (Zovirax)
Generic Name: Acyclovir
Trade Name: Zovirax
Indications: Genital herpes, Herpes Zoster, Chicken Pox
Actions: Interferes with viral DNA synthesis
Therapeutic Class: Antiviral
Pharmacological Class: Purine Analogues

Albuterol (Proventil)
Generic Name: Albuterol
Trade Name: Proventil
Indications: Bronchodilator used to prevent airway obstruction in asthma and COPD
Actions: Binds to Beta2 adrenergic receptors in the airway leading to relaxation of the smooth muscles in the airways
Therapeutic Class: Bronchodilator
Pharmacological Class: Adrenergic

Alendronate (Fosamax)
Generic Name: Alendronate
Trade Name: Fosamax
Indications: Osteoporosis (aging, menopause, corticosteroid induced)
Actions: Inhibits osteoclast activity leading to inhibition of resorption of bone
Therapeutic Class: Bone resorption inhibitor
Pharmacological Class: Bisphosphonates

Alprazolam (Xanax)
Generic Name: Alprazolam
Trade Name: Xanax
Indications: Anxiety, panic disorder, manage symptoms of PMS, insomnia, mania, psychosis
Actions: Works in CNS to produce anxiolytic effect causing CNS depression
Therapeutic Class: Antianxiety agent
Pharmacological Class: Benzodiazepine

Alteplase (t-PA)
Generic Name: Alteplase
Trade Name: t-PA
Indications: MI, acute ischemic stroke, occluded central lines
Actions: converts plasminogen to plasmin which degrades the fibrin found in clots
Therapeutic Class: Thrombolytics
Pharmacological Class: Plasminogen Activators

Amidarone (Cordarone)
Generic Name: Amiodarone
Trade Name: Cordarone
Indications: Atrial fibrillation, ventricular arrhythmias, SVT, ACLS protocol for v-fib and vTACH
Actions: Prolongs action potential, inhibits adrenergic stimulation, slows rate , decrease peripheral vascular resistance causing vasodilation
Therapeutic Class: Antiarrhytmic class III, Potassium channel blocker

Amitryptiline (Elavil)
Generic Name: Amitryptiline
Trade Name: Elavil
Indications: Depression, Anxiety, Insomnia
Actions: Increases effect of serotonin and norepinephrine in the CNS, exhibits anticholinergic effects
Therapeutic Class: Antidepressant
Pharmacological Class: Tricyclic Antidepressant

Amlodipine (Norvasc)
Generic Name: Amlodipine
Trade Name: Norvasc
Indications:Hypertension, Angina
Actions: Blocks transport or calcium into muscle cells inhibiting excitation and contraction
Therapeutic Class: Antihypertensive
Pharmacological Class: Ca Channel Blocker

Amoxicillin (Moxatag)
Generic Name: Amoxicillin
Trade Name: Moxatag
Indications: Skin infections, Respiratory infections, Sinusitis, Endocarditis Prophylaxis, Lyme disease
Actions: Inhibits synthesis of bacterial cell wall leading to cell death
Therapeutic Class: Anti-invectives, antiulcer agent
Pharmacological Class: Aminopenicillins

Ampicillin (Principen)
Generic Name: Ampicillin
Trade Name: Principen
Indications: Skin infections, soft tissue infections, otitis media, sinusitis, respiratory infections, GU infections, meningitis, septicemia
Actions: **Ampicillin** acts as an irreversible inhibitor of the enzyme transpeptidase
Therapeutic Class: Anti-infective
Pharmacological Class: Aminopenicillin

Aspart, lispro, glulisine (Novolog, humalog, apidra)
Generic Name: Aspart, Lispro, Glulisine
Trade Name: Novolog, Humalog, Apidra
Indications: Hyperglycemia with diabetes type 1 and 2, diabetic ketoacidosis
Actions: Stimulates uptake of glucose into muscle and fat cells, inhibits production of glucose in the liver, prevents breakdown of fat and protein

Route Onset Peak Duration
Aspart 10-20 min 1-3 hr 3-5 hr
Glulisine 15 min 1 hr 2-4 hr
Lispro 15 min 1-1.5 hr 3-4 hr

Therapeutic Class: Antidiabetics, hormones
Pharmacological Class: Pancreatics

Aspirin (Bayer Aspirin)
Generic Name: Aspirin
Trade Name: Bayer Aspirin
Indications: Rheumatoid Arthritis, Osteoarthritis, Ischemic stroke and MI prophylaxis
Actions: Inhibits the production of prostaglandins which leads to a reduction of fever and inflammation, decreases platelet aggregation leading to a decrease in ischemic diseases
Therapeutic Class: Antipyretics, non-opioid analgesics
Pharmacological Class: Salicylates

Atenolol (Tenormin)
Generic Name: Atenolol
Trade Name: Tenormin
Indications: Hypertension, Angina, Prevention of MI
Actions: Blocks the stimulation of beta 1 receptors in the SNS with minimal effect on beta2 receptors
Therapeutic Class: Antianginal, antihypertensive
Pharmacological Class: Beta Blocker

Atorvastatin (Lipitor)
Generic Name: Atorvastatin
Trade Name: Lipitor
Indications: Management of high cholesterol (hypercholesterolemia), primary prevention of cardiovascular disease
Actions: Lowers total cholesterol as well as LDL while slightly increasing HDL. Inhibits HMG-CoA reductase which plays a role in the liver in cholesterol formation
Therapeutic Class: Lipid Lowering agent
Pharmacological Class: HMG-CoA reductase inhibitor

Atropine (Atro-pen)
Generic Name: Atropine
Trade Name: Atro-pen
Indications: Decreases oral and respiratory secretions, Treats sinus bradycardia and heart block, Treatment of bronchospasm
Actions: Atropine is an anticholinergic which means that it inhibits the effects of the parasympathetic nervous system, specifically acetylcholine. This inhibition causes increase in HR, bronchodialation, decreased GI and respiratory secretions
Therapeutic Class: Antiarrythmic
Pharmacological Class:Anticholinergic, antimuscarinic

Azithromycin (Zithromax)
Generic Name: Azithromycin
Trade Name: Zithromax
Indications: URI, chronic bronchitis, lower respiratory infections, otitis media, skin infections, various STIs, prevention of bacterial endocarditis, treatment of cystic fibrosis
Actions: inhibits bacterial protein synthesis
Therapeutic Class: agents for atypical mycobacterium, anti-infectives
Pharmacological Class: Macrolide

Benzotropine (Cogentin)
Generic Name: Benzotropine
Trade Name: Cogentin
Indications: treatment for Parkinson's disease
Actions: Exhibits anticholinergic properties (blocks acetylcholine) in the CNS to reduce rigidity and tremors
Therapeutic Class: Antiparkinson agent
Pharmacological Class: Anticholinergic

Bisacodyl (Dulcolax)
Generic Name: Bisacodyl
Trade Name: Dulcolax
Indications: treatment of constipation, bowel regimen
Actions: stimulates peristalsis leads to fluid accumulation in the colon
Therapeutic Class: Laxatives
Pharmacological Class: stimulant laxatives

Bismuth Subsalicylate (Kaopectate, Pepto-Bismol)
Generic Name: Bismuth Subsalicylate
Trade Name: Kaopectate, Pepto-Bismol
Indications: Diarrhea, Heartburn, Indigestion, H. pylori associated ulcer
Actions: Stimulates the absorption of fluids and electrolytes in the intestinal wall, reduction in hypermotility of the stomach, and binds to toxins.

Therapeutic Class: antidiarrheal, antiulcer
Pharmacological Class: adsorbant

Bupropion (Wellbutrin)
Generic Name: Bupropion
Trade Name: Wellbutrin
Indications: Depression, Smoking cessation, Treat ADHD in adults
Actions:
Therapeutic Class: Antidepressants, Smoking deterrents
Pharmacological Class: Aminoketones

Busprione (Buspar)
Generic Name: Buspirone
Trade Name: Buspar
Indications: Management of anxiety
Actions: Relieves anxiety by binding to dopamine and serotonin receptors
Therapeutic Class: Antidepressants, Smoking deterrents
Pharmacological Class: Aminoketones

Butorphanol (Stadol)
Generic Name: Butorphanol
Trade Name: Stadol
Indications: Moderate to severe pain, Labor pain, Sedation
Actions: Alters perception and response to pain by biding to opiate receptors in CNS
Therapeutic Class: Opioid Analgesic
Pharmacological Class: Opioid agonists/ antagonists

Calcium Acetate (PhosLo)
Generic Name: Calcium Acetate
Trade Name: PhosLo
Indications: treatment of hypocalcemia, prevention of post menopausal osteoporosis, treatment of hyperkalemia and hypermagnesaemia, adjunct in cardiac arrest, control of hyperphosphatemia with ESRD. Binds to phosphate in food and prevents absorption.
Actions: calcium is essential for nervous muscular and skeletal systems, helps maintain cell membranes, aids in transmission of nerve impulses and muscle contraction, aids in blood formation and coagulation
Therapeutic Class: mineral and electrolyte replacements/ supplements
Pharmacological Class: antacids

Calcium Carbonate (Tums/ Rolaids)
Generic Name: Calcium Carbonate
Trade Name: Tums/ Rolaids
Indications: treatment of hypocalcemia, prevention of post menopausal osteoporosis, treatment of hyperkalemia and hypermagnesaemia, used as antacid
Actions: calcium is essential for nervous, muscular, and skeletal systems, helps maintain cell membranes, aids in transmission of nerve impulses and muscle contraction, aids in blood formation and coagulation
Therapeutic Class: mineral and electrolyte replacements/ supplements
Pharmacological Class: antacids

Catopril (Capoten)
Generic Name: Catopril
Trade Name: Capoten
Indications: Hypertension, Management of CHF, Decrease progression of DM neuropathy
Actions: Block conversion of angiotensin to angiotensin II, increases renin levels and decreases aldosterone leaving to vasodilation
Therapeutic Class: Antihypertensives
Pharmacological Class: ACE inhibitor

Carbamazepine (Tegretol)
Generic Name: Carbamazepine
Trade Name: Tegretol
Indications: Seizures, DM neuropathy, pain associated with trigeminal neuralgia
Actions: affects Na channels in neurons leading to decreased synaptic transmission
Therapeutic Class: anticonvulsant

Carbidopa/ Levodopa (Sinemet)
Generic Name: Carbidopa/ Levodopa
Trade Name: Sinemet
Indications: Parkinson's Disease
Actions: Levodopa is converted to dopamine and works as a neurotransmitter and carbidopa prevents the destruction of levodopa
Therapeutic Class: Antiparkinsons Agent
Pharmacological Class: Dopamine Agonist

Cefaclor (Ceclor)
Generic Name: Cefaclor
Trade Name: Ceclor
Indications: treatment of respiratory tract infections, skin infections, otitis media
Actions: Bacteriacidal, binds to bacterial cell wall causing cell death
Therapeutic Class: Anti-invectives
Pharmacological Class: Cephalosporin 2nd generations

Cefdinir (Omnicef)
Generic Name: Cefdinir
Trade Name: Omnicef
Indications: Treatment of skin infections, Otitis Media
Actions: Bactericidal, binds to bacterial cell wall causing cell death
Therapeutic Class: Anti-infectives
Pharmacological Class: Cephalosporin 2nd generations

Celecoxib (Celebrex)
Generic Name: Celecoxib
Trade Name: Celebrex
Indications: Osteoarthritis, Rheumatoid arthritis, Acute pain
Actions: Decreases pain and inflammation by inhibiting synthesis of prostaglandins
Therapeutic Class: Antirrheumatics/ NSAID
Pharmacological Class: none

Cephalexin (Keflex)
Generic Name: Cephalexin
Trade Name: Keflex
Indications: Skin infections, pneumonia, UTI, otitis media
Actions: Bactericidal: binds to bacterial cell wall leading to cell death
Therapeutic Class: Anti-infectives
Pharmacological Class: Cephalosporin 1st generations

Chlorpromazine (Thorazine)
Generic Name: Chlorpromazine
Trade Name: Thorazine
Indications: Second line treatment of schizophrenia and psychosis , nausea/ vomiting, Pre-op Sedation, Acute intermittent porphyria, Headache, Bipolar
Actions: Exhibits anticholinergic activity, alters effects of dopamine in CNS
Therapeutic Class: Antipsychotic, antiemetic
Pharmacological Class: Phenothiazines (dopamine D2 receptor antagonist)

Cimetidine (Tagamet)
Generic Name: Cimetidine
Trade Name: Tagamet
Indications: Treatment of duodenal ulcers, GERD, heartburn, Zollinger Ellison syndrome, Prevention of GI bleeding in critical patients
Actions: inhibits action of histamine leading to inhibition of gastric acid secretion
Therapeutic Class: antiulcer agent
Pharmacological Class: Histamine H2 antagonist

Ciprofloxacin (Cipro)
Generic Name: Ciprofloxacin
Trade Name: Cipro
Indications: Urinary tract infections, Gonorrhea, Respiratory tract infections, Bronchitis, Pneumonia, skin and bone infections, infectious diarrhea, abdominal infections
Actions: inhibits bacterial DNA synthesis
Therapeutic Class: anti-infectives Pharmacological Class: Fluoroquinilone

Clindamycin (Cleocin)
Generic Name: Clindamycin
Trade Name: Cleocin
Indications: Skin infections, Respiratory tract infections, Septicemia, Intra-abdominal infections, Osteomyelitis
Actions: Inhibits protein synthesis
Therapeutic Class: Anti-infectives
Pharmacological Class: none

Clopidogrel (Plavix)
Generic Name: Clopidogrel
Trade Name: Plavix
Indications: Atherosclerotic events, MI, CVA, PVD, Acute coronary syndrome
Actions: Inhibits platelet aggregation
Therapeutic Class: Antiplatelet agent
Pharmacological Class: Platelet aggregation inhibitors

Cortisone (Cortone)
Generic Name: Cortisone
Trade Name: Cortone
Indications: Management of adrenocortical insufficiency (Addison's Disease)
Actions: Replace cortisol in states of deficiency, suppress inflammation and normal immune response. The adrenal glands sit on top of the kidneys. The adrenal glands excrete steroids hormones, including cortisol that play a role in increasing blood sugars, immune suppression, and metabolism of fat, protein, and carbohydrates, as well as decreasing bone formation.
Therapeutic Class: Antiasthmatics, corticosteroids
Pharmacological Class: Corticosteroids

Cyclosporine (Cyclosporine)
Generic Name: Cyclosporine
Trade Name: Cyclosporine
Indications: Prevention of rejection in transplantation, Treatment of severe RA, Management of ulcerative colitis
Actions: Inhibits normal immune response
Therapeutic Class: Immunosuppressants, antirheumatics (DMARD)
Pharmacological Class: Polypeptides (cyclic)

Dexamethasone (Decadron)
Generic Name: Dexamethasone
Trade Name: Decadron
Indications: Manage cerebral edema, Assess for Cushing's Disease
Actions: Suppress inflammation and normal immune response. Used in inflammatory states to decrease inflammation.
Therapeutic Class: Antiasthmatics, corticosteroids
Pharmacological Class: Corticosteroids

Diazepam (Valium)
Generic Name: Diazepam
Trade Name: Valium
Indications: Anxiety, Pre-op sedation, conscious sedation, treatment of seizures, insomnia, management of alcohol withdrawal
Actions: Depresses the CNS
Therapeutic Class: Antianxiety agents, anticonvulsants, sedative/ hypnotics, skeletal muscle relaxants (centrally acting)
Pharmacological Class: Benzodiazepine

Digoxin (Lanoxin)
Generic Name: Digoxin
Trade Name: Lanoxin
Indications: CHF, A-fib, A-flutter
Actions: Positive inotropic effect (increases force of myocardial contraction), prolongs refractory period decreases conduction through SA and AV nodes. Essentially digoxin is given to increase cardiac output and slow the rate. Digoxin level (1.5-2.5)
Therapeutic Class: Antiarrhythmic, inotropics
Pharmacological Class: Digitalis glycosides

Dobutamine (Dobutrex)
Generic Name: Dobutamine
Trade Name: Dobutrex
Indications: short term management of heart failure
Actions: Dobutamine has a positive inotropic effect (increases cardiac output) with very little effect on heart rate.
Stimulates Beta 1 receptors in the heart
Therapeutic Class: inotropic
Pharmacological Class: beta-adrenergic agonist

Dopamine (Intropin)
Generic Name: Dopamine
Trade Name: Intropin
Indications: Used to improve blood pressure, cardiac output, and urine output
Actions: smaller doses result in renal vasodilation
Doses 2-10mcg/kg/min result in cardiac stimulation by acting on beta1 receptors
Doses > 10mcg/kg/min stimulate alpha receptors leading to vasoconstriction (increase SVR)
Therapeutic Class: Inotropic, vasopressor
Pharmacological Class: Adrenergic

Enalapril (Vasotec)
Generic Name: Enalapril
Trade Name: Vasotec
Indications: Hypertension, Management of CHF
Actions: Block conversion of angiotensin II, increases renin levels and decreases aldosterone leading to vasodilation
Therapeutic Class: Antihypertensive
Pharmacological Class: ACE inhibitor

Enoxaparin (Lovenox)
Generic Name: Enoxaparin
Trade Name: Lovenox
Indications:Prevention of VTE, DVT, and PE
Actions: Prevents thrombus formation by potentiating the inhibitory effect of antithrombin on factor Xa and thrombin. Enoxaparin is a low molecular weight heparin.

Therapeutic Class: Anticoagulant
Pharmacological Class: Antithrombotic

Epinephrine (Adrenalin, EpiPen)
Generic Name: Epinephrine
Trade Name: Adrenalin, EpiPen
Indications: asthma and COPD exacerbations, allergic reactions, cardiac arrest, anesthesia adjunct
Actions: Affects both beta1 and beta2 also has alpha agonist properties resulting in bronchodilation and increases in the HR and BP. Inhibits hypersensitivity reactions.
Therapeutic Class: Antiasthmatic, bronchodilator, vasopressor
Pharmacological Class: adrenergic agonist

Epoetin (Epogen)
Generic Name: Epoetin
Trade Name: Epogen
Indications: Anemia
Actions: Stimulates erythropoesis (production of RBCs)
Therapeutic Class: Antianemics
Pharmacological Class: Hormones

Erythromycin (E-Mycin)
Generic Name: Erythromycin
Trade Name: E-Mycin
Indications: Useful in place of penicillin when patient cannot take penicillin, upper and lower respiratory tract infections, otitis media, skin infections, pertussis, syphilis, rheumatic fever
Actions: Bacteriostatic: suppresses bacterial protein synthesis
Therapeutic Class: Anti-infective
Pharmacological Class: Macrolide

Escitalopram (Lexapro)
Generic Name: Escitalopram
Trade Name: Lexapro
Indications: Major depressive disorders anxiety disorder, PCD, PTSD, Social Phobia
Actions: Selectively inhibits reuptake of serotonin
Therapeutic Class: Antidepressant
Pharmacological Class: SSRI

Famotidine (Pepcid)
Generic Name: Famotidine
Trade Name: Pepcid
Indications: short term treatment of active ulcer, GERD, Treatment of heartburn, Indigestion, Management of Zollinger Ellison syndrome revention of GI bleeding in critically ill patients, Management of symptoms associated with overuse of NSAIDs, Prevention of GI bleeding in critically ill patients
Actions: Blocks action of histamine located in gastric parietal cells, inhibits gastric acid secretion
Therapeutic Class: Antiulcer agent
Pharmacological Class: Histamine H2 antagonist

Fentanyl (Sublimaze)
Generic Name: Fentanyl
Trade Name: Sublimaze
Indications: Supplement to general anesthesia, continuous IV infusion for purpose of analgesia
Actions: Binds to opiate receptors in CNS altering perception of pain, producing CNS depression
Therapeutic Class: Opioid Analgesic
Pharmacological Class: Opioid agonists

- only given in mcg

Ferrous Sulfate (Feosol)
Generic Name: Ferrous Sulfate
Trade Name: Feosol
Indications: Prevention and treatment of iron-deficiency anemia
Actions: Iron is essential for hemoglobin, myoglobin and enzymes, it is transported to organs where it becomes part of iron stores
Therapeutic Class: Antianemics
Pharmacological Class: Iron supplements

Fluoxetine (Prozac)
Generic Name: Fluoxetine
Trade Name: Prozac
Indications: depressive disorder, PCD, bulimia, panic disorder, bipolar, anorexia, ADHD, DM neuropathy, obesity
Actions: inhibits reuptake of serotonin
Therapeutic Class: antidepressant
Pharmacological Class: SSRI

Fluticasone (Flovent)
Generic Name: Fluticasone
Trade Name: Flovent
Indications: Prophylactic asthma treatment
Actions: Locally acting anti-inflammatory
Therapeutic Class: Antiasthmatics, anti-inflammatory (steroid)
Pharmacological Class: Corticosteroids, Inhalation

Furosemide (Lasix)
Generic Name: Furosemide
Trade Name: Lasix
Indications: Edema, Hypertension
Actions: Precents reabsorption of sodium and chloride in the kidneys, increase excretion of water, sodium, chloride, magnesium, potassium
Therapeutic Class: Diuretics

Pharmacological Class: loop diuretic

Gabapentine (Neurontin)
Generic Name: Gabapentine
Trade Name: Neurontin
Indications: seizure, peripheral neuropathy, neuropathic pain, prevention of migraines
Actions: exact method of action unknown, may play a role in stabilizing neural membranes
Therapeutic Class: Analgesic adjuncts, therapeutic, anticonvulsants, mood stabilizers
Pharmacological Class: none

Gentamicin
Generic Name: Gentamicin
Trade Name: Cidomycin
Indications: Treatment of gram negative infection when penicillin is ineffective
Actions: Inhibits bacterial protein synthesis
Therapeutic Class: Anti-infectives
Pharmacological Class: Aminoglycosides

Glipizide (Glucotrol)
Generic Name: Glipizide
Trade Name: Glucotrol
Indications: Type 2 diabetes mellitus
Actions: Stimulates release and sensitivity to insulin to lower blood glucose
Therapeutic Class: anti-diabetic
Pharmacological Class: Sulfonylureas

Glucagon (GlucaGen)
Generic Name: Glucagon
Trade Name: GlucaGen
Indications: Severe hypoglycemia, antidote for Beta Blockers and calcium channel blockers
Actions: Stimulates production of glucose, relaxes GI tract
Therapeutic Class: Hormones
Pharmacological Class: Pancreatics

Guaifenesin (Robitussin)
Generic Name: Guaifensin
Trade Name: Robitussin
Indications: Cough Suppression, Expectorant
Actions: Decreases viscosity of and mobilizes secretions
Therapeutic Class: Allergy, cold and cough remedies, expectorant
Pharmacological Class: none

Haloperidol (Haldol)
Generic Name: Haloperidol
Trade Name: Haldol
Indications: Schizophrenia, mania, aggressive and agitated patient
Actions: Alters the effect of dopamine
Therapeutic Class: Antipsychotic
Pharmacological Class: Butyrophenones

Heparin (Hep-Lock) Generic Name: Heparin Trade Name: Hep-Lock Indications: Venous thromboembolism prophylaxis and treatment, low dose used to ensure latency of IV catheters Actions: increases the inhibitory effect of antithrombin on factor Xa Therapeutic Class: Anticoagulant Pharmacological Class: Antithrombotic
Hydralazine (Apresoline) Generic Name: Hydralazine Trade Name: Apresoline Indications: Hypertension Actions: Arterial vasodilator Therapeutic Class: Anti-hypertensive Pharmacological Class: Vasodilator
Hydrochlorothiazide (HydroDiuril) Generic Name: Hydrochlorothiazide Trade Name: HydroDiuril Indications: Hypertension, CHF, Renal dysfunction, Cirrhosis, Glucocorticoid therapy Actions: Increases sodium and water excretion produces arterial dilation Therapeutic Class: Antihypertensives, diuretics Pharmacological Class: Thiazide diuretics
Hydrocodone-acetaminophen: Norco (opioid analgesic, allergy, cold and cough remedies, antitussive) Generic Name: Hydrocodone/ acetaminophen Trade Name: Norco Indications: Management of moderate to severe pain Actions: alters the perception and reaction to pain by binding to opiate receptors in the CNS, also suppresses the cough reflex Therapeutic Class: Opioid analgesic, allergy, cold and cough remedies, antitussive Pharmacological Class: Opioid agonists, nonopioid analgesic combinations
Hydromorphone (Dilaudid) Generic Name: Hydromorphone Trade Name: Dilaudid Indications: Moderate to severe pain Actions: Alters the perception and reaction to pain by binding to opiate receptors in the CNS, also suppresses the cough reflex Therapeutic Class: opioid analgesic, allergy, cold and cough remedies, antitussive Pharmacological Class: Opioid agonist

Ibuprofen (Advil/ Motrin)
Generic Name: Ibuprofen
Trade Name: Advil/ Motrin
Indications: Mild to moderate pain, inflammatory states
Actions: Decreases pain and inflammation by inhibiting prostaglandins
Therapeutic Class: antipyretics, antirheumatics, nonopioid analgesics, nonsteroidal anti-inflammatory agents
Pharmacological Class: Nonopioid analgesics

Indomethacin (Indocin)
Generic Name: Indomethacin
Trade Name: Indocin
Indications: Inflammatory disorders when patients do not respond to other medications
Actions: decreases pain and inflammation by inhibiting prostaglandin synthesis
Therapeutic Class: Antirhuematics, ductus arteriosus patency adjuncts (IV only), nonsteroidal anti-inflammatory agents
Pharmacological Class: none

Isoniazide
Generic Name: Isoniazide
Trade Name: INH
Indications: Tuberculosis
Actions: Inhibits synthesis of mycobacterial cell wall
Therapeutic Class: Antitubercular
Pharmacological Class: none

Ketorolac (Toradol)
Generic Name: Ketorolac
Trade Name: Toradol
Indications: pain
Actions: pain relief due to prostaglandin inhibition
Therapeutic Class: nonsteroidal anti-inflammatory agents, nonopioid analgesics
Pharmacological Class: Pyrroziline carboxylic acid

Lactulose (Kristalose)
Generic Name: Lactulose
Trade Name: Kristalose
Indications: Constipation, Portal-systemic encephalopathy , high ammonia levels
Actions: Draws water into the stool and softens stool, inhibits ammonia passing into colon
Therapeutic Class: laxative
Pharmacological Class: osmotic

Lamotrigine (Lamictal)
Generic Name: Lamotrigine
Trade Name: Lamictal
Indications: seizures r/t epilepsy, bipolar
Actions: inhibits sodium transport in neurons
Therapeutic Class: anticonvulsant

Levetiracetam (keppra)
Generic Name: Levetiracetam
Trade Name: Keppra
Indications: Seizures
Actions: Decreases severity and incidence of seizures
Therapeutic Class: Anticonvulsants
Pharmacological Class: Pyrrolidines

Levefloxacin (Levaquin)
Generic Name: Levofloxacin
Trade Name: Levaquin
Indications:Urinary tract infections, gnorrhea, respiratory tract infections, bronchitis, pneumonia, skin and bone infections
Actions: inhibits DNA synthesis in bacteria
Therapeutic Class: anti-infective
Pharmacological Class: Fluoroquinolone

Levothyroxine (Levothroid)
Generic Name: Levothyroxine
Trade Name: Levothroid
Indications: Thyroid hormone replacement in hypothyroidism
Actions: Replaces thyroid hormone increase in metabolism, promotes gluconeogenesis, stimulates protein synthesis, restores normal hormone balance and suppresses thyroid cancer
Therapeutic Class: Hormone * only given in mcg
Pharmacological Class: Thyroid Preparations

Lisinopril (Prinivil)
Generic Name: Lisinopril
Trade Name: Prinivil
Indications: Hypertension, Management of CHF
Actions: Block conversion of angiotensin I to angiotensin II, increases renin levels and decreases aldosterone leading to vasodil
Therapeutic Class: Antihypertensives
Pharmacological Class: ACE inhibitor

Lithium (Lithizine)
Generic Name: Lithium
Trade Name: Lithizine
Indications: Mania
Actions: Alters cation transport and neurotransmitter reuptake
Therapeutic Class: Mood stabilizer
Lithium level (0.6-1.2)

Loperamide (Imodium)
Generic Name: Loperamide
Trade Name: Imodium
Indications: Acute diarrhea, decrease drainage post ileostomy
Actions: Inhibits peristalsis, reduces the volume of feces while increasing the bulk and viscosity
Therapeutic Class: Antidiarrheal

Lorazepam (Ativan)
Generic Name: Lorazepam
Trade Name: Ativan
Indications: Anxiety, Sedation, Seizures
Actions: General CNS depression
Therapeutic Class: Anesthetic adjuncts, Antianxiety agents, sedative hypnotics
Pharmacological Class: Benzodiazepines

Losartan (Cozaar)
Generic Name: Losartan
Trade Name: Cozaar
Indications: Hypertension, DM neuropathy, CHF
Actions: Inhibits vasoconstriction properties of angiotensin II
Therapeutic Class: Antihypertensives
Pharmacological Class: Angiotensin II receptor antagonist

Magnesium Sulfate (MgSO4)
Generic Name: Magnesium sulfate
Trade Name: MgSO4
Indications: Treatment of hypermagnesaemia, hypertension, preterm labor, Torsade de pointes, asthma, anticonvulsant with eclampsia
Actions: Magnesium plays a role in muscle excitability
Therapeutic Class: Minerals and electrolyte replacement/supplements
Pharmacological Class: Minerals/ Electrolytes

Mannitol (Osmitrol)
Generic Name: Mannitol
Trade Name: Osmitrol
Indications: Increased ICP, Oliguric renal failure, Edema, Intraocular pressure
Actions: Inhibits reabsorption of water and electrolytes by increasing osmotic pressure, excreted by kidneys
Therapeutic Class: Diuretic
Pharmacological Class: Osmotic Diuretic

Meperidine (Demerol)
Generic Name: Meperidine
Trade Name: Demerol
Indications: Moderate to sever pain, sedation
Actions: Binds to opiate receptors in the CNS and alters perception of pain while producing a general depression of the CNS
Therapeutic Class: Opioid Analgesic
Pharmacological Class: Opioid Agonists

Metformin (Glucophage)
Generic Name: Metformin
Trade Name: Glucophage
Indications: Management of Type II DM, PCOS
Actions: Decrease glucose production in the liver, decreases absorption, increases cellular insulin sensitivity
Therapeutic Class: Antidiabetic
Pharmacological Class: Biguanide

Methadone: Mathadose (opioid analgesics)
Generic Name: Methadone
Trade Name: Mathadose
Indications: Withdrawal symptoms, pain
Actions: suppresses withdrawal symptoms. Binds to opiate receptors in the CNS and alters perception of pain while producing a general depression of the CNS. This depression also causes a decrease in the cough reflex and GI motility
Therapeutic Class: Opioid Analgesic
Pharmacological Class: Opioid Agonist

Methylergonovine (Methergine)
Generic Name: Methylergonovine
Trade Name: Methergine
Indications: Treatment of post-partum hemorrhage
Actions: Stimulates uterine muscles causing uterine contraction
Therapeutic Class: Oxytocic
Pharmacological Class: Ergot Alkaloids

Methylphenidate (Ritalin)
Generic Name: Methylphenidate
Trade Name: Ritalin
Indications: ADHA, Narcolepsy
Actions: Improves attention span in ADHD by producing CNS stimulation
Therapeutic Class: Central nervous system stimulant

Methylprednisone (Solu-medrol)
Generic Name: Methylprednisone
Trade Name: Solu-medrol
Indications: Inflammation, allergy, autoimmune disorders, prevent organ rejection
Actions: Suppress inflammation and normal immune response, the adrenal glands sit on top of the kidneys. The adrenal glands excrete steroid hormones that play a role in increasing blood sugars, immune suppression, and metabolism of fat, protein, and carbohydrates, as well as decreasing bone formation
Therapeutic Class: antiasthmatics, corticosteroids
Pharmacological Class: Corticosteroids

Metoclopramide (Reglan)
Generic Name: Metoclopramide
Trade Name: Reglan
Indications: Prevention of nausea, vomiting, hiccupsm, ,ingrained, gastric statis
Actions: accelerates gastric emptying by stimulating motility
Therapeutic Class: antiemetic
Pharmacological Class: none

Metoprolol (Lopressor)
Generic Name: Metoprolol
Trade Name: Lopressor
Indications: Tachyarrhythhmias, HTN, Angina, Prevention of MI, Heart failure management, May be used for migraine prophylaxis
Actions: Blocks the stimulation of beta1 receptors in the SNS with does not usually effect on beta2 receptors (cardioselective)
Therapeutic Class: antianginal, Antihypertensive
Pharmacological Class: beta blocker

Metronidazole (Flagyl)
Generic Name: Metrondiazole
Trade Name: Flagyl
Indications: Intra-abdominal infection, gynecoligical infections, skin infections, bone and joint infections, CNS infection, Septicemia, Endocarditis, Amebic liver abscess, Peptic ulcer disease
Actions: Inhibits DNA and protein synthesis in bacteria, Bactericidal
Therapeutic Class: Anti-infectives, antiprtozoals, antiulcer agents

Midazolam (Versed)
Generic Name: Midazolam
Trade Name: Versed
Indications: Sedation, Conscious sedation, Anesthesia, Status epileptics
Actions: Acts to produce CNS depression, may be mediated by GABA
Therapeutic Class: Antianxiety agent, sedative/ hypnotics
Pharmacological Class: Benzodiazepine

Montelukast (Singulair)
Generic Name: Montelukast
Trade Name: Singulair
Indications: Prevent or treat asthma, manage seasonal allergies, prevent exercise-induced bronchoconstriction
Actions: Disrupts the effects of leukotrienes which effect airway edema, smooth muscle constriction, and cellular activity
Therapeutic Class: allergy, cold, and cough remedies, bronchodilators
Pharmacological Class: Leukotriene Antagonist

Morphine (MS Contin)
Generic Name: Morphine
Trade Name: MS Contin
Indications: Painpulmonary edema, MI, Pulmonary edema
Actions: Binds to opiate receptors in the CNS and alters perception of pain while producing a general depression of the CNS. This depression also causes a decrease in the cough reflex and GI motility.
Therapeutic Class: Opioid Analgesic
Pharmacological Class: Opioid agonist

Nalbuphine (Nubain)
Generic Name: Nalbuphine
Trade Name: Nubain
Indications: Alters perception and response to pain, causes CNS depression
Actions: Alters perception and response to pain, causes CNS depression
Therapeutic Class: Opioid Analgesic
Pharmacological Class: Opioid agonists/ analgesics

Naproxen (Aleve)
Generic Name: Naproxen
Trade Name: Aleve
Indications: Pain, Dismenorrhea, Fever, Inflammation
Actions: Inhibits prostaglandin synthesis
Therapeutic Class: Nonsteroidal anti-inflammatory agents, nonopioid analgesics, antipyretics

Nifedipine (Procardia)
Generic Name: Nifedipine
Trade Name: Procardia
Indications: Hypertension, Angina, Migraines, CHF
Actions: Blocks calcium transport resulting in inhibition of contraction causing systemic vasodilation
Therapeutic Class: antianginal, antihypertensives
Pharmacological Class: Ca Channel Blocker

Nitroprusside (Nitropress)
Generic Name: Nitroprusside
Trade Name: Nitropress
Indications: Hypertensive crisis, Cardiogenic shock
Actions: Peripheral vasodilation of arteries and veins decreasing preload and afterload
Therapeutic Class: Antihypertensive
Pharmacological Class: Vasodilator

Norepinephrine (Levophed)
Generic Name: Norepinephrine
Trade Name: Levophed
Indications: Treatment of severe hypotension and shock
Actions: Increase blood pressure and cardiac output by stimulating alpha-adrenergic receptors in the blood vessels, demonstrates minor beta activity
Therapeutic Class: Vasopressor

NPH (Humulin N, Novolin N)
Generic Name: NPH
Trade Name: Humulin N, Novolog N
Indications: Hyperglycemia with diabetes type 1 and 2, Diabetic ketoacidosis
Actions: Stimulates uptake of glucose into muscle and fat cells, inhibits production of glucose in the liver, prevents breakdown of fat and protein
Route Onset Peak Duration
Subcutaneous 1-2hr 4-12hr 18-24hr
Therapeutic Class: Antidiabetics, hormones
Pharmacological Class: Pancreatics

Nystatin (Mycostatin)
Generic Name: Nystatin
Trade Name: Mycostatin
Indications: Candidiasis, Denture stomatitis
Actions: Causes leakage of fungal cell contents
Therapeutic Class: Antifungal

Olanzapine (Zyprexa)
Generic Name: Olanzapine
Trade Name: Zyprexa
Indications: Schizophrenia, mania, depression, anorexia nervosa, nausea/ vomiting related to chemotherapy
Actions: Antagonizes dopamine and serotonin
Therapeutic Class: Antipsychotic, mood stabilizers
Pharmacological Class: Thienobenzodiazepines

Omeprazole (Prilosec)
Generic Name: Omeprazole
Trade Name: Prilosec
Indications: GERD, Ulcers, Zollinger-Ellison syndrome, Reduce the risk of GI bleed in critically ill patients, heart burn
Actions: prevents the transport of H ion into the gastric lumen by binding to gastric parietal cells, decreases gastric acid production
Therapeutic Class: antiulcer agent
Pharmacological Class: proton-pump inhibitor

Ondanserton (Zofran)
Generic Name: Ondanserton
Trade Name: Zofran
Indications: Nausea/ vomiting
Actions: Blocks effects of serotonin on vagal nerve and CNS
Therapeutic Class: Antiemetic
Pharmacological Class: 5-HT3 antagonist

Oxycodone (OxyContin)
Generic Name: Oxycodone
Trade Name: OxyContin
Indications: pain
Actions: binds to opiate receptors in CNS altering the perception and sensation of pain
Therapeutic Class: Opioid Analgesic
Pharmacological Class: Opioid agonists, opioid agonists/ nonopioid, analgesic combinations

Oxytocin (Pitocin)
Generic Name: Oxytocin
Trade Name: Pitocin
Indications: Labor induction, Postpartum bleeding
Actions: Stimulates uterine smooth muscle
Therapeutic Class: Hormones
Pharmacological Class: Oxytocics

Pancrelipase (Creon)
Generic Name: Pancrelipase
Trade Name: Creon
Indications: Pancreatic insufficiency, Ductal obstruction
Actions: replacement of pancreatic enzymes: lipase, amylase, protease
Therapeutic Class: Digestive agent
Pharmacological Class: Pancreatic enzyme

Pantoprazole (Protonix)
Generic Name: Pantoprazole
Trade Name: Protonix
Indications: GERD, Heartburn, Reduce the risk of GI bleed in critically ill patients
Actions: Prevents the transport of H ions into the gastric lumen by binding to gastric parietal cells, decrease gastric acid production
Therapeutic Class: Antiulcer agents
Pharmacological Class: proton pump inhibitors

Paroxetine (Paxil)
Generic Name: Paroxetine
Trade Name: Paxil
Indications: major depressive disorder, OCD, anxiety, PTSD
Actions: Block reuptake of serotonin in CNS
Therapeutic Class: Antianxiety agent, antidepressant
Pharmacological Class: SSRI

Phenazopyridine (Pyridium)
Generic Name: Phenazopyridine
Trade Name: Pyridium
Indications: Urological pain
Actions: Provides analgesia to the urinary tract mucosa
Therapeutic Class: Nonopioid analgesics
Pharmacological Class: Urinary tract analgesics

Phenytoin (Dilantin)
Generic Name: Phenytoin
Trade Name: Dilantin
Indications: Tonic clinic seizures, arrhythmias, neuropathic pain
Actions: Interferes with ion transport, shortens action potentials and decreases automaticity. Blocks sustained high frequency repetitive firing of action potentials
Therapeutic Class: Antiarrhythmics, anticonvulsants
Pharmacological Class: Hydantoins

Procainamide
Generic Name: Procainamide
Trade Name:
Indications: Wide variety ventricular and atrial arrhythmias, PAC, PVC, VTach, post cardio version
Actions: Decreases excitability and slows conduction velocity
Therapeutic Class: Antiarrhythmic (Class IA Na Channel Blocker)

Promethazine (Promethacon)
Generic Name: Promethazine
Trade Name: Promethacon
Indications: allergic reactions, nausea and vomiting, sedation
Actions: blocks the effects of histamine, histamine plays a role in the immune response. Also plays an inhibitory role on the chemoreceptor trigger zone in the medulla leading to an antiemetic effect. Possess anticholinergic properties producing CNS depression
Therapeutic Class: antiemetic, antihistamine, sedative/ hypnotic
Pharmacological Class: phenothiazine

Propofol (Diprivan)
Generic Name: Propofol
Trade Name: Diprivan
Indications: Anesthesia, induction, sedation
Actions: Hypnotic, produces amnesia
Therapeutic Class: General anesthetic

Propranolol (Inderal)
Generic Name: Propanolol
Trade Name: Inderal
Indications: Hypertension, Angina, Arrythmias, Cardiomyopathy, Alcohol withdrawal, Anxiety
Actions: Blocks beta 1&2 adrenergic receptors
Therapeutic Class: Antianginal, Antiarrhythmic (class II beta blockers), antihypertensive, headache suppressant
Pharmacological Class: Beta Blocker

Propylthiouracil (PTU)
Generic Name: Propylthiouracil
Trade Name: PTU
Indications: Hyperthyroidism
Actions: Inhibits thyroid hormones
Therapeutic Class: Antithyroid agent

Quetiapine (Seroquel)
Generic Name: Quetiapine
Trade Name: Seropuel
Indications: Schizophrenia, Depressive Disorder, Mania
Actions: Dopamine and serotonin antagonist
Therapeutic Class: Antipsychotic, mood stabilizers

Radioactive Iodine
Generic Name: Radioactive Iodine
Trade Name: none
Indications: Thyroidectomy pretreatment , Thyrotoxic crisis, Radiation exposure
Actions: Inhibits the release of thyroid hormones
Therapeutic Class: Antithyroid Agent, control of hyperthyroidism

Ranitidine (Zantac)
Generic Name: Ranitidine
Trade Name: Zantac
Indications: Duodenal ulcers, GERD, Heartburn, Esophagitis, GI bleed
Actions: Inhibits action of histamine in gastric parietal cells, decreases gastric acid secretion
Therapeutic Class: antiulcer agents
Pharmacological Class: Histamine H2 antagonists

Regular (Humulin R/ Novolin R)
Generic Name: Regular
Trade Name: Humulin R/ Novolin R
Indications: Hyperglycemia with diabetes type 1 & 2, diabetic ketoacidosis
Actions: Stimulates uptake of glucose into muscle and fat cells, inhibits production of glucose in the liver, prevents breakdown of fat and protein
Therapeutic Class: antidiabetics, hormones
Pharmacological Class: Pancreatics

Rifampin (Rimactane)
Generic Name: Rifampin
Trade Name: Rimactane
Indications: Tuberculosis
Actions: Inhibits RNA synthesis
Therapeutic Class: Antitubercular
Pharmacological Class: Rifamycins

Salmeterol (Serevent)
Generic Name: Salmeferol
Trade Name: Serevent
Indications: Reversible Airway Obstruction, Exercise induced asthma
Actions: Bronchodilation through stimulation of beta 2 adrenergic receptors
Therapeutic Class: Bronchodilators
Pharmacological Class: Adrenergics

Sertraline (Zoloft)
Generic Name: Sertraline
Trade Name: Zoloft
Indications: Major depressive disorder, OCD, Anxiety
Actions: Inhibits uptake of serotonin
Therapeutic Class: Antidepressant
Pharmacological Class: SSRI

Spironolactone (Aldactone)
Generic Name: Spironolactone
Trade Name: Aldactone
Indications: Potassium loss, hypertension, edema, CHF
Actions: Inhibits sodium reabsorption while sparing potassium and hydrogen
Therapeutic Class: Diuretics
Pharmacological Class: Potassium sparing diuretics

Streptokinase (Streptase)
Generic Name: Streptokinase
Trade Name: Streptase
Indications: Pulmonary embolism, DVT, Occluded lines, Arterial thrombus
Actions: converts plasminogen to plasmin which degrades fibrin clots
Therapeutic Class: thrombolytic
Pharmacological Class: plasminogen activators

Sucralfate (Carafate)
Generic Name: Sucralfate
Trade Name: Carafate
Indications: Management of GI ulcers, GI injury prevention from high dose aspirin and NSAID treatment
Actions: reacts with gastric acid to form a paste that adheres to ulcer
Therapeutic Class: Antiulcer agent
Pharmacological Class: GI protectant

Terbutaline (Brethaire)
Generic Name: Terbutaline
Trade Name: Brethaire
Indications: Asthma, COPD, Preterm labor
Actions: Produces bronchodilation
Therapeutic Class: Bronchodilators
Pharmacological Class: Adrenergics

Tetracycline (Doxycycline)
Generic Name: Tetracycline
Trade Name: Doxycycline
Indications: treatment of infection, gonorrhea & syphilis with penicillin allergy, chronic bronchitis
Actions: Bacteriostatic by inhibiting protein synthesis
Therapeutic Class: Anti-infectives
Pharmacological Class:Tetracyclines

Trimethoprim/ Sulfamethoxazole (Bactrim/ TMP-SMZ)
Generic Name: Trimethoprim/ Sulfamethoxazole
Trade Name: Bactrim/ TMP-SMZ
Indications: Bronchitis, UTI, Diarrhea, Pneumonia, Multiple types of infection
Actions: Bacteriacidal by preventing metabolism of folic acid
Therapeutic Class: Anti-infectives, antiprotozoals
Pharmacological Class: Folate antagonists, sulfonamides

Vancomycin (Vancocin)
Generic Name: Vancomycin
Trade Name: Vancocin
Indications: Life threatening infections, Sepsis
Actions: Bactericidal
Therapeutic Class: Anti-infectives

Vasopressin (Pitressin)
Generic Name: Vasopressin
Trade Name: Pitressin
Indications: Management of diabetes insipidus, VT/VF unresponsive to initial shock, GI hemorrhage
Actions: Increases water permeability of the kidney's collecting duct and distal convoluted tubule leading to water retention, also increases peripheral vascular resistance leading to increased BP
Therapeutic Class: Hormone
Pharmacological Class: Antidiuretic hormone

Verapamil (Isoptin)
Generic Name: Verapamil
Trade Name: Isoptin
Indications: Hypertension, Angina, SVT, Migraine
Actions: Prevents transport of calcium, leading to decreased contraction, decreases SA and AV conduction
Therapeutic Class: Antianginals, antiarrhythmic, antihypertensive, vascular headache suppressants
Pharmacological Class: Ca Channel Blocker

Warfarin (Coumadin)
Generic Name: Warfarin
Trade Name: Coumadin
Indications: Venous thrombosis, Pulmonary embolism, A-fib, Myocardial infarction
Actions: Disrupts liver synthesis off Vitamin K dependent clotting factors
Therapeutic Class: Anticoagulant
Pharmacological Class: Coumarins

Dosage & Calculations Metric Table

1,000 micrograms (mcg) =1 milligram (mg)	1 milliliter (mL) = 1 cubic centimeter (cc)
1,000 grams (G) = 1 kilogram (kg)	1 teaspoon (tsp) = 5 milliliters (mL)
1,000 milligrams (mg) = 1 gram (G)	1,000 milliliters (mL) = 1 liter (L)
2.2 pounds (lbs) = 1 Kilogram (kg)	3 teaspoons (tsp) = 1 tablespoon (Tbsp)
30 milliliters (mL) = 1 ounce (oz)	1 tablespoon (Tbsp) = 15 milliliters (mL)
	2 tablespoons (Tbsp) = 1 ounce (oz)

METRIC and U.S. MEASUREMENT EQUIVALENCIES

METRIC SYSTEM OF MEASUREMENT:

Basic unit of LENGTH...METER (m) ....100cm = 1000 mm = .001 km
Basic unit of MASS (weight)...GRAM (g)........................001 kg = 1000 mg
Basic unit of CAPACITY (liquid measurement)..................LITER (L) ....1000 ml = .001 kl

Important Metric System Prefixes:

kilo	=	1,000	deci	=	0.1	tera	=	1,000,000,000,000
hector	=	100	centi	=	0.01	giga	=	1,000,000,000
deca	=	10	milli	=	0.001	mega	=	1,000,000

LENGTH

1 meter (m) = 100 centimeters (cm)
1 cm = 0.01 m
1 m = 1000 millimeters (mm)
1 mm = 0.001 m
1 cm = 10 mm
1 mm = 0.1 cm
1 kilometer = 1000 m
1 m = 0.001 km
1 megameter = 1,000,000 m
1 hectometer = 100 m
1 dekameter = 10 m
1 decimeter = 1/10 m
1 cm = 1/100 m
1 mm = 1/1000 m
1 micrometer = 1/1,000,000 m

WEIGHT

1 gram (g) = 1000 milligrams (mg)
1 kilogram (kg) = 1000 grams
1 mg = 0.001 g
1 g = 0.001 kg

CAPACITY

1 L = 1000 mL
1 mL = 0.001 L
1 k = 1000 L

U.S. CUSTOMARY SYSTEM OF MEASUREMENT:

LENGTH

1 foot = 12 inches
1 yard = 3 feet
1 yard = 36 inches
1 mile = 5,280 feet

WEIGHT

1 lb = 16 oz
1 ton = 2,000 lbs

CAPACITY

1 cup = 8 fl oz
1 pint = 2 cups
1 quart = 4 c/2 pts
1 gal = 4 quarts

AREA

1 ft^2 = 144 in^2
1 $yard^2$ = 9 ft^2
1 acre = 43,560 ft^2
1 $mile^2$ = 640 acres

APOTHECARIES' WEIGHTS and MEASURES:

1 dram	=	60 grains (gr)	1 fluid dram	=	60 minims
1 ounce	=	8 drams	1 ounce	=	8 fluid drams
1 pound (lb)	=	12 ounces	1 pint (pt)	=	16 oz
1 ounce	=	480 gr	1 quart	=	2 pints
1 fluid oz	=	480 minims	1 gallon	=	4 quarts
1minim	=	1 gr			

Drug Dosage & IV Rates Calculations

Drug Dosage Calculations

Drug dosage calculations are required when the amount of medication ordered (or desired) is *different* from what is available on hand for the nurse to administer.

Formula:

$$\frac{\textbf{Amount DESIRED (D)}}{\textbf{Amount on HAND (H)}} \textbf{ X QUANTITY (Q) = Y (Tablets Required)}$$

Note: When medication is given in tablets, the QUANTITY = 1 since the amount of medication available is specified per (one) tablet.

Example 1: Toprol XL, 50 mg PO, is ordered. Toprol XL is available as 100 mg per tablets. How many tablets would the nurse administer?

Step 1: Determine your givens.	Amount desired (D) = 50 mg Amount on hand (H) = 100 mg tablets Quantity = 1
Step 2: Plug in what you know into the formula and simplify.	$\frac{50 \text{ mg}}{100 \text{ mg}} \times 1 = \boxed{0.5 \text{ tablets}}$

Therefore, the nurse would administer 0.5 of a tablet.

Example 2: 1200 mg of Klor-Con is ordered. This medication is only available as 600 mg per tablet. How many tablets should the nurse give?

Step 1: Determine your givens.	Amount desired (D) = 1200 mg Amount on hand (H) = 600 mg Quantity = 1
Step 2: Plug in what you know into the formula and simplify.	$\frac{1200 \text{ mg}}{600 \text{ mg}} \times 1 = \boxed{2 \text{ tablets}}$

Therefore, the nurse should give 2 tablets.

The same formula can be used for dosage calculations where the medication is available as **amount per certain volume**.

In these types of calculations, the volume available on hand is the **QUANTITY**.

Example 3: Dilantin-125 is available as 125 mg/5 mL. Dilantin-125, 0.3 g PO, is ordered. How much should the nurse administer to the patient?

Step 1: Determine your givens.	Amount desired (D) = 0.3 g Amount on hand (H) = 125 mg Quantity = 5 mL
Step 2: Convert 0.3 g to mg (since the ordered dose is in grams but the drug is available on hand in milligrams).	0.3 g x 1,000 mg/g = 300 mg
Step 3: Plug in what you know into the formula and simplify.	$\frac{300 \text{ mg}}{125 \text{ mg}}$ x 5mL = $\boxed{12 \text{ mL}}$

Therefore, the nurse would administer 12 mL.

Example 4: Furosemide is available as 40 mg in 1 mL. 10 mg is ordered to be administered through an IV. What amount of furosemide should the nurse administer?

Step 1: Determine your givens.	Amount desired (D) = 10 mg Amount on hand (H) = 40 mg Quantity = 1 mL
Step 2: Plug in what you know into the formula and simplify.	$\frac{10 \text{ mg}}{40 \text{ mg}}$ x 1mL = $\boxed{0.4 \text{ mL}}$

Therefore, the nurse should administer 0.4 mL of furosemide.

Dosage Calculations based on Body Weight

Dosage calculations based on body weight are required when the dosage ordered and administered is dependent on the weight of the patient. For example, many pediatric drugs are ordered and given per weight (usually in kg).
Dosage calculations based on body weight are calculated in two main stages.

Stage 1: Using the formula below, calculate the total required dosage based on given the body weight.

Weight (kg) x Dosage Ordered (per kg) = Y (Required Dosage)

Stage 2: Apply the $\frac{D}{H}$ x Q formula to calculate the actual amount of medication to be administered.

Example 1: Medrol 4 mg/kg is ordered for a child weighing 64.8 lb. Medrol is available as 500 mg/4mL. How many milliliters of medication must the nurse administer?

Step 1: Determine your givens.	Weight: 64.8 lb Dosage ordered: 4mg/kg Available on hand: 500 mg/4mL
Step 2: Convert 64.5 lb to kg since the infant's weight is given in pounds (lb) but the dosage ordered is in mg per kilogram.	64.8 lb ÷ 2.2 lb/kg = 29.45 kg **Therefore, the infant's weight is 29.45 kg.**
Step 3: Calculate the required dosage (mg) of medication based on the child's weight.	Weight (kg) x Dosage Ordered (per kg) = Y (Required dosage) 29.45 kg x 4 mg/kg = 117.8 mg **Therefore, the required dosage of medication is 58.64 mg.**
Step 4: Calculate the volume of medication (mL) to be administered based on what's available on hand.	$\frac{\textbf{Amount Desired}}{\textbf{Amount on Hand}} \times \text{Quantity} = \boxed{Y}$ $\frac{\textbf{117.8 mg}}{\textbf{500 mg}} \times 4\text{ mL} = \boxed{0.942\text{ mL}}$

Therefore, the nurse must administer 0.942 mL of medication.

Example 2: A doctor prescribes 250 mg of Ceftin to be taken by a 20.5 lb infant every 8 hours. The medication label indicates that 75-150 mg/kg per day is the desired dosage range. Is this doctor's order within the desired range?

Step 1: Determine your givens.	Weight: 20.5 lb Dosage ordered: 250 mg Desired dosage range: 75-150 mg/kg
Step 2: Convert 20.5 lb to kg since the infant's weight is given in pounds (lb) but the medication label is in mg per kilogram.	20.5 lb ÷ 2.2 lb+/kg = 9.32 kg

Step 3: Calculate the minimum and maximum dosage for a 9.32 kg infant.	Weight (kg) x Dosage Ordered (per kg) = Y Minimum dosage: 9.32 kg x 75 mg/kg = 699 mg Maximum dosage: 9.32 kg x 150 mg/kg = 1398 mg
Step 4: Calculate the amount of medication the doctor has ordered for one day or 24 hours.	24 hr ÷ 8 hr = 3 The doctor has ordered the medication to be given 3 times per day. Every dose is 250 mg. 250 mg x 3 = 750 mg Therefore, the doctor has ordered 750 mg of medication per day.
Step 5: Compare the total amount of medication ordered for one day to the dosage range listed on the medication label.	750 mg is within the desired range of 699-1398 mg since 699 < 750 < 1398 Therefore, the doctor has ordered a dosage within the desired range.

Calculation of Intravenous Drip Rates

In these types of calculations, for a given volume, time period, and drop factor (gtts/mL), the required IV flow rate in drops per minute (gtts/min) is calculated.

Note: Since a fraction of a drop is not possible to give to a patient, it is usual to **round the answers** to the nearest whole number.

Formula:

$$\frac{\text{Volume (mL)}}{\text{Time (min)}} \times \text{Drop Factor (gtts/mL)} = Y \text{ (Flow Rate in gtts/min)}$$

Example 1: Calculate the IV flow rate for 250 mL of 0.5% dextrose to be administered over 180 minutes. The infusion set has drop factor of 30 gtts/mL.

Step 1: Determine your givens.	Volume: 250 mL Time: 180 min

	Drop factor: 30 gtts/mL
Step 2: Use the formula to calculate the IV flow rate. No unit conversions are required. Remember to round the final answer to the nearest whole number.	$\frac{Volume\ (mL)}{Time\ (\text{min})}$ x $Drop\ Factor$ $\left(\frac{\text{gtts}}{\text{mL}}\right)$ = Y (gtts/min) $\frac{250\ mL}{180\ \text{min}}$ x 30 $\left(\frac{\text{gtts}}{\text{mL}}\right)$ = 41.66 gtts/min

Therefore, the IV flow rate is 42 gtts/min.

Example 2: The infusion set is adjusted for a drop factor of 15 gtts/mL. Calculate the IV flow rate if 1500 mL IV saline is ordered to be infused over 12 hours.

Step 1: Determine your givens.	Volume: 1500 mL Time: 12 hours Drop factor: 15 gtts/mL
Step 2: Convert 8 hours into minutes.	12 h x 60 min/h = 720 min
Step 3: Use the formula to calculate the IV flow rate (gtts/min).	$\frac{Volume\ (mL)}{Time\ (\text{min})}$ x $Drop\ Factor$ $\left(\frac{\text{gtts}}{\text{mL}}\right)$ = Y (gtts/min) $\frac{1500\ mL}{720\ \text{min}}$ x 15 $\left(\frac{\text{gtts}}{\text{mL}}\right)$ = 31.25 gtts/min

Therefore, the IV flow rate is 31 gtts/min.

Calculation of Flow Rate for an Infusion Pump

Infusion pumps do not have a calibrated drop factor. The flow rate depends on the volume of fluid ordered and the time of infusion.

Formula:

$$\frac{\textbf{Volume (mL)}}{\textbf{Time (h)}} \textbf{ = Y (Flow Rate in mL/h)}$$

Example 1: 1200 mL D5W IV is ordered to infuse in 10 hours by infusion pump. Calculate the flow rate in milliliters per hour.

Step 1: Determine your givens.	Volume: 1200 mL Time: 10 h

Step 2: Since the volume is given in mL and the time is given in hours, the flow rate can be calculated in one step using the formula.	$\frac{\text{Volume (mL)}}{\text{Time (h)}} = \text{Y (Flow Rate in mL /h)}$
Step 3: Use the formula to calculate the IV flow rate (gtts/min).	$\frac{1200\ \text{mL}}{10\ \text{h}} = 120\ \text{mL/h}$

Therefore, the IV flow rate is 120 mL/hr.

Example 2: 600 mL of antibiotic is to be infused over the 180 minutes by an infusion pump. Calculate the flow rate (mL per hour).

Step 1: Determine your givens.	Volume: 600 mL Time: 180 min
Step 2: Convert 180 min into hours since the flow rate must be stated in mL/h.	180 min ÷ 60 min/h = 3 h
Step 3: Calculate the flow rate in mL/h using the formula.	$\frac{\text{Volume (mL)}}{\text{Time (h)}} = \text{Y (Flow Rate in mL /h)}$ $\frac{600\ \text{mL}}{3\ \text{h}} = 200\ \text{mL/h}$

Therefore, the flow rate is 200 mL/h.

- The following pages contain sample test questions and answers.

Instructions to ensure a correct answer

I. Round all answers to medication problems to the nearest tenth. Kilogram weights should be rounded immediately, before proceeding with the problem. Otherwise, don't round until you get to the final answer. Answers that are not correctly rounded to the nearest tenth are graded as incorrect. For example, 3.25 is rounded to 3.3.
2. I.V. flow problems are rounded to the nearest whole drop. For example, 33.3 is rounded to 33 drops.
3. If the answer is less than 1, with no whole number before the decimal point, ALWAYS place a zero in front of the decimal. This is a safety issue. An answer on the test not preceded by a zero as appropriate will be graded as an incorrect notation. For example, .7 must be written as 0.7 in order to be considered appropriate notation.
4. If the answer is 1,000 or above indicate the number with a comma.
5. ALWAYS omit terminal zeros. Answer containing terminal zeros violate patient safety standards, and will be graded as an incorrect notation. For example 12.50 must be written as 12.5 in order to be considered appropriate notation.
6. The answer must be labeled in correct terms. In incorrectly labeled answer is considered a wrong answer. For example, 7 mg is not the same as 7 mL.
7. Metric units of measure are expressed indecimals; apothecary units of measure are expressed in fractions. For example, 30 mg = *Yz* gr. Fractions must always be reduced to lowest terms.
8. On the test, circle your ONE final answer. If any answer in the circle in incorrect, the answer is graded an incorrect. Ifno answer is circled, then the question is determined to be unanswered and graded as incorrect.

Conversions

2.2 lb	=	1 kg
1 grain	=	60 mg
t oz	=	30 mL
t dram	=	4 mL
1 t	=	S mL
I T		IS mL

1 minim		1 gtt
15 minims	=	1 mL
1 mL	=	15 gtt
1 mL		I cc
t em	=	1O mm
1 inch	=	2.S cm

Roman Numerals

1	=	I
5	=	V
IO		X

Sample Problems for Basic Dosage Calculation

1. Order: Amoxicillin 0.25 g p.o. every 8 hours.
   Available: Amoxicillin 125 mg tablets.
   How many tablets will the nurse give per dose?

2. Order: Zofran 8 mg p.o.t.i.d.
   Available: Zofran in a 100 mL bottle labeled 4 mg/tsp.
   How many mL will the nurse administer for each dose?

3. Order: Morphine gr 1/10
   Available: Morphine 10 mg/mL
   How many mL will the nurse give?

Answers at the end of study guide.

Sample Problems for Pediatric Dose Calculation Based on Weight and BSA

4. Give Fortaz 50 mg/kg p.o. t.i.d. to a child who weighs 25.5 kg. Fortaz is available in an oral suspension labeled 100 mg/mL. How many mL would the nurse administer per dose?

5. Give Ceclor 45 mg/kg/day p.o. in 3 divided doses for a patient who weighs 66 pounds. A 75 mL stock medication is labeled Ceclor 125 mg/mL. How many mL would the nurse administer per dose?

6. Give Biaxin for a child whose BSA is 0.55 m^2. The usual adult dose is 500 mg. Biaxin is available in an oral suspension. The 100 Ml bottle is labeled 50 mg/mL. How many mL would the nurse give per dose?

7. Give Phenergan for a child whose BSA is 1.2 m^2. The usual adult dose is 25 mg. How many milligrams would the nurse administer for the dose?

Answers at the end of study guide.

Sample Problems for I.V. Drip Rate Calculations and Infusion Times

8. LR 125 mL/hr via gravity flow using tubing calibrated at 15 gtt/mL. Calculate the flow rate.

9. One liter NS to infuse over 24 hours using a microdrip (gravity flow). Calculate the flow rate.

10. At the change of shift you notice 200 mL left to count in the I.V. bag. The I.V. is infusing at 80 mL/hr. How much longer will the I.V. run? (Express your answer in hours and minutes.)

11. Keflin 2 g in 100 mL D_5W IVPB over 20 minutes. The I.V. tubing is 15 gtt/mL. Calculate the flow rate.

Answers at the end of study guide.

Sample Problems for Continuous I.V. Heparin Drip Calculations

12. The physician writes an order for heparin 900 units/hr. The label on the I.V. bag reads: Heparin 10,000 units in 500 mL D_5W. How many mL/hr will deliver the correct dose?

13. Administer Heparin 1,000 units/hr from an I.V. bag mixed 40,000 units in 1 L D_5W. How many mL/hr will deliver the correct amount of heparin?

14. The patient's heparin is infusing at 28 mL/hr on an infusion pwnp. The bag of fluid is mixed 20,000 units of heparin in 500 mL D_5W. What hourly dose of heparin is the patient receiving?

15. The patient's heparin drip is infusing at 11 mL/hr on an infusion pwnp. The bag of fluid is mixed 25,000 units of heparin in 250 mL D_5W. What hourly dose of heparin is the patient receiving?

Answers at the end of study guide.

Sample Problems for Critical Care Calculations for I.V. Infusions

Calculating the m/hr Rate

16. Give Regular insulin by continuous I.V. infusion at 20 units/hr. The solution is 250 mL NS with 100 units of Regular insulin. What rate on the infusion pump will deliver the correct dose?

17. Administer a Theophylline drip at 40 mg/hr I.V. The solution is 250 mL D_5W + Theophylline 500 mg. What rate on the infusion pump will deliver the correct dose?

Calculating the pose per Minute or per Hour

18. Give Tridil 15 mcg/minute. Tridil is mixed 50 mg in 500 mL D_5W. What rate on the infusion pump will deliver the correct dose?

19. Give propofol 10 mcg/kg/minute. The infusion is mixed propofol 250 mg in 250 mL D_5W. The patient weighs 168 pounds. What rate on the infusion pump will deliver the correct dose?

20. Give Nitroprusside 5 mcg/kg/minute via continuous infusion for a patient weighing 205 lbs. Nitroprusside is available in a solution of 200 mg in 250 mL D_5W. What rate on the infusion pwnp will deliver the correct dose?

Calculating the Dose Based on Infusion Rate

21. Tridil is infusing at 15 mL/hr on an infusion pump. The drug is mixed 50 mg in 500 mL D_5W. How many mcg/minute is the patient receiving?

22. A lidocaine drip is infusing at 30 mL/hr on an infusion device. The drug is mixed 2 g in 500 mL D_5W. How many mg/minute is the patient receiving?

23. Aminophylline is infusing at 30 mL/hr. The drug is mixed 250 mg in 500 mL D_5W. How many mg/hr is the patient receiving?

Answers at the end of study guide.

Answers in Sample Test Questions

formula: $\frac{\text{desired Amt.} \times \text{quantity}}{\text{have on hand}}$ } $\frac{D}{H} \times Q = X$

1. 0.25g = 250mg ⇒ $\frac{250mg}{125mg} \times 1 \text{ tab} =$ (2 tabs)

2. 1 tsp = 5mL ⇒ $\frac{8mg}{4mg} \times 5mL =$ (10mL)

3. gr 1/10 = 6mg ⇒ $\frac{6mg}{10mg} \times 1mL =$ (0.6mL)

4. 50mg/kg × 25.5 kg = 1,275 mg $\frac{1,275mg}{100mg} \times 1mL = 12.75$ → (12.8mL)

5. 66 lbs = 30 kg $\left(\frac{2.2 lb}{1kg} = \frac{66 lb}{x kg}\right)$
45mg/kg/day × 30 kg = 1,350 mg/day ÷ 3 doses = 450mg per dose
$\frac{450mg}{125mg} \times 1mL =$ (3.6mL)

6. BSA formula: $\frac{\text{child's BSA } [m^2] \times \text{usual adult dose}}{1.7m^2} = \text{child's dose}$

$\frac{0.55m^2 \times 500mg}{1.7m^2} = 161.76$ ⇒ $\frac{161.76mg}{50mg} \times 1mL = 3.236$ → (3.2mL)

7. $\frac{1.2m^2 \times 25mg}{1.7m^2} = 17.64$ ⇒ (17.6mg)

8. IV flow formula: $\frac{\text{vol to be infused (mL)} \times \text{calibration (gtt/mL)}}{\text{time (minutes)}}$ = flow rate (gtt/min)

$\frac{125\text{mL} \times 15\text{gtt/mL}}{60\text{min.}} = 31.25 \Rightarrow$ **31gtt/min**

9. $\frac{1000\text{mL} \times 60\text{gtt/mL}}{1440\text{min}} = 41.6\overline{6}.. \Rightarrow$ **42gtt/min**

10. $80\overline{)200}$ = 2.5 = **2hr and 30min**

11. $\frac{100\text{mL} \times 15\text{gtt/mL}}{20\text{min}} =$ **75gtt/min**

12. you desire / you have $\frac{900\text{units/hr}}{10{,}000\text{units}} \times 500\text{mL} =$ **45mL/hr**

13. $\frac{1{,}000\text{units/hr} \times 1000\text{mL}}{40{,}000\text{units}} =$ **25mL/hr**

14. $\frac{20{,}000\text{units}}{500\text{mL}} = \frac{X\text{units}}{28\text{mL/hr}} \Rightarrow X =$ **1,120 units/hr**

15. $\frac{25{,}000\text{units}}{250\text{mL}} = \frac{X\text{units}}{11\text{mL/hr}} \Rightarrow$ **1,100 units/hr**

16. you desire / you have $\frac{20\text{units/hr} \times 250\text{mL}}{100\text{units}} \rightarrow$ **50mL/hr**

17. $\frac{40\,mg/hr \times 250\,mL}{500\,mg} \Rightarrow$ (20 mL/hr)

18. (a) infusion device is set at hourly rate, so convert (whole numbers) mcg/min to mcg/hr → 15 mcg/min = 900 mcg/hr (15×60)

(b) drug is expressed in mg → convert mcg to mg → 900 mcg/hr = 0.9 mg/hr

(c) $\frac{D}{H} \times Q = \frac{0.9\,mg/hr \times 500\,mL}{50\,mg} \Rightarrow$ (9 mL/hr)

19. a) convert lbs to kg → 168 ÷ 2.2 = 76.36 → 76.4 kg

b) calculate the minute rate → 76.4 kg × 10 mcg/kg/min = 764 mcg/min

c) calculate hourly rate → 764 mcg/min × 60 min/hr = 45,840 mcg/hr

d) drug is expressed in mg → convert mcg to mg → 45,840 mcg = 45.84 mg

e) $\frac{D}{H} \times Q = \frac{45.84\,mg \times 250\,mL}{250\,mg} = 45.84 \Rightarrow$ (46 mL/hr)

20. 205 lbs = 93.8 = 93.2 kg

× 5 mcg/kg/min

466 mcg/min

× 60 min/hr

27,960 mcg/hr ⇒ $\frac{27.96\,mg \times 250\,mL}{200\,mg}$ = 34.95

(35 mL/hr)

21. a) convert 50mg to mcg = 50,000mcg
b) use ratio/proportion to solve

$$\frac{50{,}000\,mcg}{500\,mL} = \frac{X\,mcg}{15\,mL/hr} \qquad x = 1500\ mcg/hr$$

c) calculate the minute rate
1500 mcg/hr ÷ 60 min/hr = 25 mcg/min

22. ⓐ 2g = 2000mg
ⓑ $$\frac{2{,}000\,mg}{500\,mL} = \frac{X\,mg}{30\,mL/hr} \qquad x = 120\,mg/hr$$
ⓒ 120mg/hr ÷ 60min/hr = 2mg/min

23. $$\frac{250\,mg}{500\,mL} = \frac{X\,mg}{30\,mL/hr} \qquad x = 15\,mg/hr$$

LABORATORY VALUES

U.S. traditional units are followed in parentheses by equivalent values expressed in S.I. units.

Hematology

Absolute neutrophil count
Male — **1780-5380/µL (1.78-5.38 x 10^9/L)**
Female — **1560-6130/µL (1.56-6.13 x 10^9/L)**
Activated partial thromboplastin time — 25-35 s
Bleeding time — less than 10 min
Erythrocyte count — 4.2-5.9 x 10^6/µL (4.2-5.9 x 10^{12}/L)
Erythrocyte sedimentation rate
Male — 0-15 mm/h
Female — 0-20 mm/h
Erythropoietin — less than 30 mU/mL (30 units/L)
D-Dimer — less than 0.5 µg/mL (0.5 mg/L)
Ferritin, serum — 15-200 ng/mL (15-200 µg/L)
Haptoglobin, serum — 50-150 mg/dL (500-1500 mg/L)
Hematocrit
Male — 41%-51%
Female — 36%-47%
Hemoglobin, blood
Male — 14-17 g/dL (140-170 g/L)
Female — 12-16 g/dL (120-160 g/L)
Leukocyte alkaline phosphatase — 15-40 mg of phosphorus liberated/h per 10^{10} cells; score = 13-130/100 polymorphonuclear neutrophils and band forms
Leukocyte count — 4000-10,000/µL (4.0-10 x 10^9/L)
Mean corpuscular hemoglobin — 28-32 pg
Mean corpuscular hemoglobin concentration — 32-36 g/dL (320-360 g/L)
Mean corpuscular volume — 80-100 fL
Platelet count — 150,000-350,000/µL (150-350 x 10^9/L)
Prothrombin time — 11-13 s
Reticulocyte count — 0.5%-1.5% of erythrocytes; absolute: 23,000-90,000/µL (23-90 x 10^9/L)

Blood, Plasma, and Serum Chemistry Studies

Albumin, serum — 3.5-5.5 g/dL (35-55 g/L)
Alkaline phosphatase, serum — 36-92 units/L
α-Fetoprotein, serum — 0-20 ng/mL (0-20 µg/L)
Aminotransferase, alanine (ALT) — 0-35 units/L
Aminotransferase, aspartate (AST) — 0-35 units/L
Ammonia, plasma — 40-80 µg/dL (23-47 µmol/L)
Amylase, serum — 0-130 units/L
Bicarbonate, serum — 23-28 meq/L (23-28 mmol/L)
Bilirubin, serum
Total — 0.3-1.2 mg/dL (5.1-20.5 µmol/L)
Direct — 0-0.3 mg/dL (0-5.1 µmol/L)
Blood gases, arterial (ambient air)
pH — 7.38-7.44
P_{CO_2} — 35-45 mm Hg (4.7-6.0 kPa)
P_{O_2} — 80-100 mm Hg (10.6-13.3 kPa)
Oxygen saturation — 95% or greater
Blood urea nitrogen — 8-20 mg/dL (2.9-7.1 mmol/L)
C-reactive protein — 0.0-0.8 mg/dL (0.0-8.0 mg/L)
Calcium, serum — 9-10.5 mg/dL (2.2-2.6 mmol/L)
Carbon dioxide, serum — See Bicarbonate
Chloride, serum — 98-106 meq/L (98-106 mmol/L)
Cholesterol, plasma
Total — 150-199 mg/dL (3.88-5.15 mmol/L), desirable
Low-density lipoprotein (LDL) — less than or equal to 130 mg/dL (3.36 mmol/L), desirable
High-density lipoprotein (HDL) — greater than or equal to 40 mg/dL (1.04 mmol/L), desirable
Complement, serum
C3 — 55-120 mg/dL (550-1200 mg/L)
Total (CH_{50}) — 37-55 U/mL (37-55 kU/L)
Creatine kinase, serum — 30-170 units/L
Creatinine, serum — 0.7-1.3 mg/dL (61.9-115 µmol/L)
Electrolytes, serum
Sodium — 136-145 meq/L (136-145 mmol/L)
Potassium — 3.5-5.0 meq/L (3.5-5.0 mmol/L)
Chloride — 98-106 meq/L (98-106 mmol/L)
Bicarbonate — 23-28 meq/L (23-28 mmol/L)
Fibrinogen, plasma — 150-350 mg/dL (1.5-3.5 g/L)
Folate, red cell — 160-855 ng/mL (362-1937 nmol/L)
Folate, serum — 2.5-20 ng/mL (5.7-45.3 nmol/L)
Glucose, plasma — fasting, 70-100 mg/dL (3.9-5.6 mmol/L)
γ-Glutamyltransferase, serum — 0-30 units/L
Homocysteine, plasma
Male — 0.54-2.16 mg/L (4-16 µmol/L)
Female — 0.41-1.89 mg/L (3-14 µmol/L)
Immunoglobulins
Globulins, total — 2.5-3.5 g/dL (25-35 g/L)
IgG — 640-1430 mg/dL (6.4-14.3 g/L)
IgA — 70-300 mg/dL (0.7-3.0 g/L)
IgM — 20-140 mg/dL (0.2-1.4 g/L)
IgD — less than 8 mg/dL (80 mg/L)
IgE — 0.01-0.04 mg/dL (0.1-0.4 mg/L)
Iron studies
Ferritin, serum — 15-200 ng/mL (15-200 µg/L)
Iron, serum — 60-160 µg/dL (11-29 µmol/L)
Iron-binding capacity, total, serum — 250-460 µg/dL (45-82 µmol/L)
Transferrin saturation — 20%-50%
Lactate dehydrogenase, serum — 60-100 units/L
Lactic acid, venous blood — 6-16 mg/dL (0.67-1.8 mmol/L)
Lipase, serum — less than 95 units/L
Magnesium, serum — 1.5-2.4 mg/dL (0.62-0.99 mmol/L)
Methylmalonic acid, serum — 150-370 nmol/L
Osmolality, plasma — 275-295 mosm/kg H_2O
Phosphatase, alkaline, serum — 36-92 units/L
Phosphorus, serum — 3-4.5 mg/dL (0.97-1.45 mmol/L)
Potassium, serum — 3.5-5.0 meq/L (3.5-5.0 mmol/L)
Prostate-specific antigen, serum – less than 4 ng/mL (4 µg/L)
Protein, serum
Total — 6.0-7.8 g/dL (60-78 g/L)
Albumin — 3.5-5.5 g/dL (35-55 g/L)
Globulins, total — 2.5-3.5 g/dL (25-35 g/L)
Rheumatoid factor — less than 40 U/mL (40 kU/L)
Sodium, serum — 136-145 meq/L (136-145 mmol/L)
Transferrin saturation — 20%-50%
Triglycerides — less than 150 mg/dL (1.69 mmol/L), desirable
Troponins, serum
Troponin I — 0-0.5 ng/mL (0-0.5 µg/L)
Troponin T — 0-0.10 ng/mL (0-0.10 µg/L)
Urea nitrogen, blood — 8-20 mg/dL (2.9-7.1 mmol/L)
Uric acid, serum — 2.5-8 mg/dL (0.15-0.47 mmol/L)
Vitamin B_{12}, serum — 200-800 pg/mL (148-590 pmol/L)

Endocrine

Adrenocorticotropic hormone (ACTH), serum — 9-52 pg/mL (2-11 pmol/L)
Aldosterone, serum
Supine — 2-5 ng/dL (55-138 pmol/L)
Standing — 7-20 ng/dL (194-554 pmol/L)
Aldosterone, urine — 5-19 μg/24 h (13.9-52.6 nmol/24 h)
Catecholamines
Epinephrine, plasma (supine) — less than 75 ng/L (410 pmol/L)
Norepinephrine, plasma (supine) — 50-440 ng/L (296-2600 pmol/L)
Catecholamines, 24-hour, urine — less than 100 μg/m^2 per 24 h (591 nmol/m^2 per 24 h)
Cortisol, free, urine – less than 50 μg/24 h (138 nmol/24 h)
Dehydroepiandrosterone sulfate (DHEA), plasma
Male — 1.3-5.5 μg/mL (3.5-14.9 μmol/L)
Female — 0.6-3.3 μg/mL (1.6-8.9 μmol/L)
Epinephrine, plasma (supine) — less than 75 ng/L (410 pmol/L)
Estradiol, serum
Male — 10-30 pg/mL (37-110 pmol/L);
Female — day 1-10, 14-27 pg/mL (50-100 pmol/L); day 11-20, 14-54 pg/mL (50-200 pmol/L); day 21-30, 19-41 pg/mL (70-150 pmol/L)
Follicle-stimulating hormone, serum
Male (adult) — 5-15 mU/mL (5-15 units/L)
Female — follicular or luteal phase, 5-20 mU/mL (5-20 units/L); midcycle peak, 30-50 mU/mL (30-50 units/L); postmenopausal, greater than 35 mU/mL (35 units/L)
Growth hormone, plasma — after oral glucose: less than 2 ng/mL (2 μg/L); response to provocative stimuli: greater than 7 ng/mL (7 μg/L)
Luteinizing hormone, serum
Male — 3-15 mU/mL (3-15 units/L)
Female — follicular or luteal phase, 5-22 mU/mL (5-22 units/L); midcycle peak, 30-250 mU/mL (30-250 units/L); postmenopausal, greater than 30 mU/mL (30 units/L)
Metanephrine, urine — less than 1.2 mg/24 h (6.1 mmol/24 h)
Norepinephrine, plasma (supine) — 50-440 ng/L (296-2600 pmol/L)
Parathyroid hormone, serum — 10-65 pg/mL (10-65 ng/L)
Progesterone, blood
Male (adult) — 0.27-0.9 ng/mL (0.9-2.9 nmol/L)
Female —
follicular phase, 0.33-1.20 ng/mL (1.0-3.8 nmol/L);
luteal phase, 0.72-17.8 ng/mL (2.3-56.6 nmol/L);
postmenopausal, <0.2-1 ng/mL (0.6-3.18 nmol/L);
oral contraceptives, 0.34-0.92 ng/mL (1.1-2.9 nmol/L)
Prolactin, serum
Male — less than 15 ng/mL (15 μg/L)
Female — less than 20 ng/mL (20 μg/L)
Testosterone, serum
Male (adult) — 300-1200 ng/dL (10-42 nmol/L)
Female — 20-75 ng/dL (0.7-2.6 nmol/L)
Thyroid function tests
Thyroid iodine (^{131}I) uptake — 10%-30% of administered dose at 24 h
Thyroid-stimulating hormone (TSH) — 0.5-5.0 μU/mL (0.5-5.0 mU/L)
Thyroxine (T_4), serum
Total — 5-12 μg/dL (64-155 nmol/L)
Free — 0.9-2.4 ng/dL (12-31 pmol/L)
Free T_4 index — 4-11
Triiodothyronine, free (T_3) — 3.6-5.6 ng/L (5.6-8.6
Triiodothyronine, resin (T_3) — 25%-35%
Triiodothyronine, serum (T_3) — 70-195 ng/dL (1.1-3.0 nmol/L)
Vanillylmandelic acid, urine — less than 8 mg/24 h (40.4 μmol/24 h)
Vitamin D
1,25-dihydroxy, serum — 25-65 pg/mL (60-156 pmol/L)
25-hydroxy, serum — 25-80 ng/mL (62-200 nmol/L)

Urine

Albumin-creatinine ratio — less than 30 mg/g
Calcium — 100-300 mg/24 h (2.5-7.5 mmol/24 h) on unrestricted diet
Creatinine — 15-25 mg/kg per 24 h (133-221 nmol/kg per 24 h)
Glomerular filtration rate (GFR)
Normal
Male — 130 mL/min/1.73 m^2
Female — 120 mL/min/1.73 m^2
Stages of Chronic Kidney Disease
Stage 1 — greater than or equal to 90 mL/min/1.73 m^2
Stage 2 — 60-89 mL/min/1.73 m^2
Stage 3 — 30-59 mL/min/1.73 m^2
Stage 4 — 15-29 mL/min/1.73 m^2
Stage 5 — less than 15 mL/min/1.73 m^2
5-Hydroxyindoleacetic acid (5-HIAA) — 2-9 mg/24 h (10.4-46.8 μmol/24 h)
Protein–creatinine ratio – less than or equal to 0.2 mg/mg
Sodium — 100-260 meq/24 h (100-260 mmol/24 h) (varies with intake)
Uric acid — 250-750 mg/24 h (1.48-4.43 mmol/24 h) (varies with diet)

Gastrointestinal

Gastrin, serum — 0-180 pg/mL (0-180 ng/L)
Stool fat — less than 5 g/d on a 100-g fat diet
Stool weight — less than 200 g/d

Pulmonary

Forced expiratory volume in 1 second (FEV_1) — greater than 80% of predicted
Forced vital capacity (FVC) — greater than 80% of predicted
FEV_1/FVC — greater than 75%

Cerebrospinal Fluid

Cell count — 0-5/μL (0-5 x 10^6/L)
Glucose — 40-80 mg/dL (2.2-4.4 mmol/L); less than 40% of simultaneous plasma concentration is abnormal
Pressure (opening) — 70-200 mm H_2O
Protein — 15-60 mg/dL (150-600 mg/L)

Hemodynamic Measurements

Cardiac index — 2.5-4.2 L/min/m^2
Left ventricular ejection fraction — greater than 55%
Pressures
Pulmonary artery
Systolic — 20-25 mm Hg
Diastolic — 5-10 mm Hg
Mean — 9-16 mm Hg
Pulmonary capillary wedge — 6-12 mm Hg
Right atrium — mean 0-5 mm Hg
Right ventricle
Systolic — 20-25 mm Hg
Diastolic — 0-5 mm Hg

Lab Values and Indications

Potassium (3.5-5.0)

↑	Tachycardic dysthymias Flaccid muscle paralysis Tall T-Waves Numbness Tingling Increased bowel motility
↓	Muscle Weakness Constipation Flat T-Waves on EKG

Calcium (8.5-10.2)

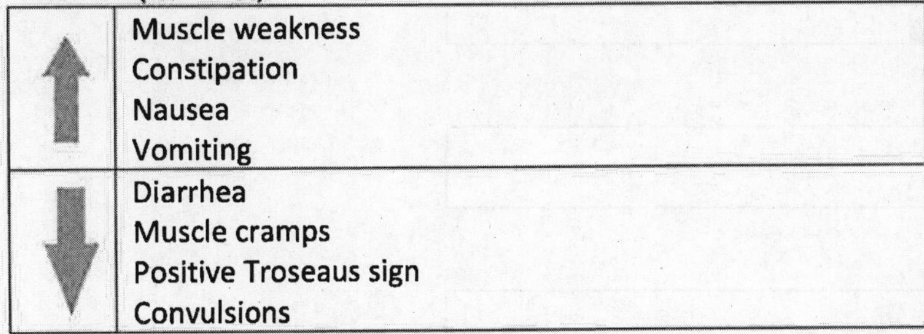

↑	Muscle weakness Constipation Nausea Vomiting
↓	Diarrhea Muscle cramps Positive Troseaus sign Convulsions

Chloride (96-108)

↑	Kidney Dysfunction Dehydration
↓	Low Sodium

Creatinine (0.6-1.2)

↑	Impaired kidney function
↓	Muscle waiting Malnutrition

BUN (Blood Urea Nitrogen) (7-20)

↑	Impaired kidney function Heart Failure Dehydration
↓	Liver disease

Albumin (3.5-5.0)

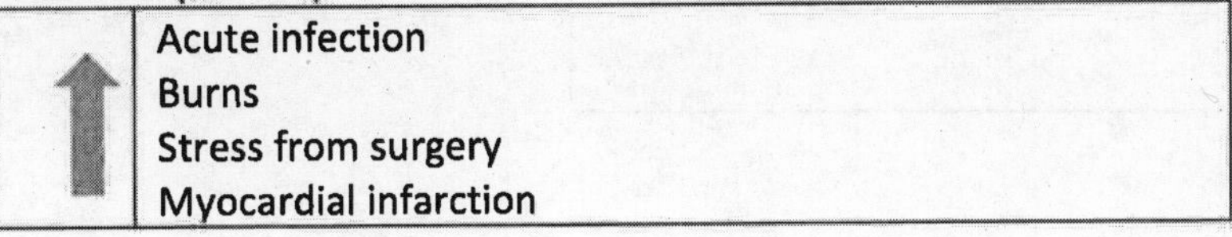

↑	Acute infection Burns Stress from surgery Myocardial infarction

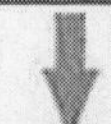 ↓	Malnutrition

Pre Albumin (19-38)

↑	Kidney disease Steroid use Alcoholism
↓	Malnutrition Liver disease

Platelets (150,000-450,000)

↑	Thrombocytosis Elevated rise for blood clots
↓	Thrombocytopenia Elevated risk for bleeding

Cholesterol (>200)

↑	Obesity Vascular disease

Sodium (135-145)

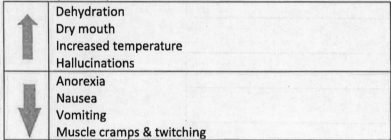

↑	Dehydration Dry mouth Increased temperature Hallucinations
↓	Anorexia Nausea Vomiting Muscle cramps & twitching

WBC (White Blood Cell Count) (5,000-10,000)

↑	Infection
↓	Immunocompromised

Magnesium (1.6-2.6)

↑	Hypotension Bradycardia Lethargy Hypo... reflex
↓	Anorexic Abdominal distension Depression Disorientation

Lactic Acid (0.5-2.2)

↑	Muscle cramps Burning Nausea Shock

RBC (Red Blood Call Count) (male 4.7-6.1 female 4.2-5.4)

↑	Polycythemia treated with phlebotomy
↓	Fatigue Dyspnea Dizziness Tachycardia Pale

Triglycerides (<150)

↑	Indicates high fat content in blood Vascular disease

UGS (Urine Specific Gravity) (1.010-1.030)

↑	Dehydration Impaired kidney function

Hemoglobin (male 13.5-17.5 female 12-16)

↓	Anemia (02 recommended) if below 8 A red blood cell infusion is recommended

Hematocrit (male 42-52 female 37-47)

↑	Dehydration Low oxygen Erythocytosis
↓	Anemia Bleeding Splenomegaly Bone marrow suppression

Blood Osmolality (275-295)

——	Increases with dehydration and lowers with fluid overload

Neutrophils (2300-7400)

↑	Infection
↓	Decreased immunity (neutropenic)

Eosinophils (0-6% 0-450)

↑	Infection Inflammation
↓	Immunocompromised

Phosphorus (2.5-4.5)

↑	Tetany Seizures
↓	Muscle pain & weakness Respiratory failure
*	Phosphorous moves in the opposite direction of calcium

PT (Prothrombin Time) (11-13)

↑	Risk for bleeding
↓	Risk for blood clot

INR (International Normalized Ratio) (0.8-1.2 normal person, 2-3 pt. on warfarin therapy)

↑	Risk for bleeding
↓	Risk for clotting

PTT (Partial Thromboplastin Time) (60-70)

↑	Risk for bleeding
↓	Risk for clotting

APTT (Actirated Partial Thromboplastin Time) (30-40)

↑	Risk for bleeding
↓	Risk for clotting

Basophils (0-2% 0-300)

↑	Infection Allergic reaction Hyperthyroid

HDL (High Density Lipoprotein) (40-59)

*	Good cholesterol

LDL (Low Density Lipoprotein) (100-129)

*	Bad cholesterol

Bilirubin (0.2-1.9)

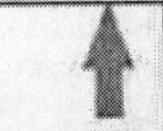	Liver damage

GFR (Glomerular Filtration Rate) (90-120)

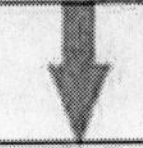	Poor kidney function Peripheral edema

LABS

LABS – ALCOHOL ABUSE

Lab	Lab – Full Text	Explanation
AST ALT	Aspartate aminotransferase Alanine aminotransferase	Enzymes that can indicate liver damage, which is often related to alcohol use.
BAL	Ethanol test Blood alcohol level	Used to determine if a person has been drinking alcohol recently but does not diagnose alcoholism.
CDT	Carbohydrate-deficient transferrin	Can indicate relapse to heavy drinking following a period of abstinence but may be less sensitive for women and younger people.
CMP	Comprehensive metabolic panel	Groups of tests that are used to evaluate organ and liver function.
EtG EtS	Ethyl glucuronide Ethyl sulfate	Biomarkers and direct analytes of the breakdown of alcohol; commonly found in urine testing.
GGT	Gamma-glutamyl transferase	Liver enzyme that is increased by heavy alcohol intake and/or other conditions that affect the liver.
MCV	Mean corpuscular volume	May increase over time in those who are heavy drinkers but may also be affected by many other conditions.
Mg	Magnesium	Which can be low in those who are alcoholic due to insufficient dietary intake and loss by the kidneys
PEth	Phosphatidyl ethanol	A marker, typically measured in blood, that is used to indicate moderate to heavy drinking.

LABS - DIABETIC PATIENTS

Lab	Lab – Full Text	Explanation
GSP	Glycated Serum Protein Fructosamine	Evaluates average glucose levels over the past 2 to 3 weeks. Helpful if the pt has received a transfusion in the recent months.
BG	Blood glucose	The amount of glucose present in a whole blood sample. > 200 mg/dL – Diabetes.
C-Peptide	Insulin C-peptide	Evaluate insulin production by the beta cells in the pancreas or to help determine the cause of low blood glucose.
CBG	Capillary Blood Glucose	Current level of glucose present in the blood in a capillary glucose sample.
CHOL HDL-C LDL-C TRIG/TG Lipids	Cholesterol High-Density Lipoprotein Cholesterol Low-Density Lipoprotein Cholesterol Triglycerides Lipid Profile	To monitor lipids/cholesterol- complications of diabetes can be related to unhealthy lipid levels, which causes damage to blood vessels throughout the body.
FBG	Fasting blood glucose	The level of glucose in the blood after an 8-12 hour fast. 70-99 mg/dL – Normal 100-125 mg/dL – Prediabetes > 126 - Diabetes
HA1C	hemoglobin A1c or glycohemoglobin	The average amount of glucose in the blood over the last 2 to 3 months. 5.7% - Normal 5.7-6.4 Prediabetes > 6.5% - Diabetes
ICA IAA GADA IA-2A	Islet Cell Cytoplasmic Autoantibodies Insulin Autoantibodies Glutamic Acid Decarboxylase Autoantibodies Insulinoma-Associated-2 Autoantibodies	Diabetes-related Autoantibodies – help determine whether the DM is autoimmune related or not.
Microalbumin CRCL eGFR CMP BUN Cr CYSC	Urinary Albumin Creatinine Clearance Est. Glomerular Filtration Rate Comprehensive Metabolic Panel Blood Urea Nitrogen Creatinine Cystatin C	To monitor kidney function – Poorly managed diabetes can cause damage to the organs, specifically the kidneys. It is important to monitor kidney function closely.
UA	Urine Analysis	Urine samples are tested for glucose, protein, and ketones. The presence of glucose and ketones in the urine is a result of diabetic ketoacidosis.

LABS – THYROID DISORDERS

Lab	Lab – Full Text	Explanation
Free T3 Free T4	Free Triiodothyroine Free Thyroxine	Test for hyperthyroidism, especially when the free T4 is not elevated; when people are iodine-deficient, the thyroid makes much more T3 than T4.
TBII	Thyroid binding inhibitory immunoglobulin	Measures the ability of a person's serum to block TSH from binding to receptors.
Tg TGB	Thyroglobulin antibody	Monitor the treatment of thyroid cancer and to detect recurrence.
Total T3 Total T4	Total Triiodothyroine Total Thyroxine	Triiodothyronine (T3) and thyroxine (T4) help control the rate at which the body uses energy. Almost all of the body's T3 and T4 is to protein. The rest is free (unbound) and is the active form of the hormone. Tests can measure the amount of free T3 or the total (bound plus unbound) in the blood.
TPO	Thyroid peroxidase	Autoimmune marker - Detected in Graves disease or Hashimoto thyroiditis. It is very helpful in early Hashimoto thyroiditis when the TSH is elevated but the remaining thyroid is still able to maintain normal free T4 level.
TSH	Thyroid Stimulating Hormone	To test for hypothyroidism, hyperthyroidism, screen newborns for hypothyroidism, and monitor treatment for thyroid disorders.
TSHR	Thyroid stimulating hormone receptor antibodies	A marker for Graves disease; these may be measured in two different ways:
TSI	Thyroid stimulating immunoglobulin	Measures the stimulation of thyroid cells in a culture dish.

LABS – CONGESTIVE HEART FAILURE (CHF)

Lab	Lab – Full Text	Explanation
BMP	Basic Metabolic Panel	Check for electrolyte imbalance, kidney failure (symptoms are similar to those of CHF) and liver disease.
TBII	Thyroid binding inhibitory immunoglobulin	Measures the ability of a person's serum to block TSH from binding to receptors.
NT-proBNP BNP	B-type Natriuretic Peptide Brain Natriuretic Peptide Natriuretic Peptides	Substances that are produced in the heart and released when it is stretched and over worked.
CBC	Complete blood count	Check for anemia, which can cause similar symptoms to CHF as well as contribute to CHF.
TSH T3 T4	Thyroid Panel	Check the level of thyroid hormone in the blood; untreated hyperthyroidism and hypothyroidism can cause heart failure.
Gal-3 ST2	Galectin-3 ST2 cardiac biomarker	Measure these proteins in the blood. Used to predict the course and prognosis of the disease. When these biomarkers are elevate it may indicate that this pt is at risk for complications and needs more aggressive treatment.

CHEMISTRY TESTS

Alanine Aminotransferase (ALT)

Normal Findings:

Elderly: may be slightly higher than adult values

Adult/child: 4 – 36 units/L (SI units)[1]

Indications:

This test is used to identify hepatocellular diseases of the liver. It is also an accurate monitor of improvement or worsening of these diseases.

Test Explanation:

ALT is found predominately in the liver; lesser quantities are found in the kidneys, heart, and skeletal muscle. Injury or disease affecting the liver functioning part of the organ (parenchyma) will cause a release of this hepatocellular enzyme into the bloodstream, thus elevating the ALT serum levels. Most ALT serum level increases are due to liver dysfunction. ALT serum levels are quite specific for hepatocellular disease indicators. In viral hepatitis the ALT/AST ratio is greater than 1, in hepatocellular disease the ratio is less than 1 u/L.

Test Results and Clinical Significance

Mildly Increased Levels:

- Myositis
- Pancreatitis
- Myocardial infarction
- Infectious mononucleosis
- Shock: *injury or disease affecting the liver, heart, or muscles will cause a release of this enzyme into the bloodstream.*

[1] Values may be higher in men and in African Americans

Moderately Increased Levels:

- Cirrhosis
- Hepatic tumor
- Cholestasis (obstructive jaundice)
- Hepatotoxic drugs
- Severe burns

Significantly increased levels:

- Hepatitis
- Hepatic necrosis
- Hepatic ischemia

Alkaline Phosphatase (ALP or ALK Phos)

Normal Findings:

Elderly: slightly higher than adult

Adult: 30 120 units/L

Indications:

ALK Phos is used to detect and monitor diseases of the liver or bone.

Test Explanation:

Although ALK Ph. Is found in many tissues, the highest concentrations are found in the liver, biliary tract and bone. The intestinal mucosa and placenta also contain ALK Ph. The ALK Ph enzyme functions as an alkaline. It increases in an alkaline environment (pH of 9 -10). This enzyme test is important for detecting liver and bone disorders. This enzyme is excreted into the bile and increased levels can be indicators of extrahepatic and intrahepatic obstructive biliary disease and cirrhosis. Other liver abnormalities, such as hepatic tumors, hepatotoxic drugs, and hepatitis, cause smaller elevations. Evidence has indicated that the most sensitive test to indicate tumor metastasis to the liver is the ALK Ph test.

Bone is the most frequent extrahepatic source of ALK Ph.; new bone growth is associated with elevated levels. Diseases causing new bone growth due to osteoblastic metastatic tumors (ie: breast, prostate). Paget disease, healing fractures, rheumatoid arthritis, hyperparathyroidism, and normal-growing bones are all sources of elevated ALK Ph.

Interfering Factors:

- Recent ingestion of a meal can increase the ALK Ph level
- Age: young children with rapid bone growth. This is magnified during the growth spurt.
- Drugs that may cause increased ALK Ph levels (ie: albumin made from placental tissues, allopurinol, antibiotics, methyldopa, tetracycline)

Test Results and Clinical Significance

Increased Levels:

- Primary cirrhosis
- Intrahepatic or extrahepatic biliary obstruction
- Primary or metastatic liver tumor
- Normal pregnancy (third trimester, early postpartum period)
- Normal bones of growing children
- Metastatic tumor to the bone
- Healing fracture
- Hyperparathyroidism
- Paget disease
- Rheumatoid arthritis
- Intestinal ischemia or infarction
- Myocardial Infarction

Decreased Levels:

- Malnutrition
- Milk-alkali syndrome
- Pernicious anemia
- Scurvy (vitamin C deficiency)

Ammonia (or NH_3)

Normal Findings:

Adults: **15-60 micrograms per deciliter (mcg/dL) or**
21-50 micromoles per liter (mcmol/L)

Indications:

Ammonia is used to support the diagnosis of severe liver diseases, and for surveillance of these diseases. Ammonia levels are also used in the diagnosis and follow-up of hepatic encephalopathy.

Test Explanation:

Ammonia is a by-product of the breakdown of protein. Most ammonia in the body forms when protein is broken down by bacteria in the intestinal tract. By way of the portal vein it goes to the liver, where it is normally converted into urea and then secreted by the kidneys. Impaired renal function diminishes excretion of ammonia and the blood levels rise. High levels of ammonia in the liver may be caused by diseases of the liver (Cirrhosis or severe hepatitis). Ammonia then crosses the blood/brain barrier and could result in encephalopathy or neurological dysfunction.

Interfering Factors:

- Hemolysis increases ammonia levels because the RBCs have about three times the ammonia level content of plasma.
- Muscular exertion can increase ammonia levels.
- Cigarette smoking can produce significant increases in ammonia levels within 1 hour of inhalation.
- Drugs that may cause ***increased*** ammonia levels include acetazolamide, alcohol, barbiturates, narcotics, parenteral nutrition and diuretics (loop, thiazide).

- Drugs that may cause ***decreased*** ammonia levels include broad-spectrum antibiotics (neomysin), lactulose, levodopa, lactobacillus, and potassium salts.

Test Results and Clinical Significance

Increased Levels:

- Primary hepatocellular disease
- Reyes Syndrome
- Portal Hypertension
- Severe heart failure with congestive hepatomegaly:
  The portal blood flow from the gut to the liver is altered. The ammonia cannot get to the liver to be metabolized for excretion. Furthermore the ammonia from the gut is rapidly shunted around the liver (by way of gastroesophageal varices) and into the systemic circulation.
- GI bleeding with mild liver disease
- GI obstruction with mild liver disease:
  Ammonia production is increased because the bacteria have more protein (blood) to catabolize. An impaired liver may not be able to keep up with the increased load of ammonia presented to it.

Decreased Levels:

- Essential or malignant hypertension
- Hyperornithinemia

Amylase *cross reference "Lipase"* [2]

Normal Findings:

Adult: < 100 u/L

Indications:

This test is used to detect and monitor the clinical course of pancreatitis. It is frequently ordered when a patient presents with acute abdominal pain.

Test Explanation:

The serum amylase test, which is easy and rapidly performed, is most specific for pancreatitis. Amylase is normally secreted from pancreatic acinar cells into the pancreatic duct and then into the duodenum. Once in the intestine it aides in the breakdown of carbohydrates (starch) to their component simple sugars. Damage to pancreatic acinar cells (as in pancreatitis) or obstruction of the pancreatic duct flow (as in pancreatic carcinoma or common bile duct gallstones) causes an outpouring of this enzyme into the intrapancreatic lymph system and the free peritoneum.

Interfering Factors:

- IV dextrose solutions can lower amylase levels and cause a false-negative result.
- Drugs that may cause ***increased*** serum amylase levels include aminosalicylic acid, aspirin, azathioprine, corticosteroids, dexamethasone, ethyl alcohol, glucocorticoids, loop diuretics (eg: furosemide), methyldopa, narcotic analgesics, oral contraceptives and prednisone.
- Drugs that may cause ***decreased*** levels include citrates, glucose and oxalates.

[2] Lipase is becoming the preferred lab value depending on the physicians order for diagnostic purposes

Test Results and Clinical Significance

Increased Levels:

- Acute pancreatitis
- Chronic relapsing pancreatitis:

  Damage to pancreatic acinar cells as in pancreatitis causes an outpouring of amylase into the intrapancreatic lymph system and the free peritoneum. Blood vessels draining the free peritoneum and absorbing the lymph pick up the excess amylase.
- Penetrating peptic ulcer into the pancreas:

  The peptic ulcer penetrates the posterior wall of the duodenum into the pancreas. This causes a localized pancreatitis with elevated amylase levels.
- GI disease:

  In patients with perforated peptic ulcer, necrotic bowel, perforated bowel, or duodenal obstruction, amylase leaks out of the gut and into the free peritoneal cavity.
- Acute cholecystitis
- Parotiditis (mumps)
- Renal failure

  Amylase is cleared by the kidney. Renal diseases will reduce excretion of amylase.
- Diabetic Ketoacidosis
- Pulmonary infarction

Urea or (Blood Urea Nitrogen) Serum

Critical Values: indicates serious impairment of renal function

Normal Findings:

Adult: 2-9 mmol/L

Indications:

Urea (BUN) is an indirect and rough measurement of renal function and glomerular filtration rate (if normal liver function exists). It is also a measurement of liver function. It is performed on patients undergoing routine laboratory testing. It is usually performed as a part of a multiphase automated testing process.

Test Explanation:

The Urea measures the amount of urea nitrogen in the blood. Urea is formed in the liver as the end product of protein metabolism and digestion. During ingestion, protein is broken down into amino acids. In the liver these amino acids are broken down and free ammonia is formed. The ammonia molecules are combined to form urea, which is then deposited in the blood and transported to the kidneys for excretion. Therefore the Urea is directly related to the metabolic function of the liver and the excretory function of the kidney. It serves as an index of the function of these organs.

Nearly all renal diseases cause an inadequate excretion of urea, which causes the blood concentration to rise above normal. The Urea is interpreted in conjunction with the creatinine test. These tests are referred to as ***"renal function studies"***. The Urea is less accurate than creatinine as an indicator of renal disease.

Test Results and Clinical Significance

Increased Levels:

- Shock
- Burns
- Dehydration:

  With reduced blood volume, renal blood flow is diminished. Therefore renal excretion of Urea is decreased and Urea levels rise.

- Congestive Heart Failure
- Myocardial Infarction

  With reduced cardiac function, renal blood flow is diminished. Therefore renal excretion of urea is decreased and urea levels rise.

- GI bleeding
- Starvation

  As protein is broken down to amino acids at an accelerated rate, urea is formed at a higher rate and urea accumulates.

- Sepsis

  As sepsis increases in severity, renal blood flow and primary renal function are reduced due to hypoperfusion. Urea levels rise.

Decreased Levels:

- Liver failure:

  Urea is made in the liver from urea. Reduced liver function is associated with reduced urea levels.

Brain Natriuretic Peptide (BNP)

Normal Findings:

BNP < 100 pg/mL

Indications:

Natriuretic peptides are used to identify and stratify patients with congestive heart failure[3] (CHF).

Test Explanation:

Natriuretic peptides are neuroendocrine peptides that prevent the activity of the renin-angiotensin[4] system. There are three major natriuretic peptides (NPs).

- ANP – is synthesized in the cardiac atrial muscle.
    - (Normal range: 22-77 pg/mL)
- BNP – the main source of BNP is the cardiac ventricle.
- C-type – is produced by the endothelial cells.

The cardiac peptides are continuously released by the heart muscle cells in low levels. The rate of release can be increased by a variety of physiological factors including hemodynamic load[5] to regulate cardiac reload and afterload. BNP and ANP have been used in the pathophysiology of hypertension, CHF and atherosclerosis. Both BNP and ANP are released in response to atrial and ventricular stretch causing vasorelaxation, inhibition of aldosterone secretion from the adrenal gland and renin from the kidney, resulting in increasing the natriuresis and reduction in blood volume.

BNP correlates to the left ventricular pressures so is a good indicator for CHF. The increasing levels of BNP the more severe the CHF. This test is becoming increasingly used in urgent care

---

[3] Congestive heart failure is a condition in which the heart can no longer pump enough blood to the rest of the body.

[4] The **renin-angiotensin** system is a complex biologic system between the heart, brain, blood vessels, and kidneys that leads to the production of biologically active agents, including **angiotensin** I and II and aldosterone

[5] **Hemodynamics**, meaning literally "blood movement" is the study of blood flow or the circulation

settings to aid in the differential diagnosis of shortness of breath (SOB).[6] If the BNP is elevated, the SOB is related to CHF. If BNP levels are normal then SOB is pulmonary and not cardiac in nature. This is particularly useful in assessing patients with medical histories of both cardiac and chronic lung disease.

Interfering Factors

- BNP levels are generally higher in healthy women than healthy men
- BNP levels are higher in older patients

Test Results and Clinical Significance

Increased levels

- Congestive Heart Failure
- Myocardial infarction
- Systemic hypertension

[6] Note: The range of normal is wide, and the range of test in true pathology is also wide. A VERY high value may be helpful, but most results are indeterminate. Dr. A. Lund

Chloride, blood (Cl)

Normal Findings:

Adult: 98-108 mmol/L

Indications:

This test is performed as a part of multiphase testing for what is usually called "electrolytes". By itself, this test does not provide much information. However, with interpretation of the other electrolytes, chloride can give an indication of acid-base balance and hydration status.

Test Explanation:

Chloride is the major extracellular anion. Its primary purpose is to maintain electrical neutrality, mostly as a salt with sodium. It follows sodium losses and accompanies sodium excesses in an attempt to maintain electrical neutrality. Because water moves with sodium and chloride, chloride also affects water balance. Finally, chloride also serves as a buffer to assist in acid-base balance. As carbon dioxide increases, bicarbonate must move from the intracellular space to the extracellular space. To maintain electrical neutrality, chloride will shift back into the cell.

Hypochloremia and hyperchloremia rarely occur alone and usually are part of parallel shifts in sodium or bicarbonate levels. Signs and symptoms of hypochloremia include hyperexcitability of the nervous system and muscles, shallow breathing, hypotension and tetany. Signs and symptoms of hyperchloremia include lethargy, weakness and deep breathing.

Interfering Factors:

- Excessive infusions of saline solutions can results in increased chloride levels.
- Drugs that may cause ***increased*** serum chloride levels include androgens, chlorothiazide, cortisone preparations, estrogens, hydrochlorothiazide, methyldopa, and nonsteroidal anti-inflammatory.
- Drugs that may cause ***decreased*** levels include aldosterone, bicarbonates, corticosteroids, cortisone, hydrocortisone, loop diuretics, thiazide diuretics and triamterene.

Test Results and Clinical Significance

Increased Levels (Hyperchloremia):

- Dehydration

  Chloride ions are more concentrated in the blood.
- Excessive infusion of normal saline solution

  Intake of chloride exceeds output, and blood levels rise.
- Kidney dysfunction

Decreased Levels (Hypochloremia):

- Over-hydration
- Congestive heart failure

  Chloride is retained with sodium retention but is diluted by excess total body water.
- Vomiting or prolonged gastric suction
- Chronic diarrhea

  Chloride is high in the stomach and GI tract because of HCl acid produced in the stomach.
- Chronic respiratory acidosis
- Burns

  Sodium and Chloride losses from massive burns can be great.

Creatine Kinase (CK) *cross reference "Troponins"*

Normal Findings:

Adult: < 165 U/L

Indications:

This test is used to support the diagnosis of myocardial muscle injury (Infarction). It can also indicate neurologic or skeletal muscle diseases.[7]

Test Explanation:

CK is found predominantly in the heart muscle, skeletal muscle, and brain. Serum CK levels are elevated when these muscle or nerve cells are injured. CK levels can rise within 6 hours after damage. If damage is not persistent, the levels peak at 18 hours after injury and return to normal in 2 to 3 days. When the total CK level is elevated injury to or disease of the skeletal muscle is present. Examples of this include myopathies, vigorous exercise, multiple intramuscular (IM) injections, ETC, cardioversion, chronic alcoholism, or surgery. Because CK is made only in the skeletal muscle, the normal value of total CK varies according to a person's muscle mass. Large muscular people may normally have a CK level in the high range of normal. This is important because high normal CK levels in these patients can mask a MI.

CK is the main cardiac enzyme studied in patients with heart disease. Because its blood clearance and metabolism are well known, its frequent determination (on admission and at 12 hours & 24 hours) can accurately reflect timing, quantity, and resolution of a MI. New blood

[7] Note: CK is now rarely used in the context of ruling out myocardial injury, in favour of the more sensitive and specific Troponin tests. However, CK remains an important test in evaluating myonecrosis from crush injuries, compartment syndromes, and rhabdomyolysis. Dr. A. Lund

assays for cardiac markers have promised to rapidly and accurately detect acute MI in the emergency room.

***Troponin*.**

Both Troponin T and Troponin I are specific to cardiac tissue and are released following an MI. Troponins will be discussed in more detail in a later section (see pg 34).

Timing of Commonly Used Cardiac Enzymes

Enzyme	Elevation begins	Peaks	Returns to Normal
Total CK	4-6 hours	24 hours	3-4 days
CK- MB	4 hours	18 hours	2 days
Troponin T	4-6 hours	10-24 hours	10 days
Troponin I	4-6 hours	10-24 hours	4 days

Interfering Factors:

- IM injections can cause elevated CK levels
- Strenuous exercise and recent surgery may cause increased levels
- Muscle mass is directly related to a patient's normal CK level
- Drugs that may cause ***increased*** levels include ampicillin, some anesthetics, anticoagulants, aspirin, dexamethasone (Decadron), furosemide (Lasix), captopril, alcohol, lovastatin, lithium, lidocaine, propranolol, and morphine.

Test Results and Clinical Significance

Increased Levels of Total CK:

- Diseases or injury affecting the heart muscle, skeletal muscle, and brain

Increased Levels of CK-MB Isoenzyme:

- AMI
- Cardiac aneurysm surgery
- Cardiac defibrillation
- Myocarditis
- Ventricular arrhythmias
- Cardiac ischemia

Any disease or injury to the myocardium causes CK-MB to spill out of the damaged cells and into the bloodstream, producing elevated CK-MB isoenzyme levels.

Creatinine, Blood

Critical Values: indicates serious impairment in renal function

Normal Findings:

Adult: 45-110 umol/L

Indications:

Creatinine is as part of a complete renal function panel including Urea and the eGFR which will be calculated to assist in the diagnosis of impaired renal function.

Test Explanation:

This test measures the amount of creatinine in the blood. Creatinine is a catabolic product of creatine phosphate, which is used in skeletal muscle contraction. The daily production of creatine, and subsequently creatinine, depends on muscle mass, which fluctuates very little. Creatinine, as Urea is excreted entirely by the kidneys and therefore is directly proportional to renal excretory function. Thus, with normal renal excretory function, the serum creatinine level should remain constant and normal. Only renal disorders, such as glomerulonephritis, pylonephritis, acute tubular necrosis, and urinary obstruction, will cause an abnormal elevation in creatinine. There are slight increases in creatinine levels after meals, especially after ingestion of large quantities of meat. The serum creatinine test, as with the Urea is used to diagnose impaired renal function. The creatinine level is interpreted in conjunction with Urea and GFR. These tests are referred to as ***renal function studies***.

Age Related Concerns:

The elderly normally have lower creatinine levels due to reduced muscle mass. This may potentially mask renal disease in patients of this age group.

Interfering Factors:

- A diet high in meat content can cause transient elevations of serum creatinine.
- Drugs that may ***increase*** creatinine values include aminoglycosides (ie: getamicin), cimetidine, and other nephrotoxic drugs such as cephalosporins (ie: cefoxitin)

Test Results and Clinical Significance

Increased Levels:

Diseases affecting renal function include:

- Glomerulonephritis
- Pyelonephritis
- Acute tubular necrosis
- Urinary tract obstruction
- Reduced renal blood flow (ie: shock, dehydration, congestive heart failure, atherosclerosis)
- Diabetic nephropathy
- Nephritis

With these illnesses, renal function is impaired and creatinine levels rise.

- **Note:** Patients with impaired renal function (i.e. high urea, creatinine, or low eGFR) are at increased risk of total renal failure after CT with contrast.
- Reference the "Contrast Induced Nephropathy" order set

D-dimer (Fibrin Degradation Product, FDP)

Normal Findings:

Adult: < 500 ug FEU/L

Indications:

A d-dimer test is a blood test that measures a substance released as a blood clot breaks up. D-dimer levels are often higher than normal in people who have a blood clot.

In current practice, the most common indication for this test would be to rule out Pulmonary Embolus[8] (PE) or Deep Vein Thrombosis (DVT)[9].

Test Explanation:

The fragment D-dimer assesses both thrombin and plasmin activity. D-dimer is a fibrin degradation fragment that is made through fibrinolysis. As plasmin acts on the fibrin polymer clot, FDP's and D-dimer are produced. D-dimer is a highly specific measurement of the amount of fibrin degradation that occurs. Normal plasma does not have detectable amounts of fragment D-dimer. Levels of D-dimer can also increase when a fibrin clot is lysed by thrombolytic therapy. Thrombotic problems such as deep-vein thrombosis, pulmonary embolism, can be part of the complex clinical assessment using the D-dimer levels.

[8] A pulmonary embolism is a blockage in an artery in the lung. It is usually due to a blood clot that has traveled to the lung from another part of the body, usually the leg (DVT).

[9] Deep vein thrombosis is a condition in which a blood clot (thrombus) forms in the deep veins of the legs, pelvis, or arms. These veins are located near the bones and are surrounded by muscle.

Test Results and Clinical Significance

Increased Levels:

- Disseminated intravascular coagulation (DIC):

  This is a serious bleeding disorder resulting from abonormally initiated and accelerated clotting. The ensuing depletion of clotting factors and platelets may lead to uncontrollable hemorrhage.

  DIC is always caused by an underlying disease (e.g. Multiple organ failure, mass transfusions). The underlying disease must be treated for the DIC to resolve.
- Primary fibrinolysis
- Deep-vein thrombosis
- Pulmonary embolism
- Vasoocclusive crisis of sickle cell anemia
- Surgery:

  These clinical situations are associated with varying degrees of clotting and fibrinolysis. D-dimer is produced by the action of plasmin on the fibrin polymer clot.

Digoxin Level

Therapeutic range:

Heart failure - **0.5-2.0 ng/ml**
Arrhythmia - **1.5-2.0 ng/ml**

Indications:

A digoxin test is used to monitor the concentration of the drug in the blood. The dose of digoxin prescribed may be adjusted depending on the level measured.

Test Explanation:

A doctor may order one or more digoxin tests when a person begins treatment to determine if the initial dosage is within therapeutic range and then order it at regular intervals to ensure that the therapeutic level is maintained. A digoxin test may also be used to determine if symptoms are due to an insufficient amount of the drug or due to **digoxin toxicity**[10]**.** Digoxin takes approximately one to two weeks to reach a steady level in the blood and in the target organ, the heart. Once the dosage level is determined, digoxin levels are monitored routinely, at a frequency determined by the doctor, to verify correct dosage and if any changes occur in drug source, dosage, or other medications taken at the same time.

Test Results and Clinical Significance

Digoxin is primarily cleared from your system by the kidneys. When someone has kidney problems, their doctor may want to monitor kidney function and blood potassium levels since kidney dysfunction and low levels of potassium can result in symptoms of digoxin toxicity.

[10] **Digoxin toxicity** is a poisoning that occurs when excess doses of digoxin are consumed acutely or over an extended period.

The test may be done when toxicity is suspected and the affected person has signs and symptoms such as:

- Dizziness
- Blurred vision or seeing yellow or green halos
- Vomiting
- Diarrhea
- Irregular heartbeat
- Difficulty breathing
- Fatigue
- Shortness of breath
- Swelling in the hands and feet (edema)
- Characteristic EKG changes include bradycardia[11] (the most frequent vital sign abnormality in toxicity), a prolonged PR interval

Changes in health status can affect levels of digoxin and its ability to control symptoms. Digoxin tests may be done and the dose adjusted if necessary when someone experiences a physiologic change that may affect blood levels and effectiveness of digoxin. This may be when someone develops, for example, kidney or thyroid problems, cancer, or stomach or intestinal illness.

[11] **Bradycardia** in the context of adult medicine, is the resting heart rate of under 60 beats per minute

Glomerular Filtration Rate (GFR)

Normal Range:

Adult: 90-120 ml/min

Indications:

The GFR test is used to screen for and detect early kidney damage and to monitor kidney status. Glomerular filtration rate (GFR) is a calculation that determines how well the blood is filtered by the kidneys, which is one way to measure remaining kidney function. Glomerular filtration rate is usually calculated using a mathematical formula that compares a person's size, age, sex, and race to serum creatinine levels.

Test Explanation:

It is performed by ordering a creatinine test and calculating the eGFR. The creatinine test is ordered frequently as part of a routine Comprehensive Metabolic Panel (CMP) or Basic Metabolic Panel (BMP), or along with a Urea (or BUN) test whenever a doctor wants to evaluate the status of the kidneys. It is ordered to monitor those with known kidney disease and those with conditions such as diabetes and hypertension that may lead to kidney damage.

Test Results and Clinical Significance

The GFR is used to monitor or evaluate kidney function early warning signs of kidney disease may include:

- Swelling or puffiness, particularly around the eyes or in the face, wrists, abdomen, thighs, or ankles
- Urine that is foamy, bloody, or coffee-colored
- A decrease in the amount of urine
- Problems urinating, such as a burning feeling or abnormal discharge during urination, or a change in the frequency of urination, especially at night

- Mid-back pain (flank), below the ribs, near where the kidneys are located
- High blood pressure (hypertension)

As kidney disease worsens, symptoms may include:

- Urinating more or less often
- Feeling itchy
- Tiredness, loss of concentration
- Loss of appetite, nausea and/or vomiting
- Swelling and/or numbness in hands and feet
- Darkened skin
- Muscle cramps

A person's GFR decreases with age and some illnesses. There is different equation that should be used to calculate the GFR for those under the age of 18.

A GFR test may not be as useful for those who differ from normal creatinine concentrations. This may include people who have significantly more muscle (such as a body builder) or less muscle (such as a muscle-wasting disease) than the norm, those who are extremely obese, malnourished, follow a strict vegetarian diet, ingest little protein, or who take creatine dietary supplements.

Important to note GFR equations are not valid for those who are 75 year of age or older because muscle mass normally decreases with age.

Glucose, Blood (Blood Sugar, Fasting Blood Sugar, FBS)

Normal Findings:

Adult: 4.0 – 8.3 mmol/L

Elderly: Increase in normal range after age 50 years

Indications:

This test is a direct measurement of the blood glucose level. It is most commonly used in the evaluation of diabetic patients, septic patients or any patient with an altered level of consciousness. Blood glucose testing is a vital part of the data gathering process of patient comprehensive assessments (ie: blood pressure, pulse, respirations, temperature) to help assist with diagnosis.

Test Explanation:

Through multiple feedback mechanisms, glucose levels are primarily controlled by insulin and glucagons, though many other things can affect the glucose level in the blood. Glucagon[12] breaks glycogen down to glucose in the liver and glucose levels rise. Glucose levels are elevated after eating. Insulin, which is made in the beta cells of the pancreatic islets of Langerhans, is secreted. Insulin attaches to insulin receptors in muscle, liver and fatty cells in which it drives glucose into these target cells to be metabolized to glycogen, amino acids and fatty acids. Blood glucose levels diminish.

[12] **Glucagon**, a hormone secreted by the pancreas, raises blood glucose levels. Its effect is opposite that of insulin, which lowers blood glucose levels

In general, true glucose elevations indicate diabetes mellitus (DM), however, there are many other possible causes of hyperglycemia[13]. Similarly, hypoglycemia[14] has many causes. Fingerstick blood glucose determinations are often performed before meals and at bedtime. Results are compared with a sliding-scale insulin chart ordered by the physician to provide coverage with subcutaneous regular insulin.

Interfering Factors:

- Many forms of stress (ie: trauma, general anesthesia, infection, burns, MI, can cause increased serum glucose levels).
- Caffeine may cause increased levels.
- Most IV fluids contain dextrose, which is quickly converted to glucose. Most patients receiving IV fluids will have increased glucose levels.
- Drugs that may cause increased levels include antidepressants (tricyclics), beta-adrenergic blocking agents, corticosteroids, IV dextrose infusion, diuretic, Epinephrine, estrogens, glucagons, lithium, phenothiazines, phenytoin, and salicylates (acute toxicity).

Test Results and Clinical Significance

Increased Levels (Hyperglycemia):

- Diabetes mellitus (DM)

  This disease is defined by glucose intolerance.

- Acute stress response

  Severe stress, including infection, burns and surgery stimulates catecholamine release. This in turn stimulates glucagon secretion which causes hyperglycemia.

- Chronic renal failure

  Glucagon is metabolized by the kidney. With loss of kidney function, glucagon and glucose levels rise.

- Acute pancreatitis

---

[13] See signs and symptoms at end of text
[14] See signs and symptoms at end of text

As cells are injured during the inflammation process, the contents of the pancreatic cells (including glucagon) are spilled into the bloodstream. The glucagon causes hyperglycemia.

- Diuretic therapy

  Certain diuretics cause hyperglycemia.

- Corticosteroid therapy

  Cortisol causes hyperglycemia (response to stress and to sepsis).

Decreased Levels (Hypoglycemia):

- Insulin overdose

  This is the most common cause of hypoglycemia. Insulin is administered at too high of a dose (especially in brittle diabetes) and glucose levels fall.

- Insulinoma

  Insulin is autonomously produced without regard to biofeedback mechanisms.

- Hypothyroidism

  Thyroid hormones affect glucose metabolism. With diminished levels of this hormone, glucose levels fall.

- Addison disease

  Cortisol affects glucose metabolism. With diminished levels of this hormone glucose levels fall.

- Extensive liver disease

  Most glucose metabolism occurs in the liver. With decreased liver function, glucose levels decrease.

- Starvation

  With decreased carbohydrate ingestion, glucose levels diminish.

Signs and Symptoms:

Hyperglycemia

The following symptoms may be associated with acute or chronic hyperglycemia, with the first three composing the classic hyperglycemic triad:

- *Polyphagia - frequent hunger, especially pronounced hunger*
- *Polydipsia - frequent thirst, especially excessive thirst*
- *Polyuria - frequent urination*
- *Blurred vision*
- *Fatigue (sleepiness).*
- *Weight loss*
- *Poor wound healing (cuts, scrapes, etc.)*
- *Dry mouth*
- *Dry or itchy skin*
- *Tingling in feet or heels*
- *Erectile dysfunction*
- *Cardiac arrhythmia*
- *Stupor*
- *Coma*

Hypoglycaemia causes symptoms such as:

- hunger
- shakiness
- nervousness
- sweating
- dizziness or light-headedness
- sleepiness
- confusion
- difficulty speaking
- anxiety
- weakness

Lactic Acid (Lactate)

Normal Findings:

Venous blood: 5-20 mg/dL or 0.6 – 2.2 mmol/L (SI units)

Indications:

This test is a measurement of the lactic acid in the tissues associated with shock or localized vascular occlusion. Lactic acid is produced when oxygen levels in the body drop, and the tissues switch from aerobic to anaerobic means of energy production. Lactic acidosis is when lactic acid builds ups in the bloodstream faster than it can be removed.

Test Explanation:

When tissues have normal oxygenation to the tissues, glucose is metabolized to CO2 and H2O for energy. When the tissues experience oxygen deprivation or hypoxemia then the glucose is converted to lactate (lactic acid) instead of CO2 and H2O and lactic acid buildup occurs causing lactic acidosis (LA). Therefore, blood lactate is a fairly sensitive and reliable indicator of tissue hypoxia. The hypoxia may be caused by local tissue hypoxia such as tissue hypoxia (ie: extremity ischemia) or generalized tissue hypoxia such as exists in shock.

Test Results and Clinical Significance

Increased Levels:

- **Shock (total body state)**
- **Tissue Ischemia**: Anaerobic metabolism [15] occurs in hypoxemic organs and tissues. As a result, lactic acid is formed, causing increased blood levels.

---

[15] Anaerboic describing a type of cellular respiration in which usually carbohydrates are never completely oxidized because molecular oxygen is not used.

- **Carbon monoxide poisoning**: Carbon monoxide binds hemoglobin more tightly than oxygen resulting in lack of oxygen available to tissues for normal aerobic metabolism – anaerobic metabolism occurs.
- **Severe Liver Disease**
- Diabetes mellitus[16] (nonketotic): Lactic Acid levels rise in patients with poorly controlled diabetes most likely because of inefficient aerobic glucose metabolism, causing increased production of this lactic acid.

---

[16] **Diabetes mellitus**, often simply referred to as **diabetes**, is a group of metabolic diseases in which a person has high blood sugar, either because the body does not produce enough insulin, or because cells do not respond to the insulin that is produced

- Type 1 diabetes: results from the body's failure to produce insulin, and presently requires the person to inject insulin. (Also referred to as *insulin-dependent* diabetes mellitus, *IDDM* for short, and *juvenile* diabetes.)
- Type 2 diabetes: results from insulin resistance, a condition in which cells fail to use insulin properly, sometimes combined with an absolute insulin deficiency. (Formerly referred to as *non-insulin-dependent* diabetes mellitus, *NIDDM* for short, and *adult-onset* diabetes.)

Lipase

Normal Findings:

0-160 units/L (Normal value ranges may vary slightly among different laboratories)

Indications:

This test is used in the evaluation of pancreatic disease. In acute pancreatitis, elevated lipase levels usually parallel blood amylase concentrations, although amylase levels tend to rise and fall a bit sooner than lipase levels.

Test Explanation:

Lipase is a protein (enzyme) released by the pancreas into the small intestine (duodenum). It helps the body absorb fat by breaking the fat (triglycerides)down into fatty acids. As with amylase, lipase appears in the bloodstream following damage to or disease affecting the pancreatic acinar[17] cells. Lipase is excreted through the kidneys so it is now apparent that other conditions can be associated with elevated lipase levels. Therefore elevated lipase levels are often found in patients with renal failure, intestinal infarction of obstruction also can be associated with lipase elevation.

In acute pancreatitis, elevated lipase levels usually parallel serum amylase levels. The lipase levels usually rise slightly later than amylase levels (24 – 48 hours after onset of pancreatitis) and remain elevated in the blood stream for 5 to 7 days. Due to Lipase peaking later and remaining elevated longer than amylase the usage of serum lipase levels are deemed more useful in the lat diagnosis of acute pancreatitis. Lipase levels are less useful in more chronic pancreatic diseases (if: chronic pancreatitis, pancreatic carcinoma).

[17] An **acinus** (adjective: **acinar**, plural **acini**) refers to any cluster of cells that resembles a many-lobed cluster

Interfering Factors

- Drugs that may cause ***increased*** lipase levels include: codeine, meperidine, morphine, cholinergics, indomethacin, methacholine and bethanechol.
- Drugs that may cause ***decreased*** levels include: calcium ions

Test Results and Clinical Significance

Increased Levels:

- Pancreatic diseases (ie: acute pancreatitis, chronic relapsing pancreatitis, pancreatic cancer) Lipase exists in the pancreatic cell and is released into the bloodstream when disease or injury affects the pancreas.
- Biliary disease (ie: acute cholecystitis, cholangitis, extrahepatic duct obstruction) Although the pathophysiology of these observations is not well understood it is suspected that lipase exists inside the cells of the hepatobiliary system. Disease or injury of these tissues would cause the lipase to leak into the bloodstream and cause levels to be elevated.
- Renal failure: Lipase is excreted by the kidney. If excretin is poor, as in renal failure, lipase levels will rise.
- Intestinal diseases (ie: bowel obstruction, infarction) Lipase exists in the mucosal cells lining the bowel (mostly in the duodenum). Injury through obstruction or ischemia will cause the cells to lyse[18]. Lipase will leak into bloodstream and cause levels to be elevated.
- Salivary gland inflammation or tumor: Like amylase, salivary glands contain lipase, although to a much lesser degree. Tumors, inflammation, or obstruction of salivary ducts will cause the cells to lyse. Lipase will leak into the bloodstream and cause levels to be elevated.

---

[18] To induce lysis, or to cause dissolution or destruction of a cell membrane with lysin

Potassium, Blood (K)

Normal Findings:

Adult: 3.5 - 5.0 mmol/L

Indications:

This test is routinely performed in most patients investigated for any type of serious illness. Furthermore, because this electrolyte is so important to cardiac function, it is a part of all complete routine evaluations, especially in patients who take diuretics or heart medications.

Test Explanation:

Potassium is the major cation within the cell. The intracellular potassium concentration is approximately 150 mEq/L, whereas the normal serum potassium concentration is approximately 4 mEq/L. This ratio is the most important determinant in maintaining membrane electrical potential, especially in neuromuscular tissue. Because the serum concentration of potassium is so small, minor changes in concentration have significant consequences. Potassium is excreted by the kidneys. Potassium is an important part of protein synthesis and maintenance of normal metabolic portion of acid-base balance in that the kidneys can shift potassium or hydrogen ions to maintain a physiologic pH.

Symptoms of ***hyperkalemia*** include irritability, nausea, vomiting, intestinal colic, and diarrhea. Signs of ***hypokalemia*** are related to a decrease in contractility of smooth, skeletal, and cardiac muscles, which results in weakness, paralysis, hyporeflexia[19], ileuses, increased cardiac sensitivity to digoxin, cardiac arrhythmias. This electrolyte has profound effects on the heart rate and contractility.

[19] **Hyporeflexia** is the condition of below normal or absent reflexes

The potassium level should be carefully followed in patients with uremia, Addison disease, and vomiting & diarrhea and in patients taking potassium-depleting diuretics or steroid therapy. Potassium must be closely monitored in patients taking digitalis-like drugs, because cardiac arrhythmias may be induced by hypokalemia and digoxin.

Interfering Factors:

- Drugs that may cause ***increased*** potassium levels include aminocaproic acid, antibiotics, antineoplastic drugs, captopril, epinephrine, heparin, histamine, lithium, mannitol, potassium-sparing diuretics, and potassium supplements.
- Drugs that may cause ***decreased*** levels include acetazolamide, aminosalicylic acid, glucose infusions, carbenicillin, cisplatin, diuretics (potassium wasting), insulin, laxatives, lithium carbonate, penicillin G sodium (high doses), phenothiazines, salicylates (aspirin).

Test Results and Clinical Significance

Increased Levels (Hyperkalemia):

- Excessive dietary intake
- Excessive IV intake

  Because the amount of potassium in the serum is so small, minimal but significant increases in potassium intake can cause elevations in the serum level.
- Acute or chronic renal failure

  This is the most common cause of hyperkalemia. Potassium excretion is diminished and potassium levels rise.
- Crush injury to tissues

- Infection

  Potassium exists in high levels in the cell. With cellular injury and lysis, the potassium within the cell is released into the bloodstream.

- Dehydration

  Potassium becomes more concentrated in dehydrated patients, and serum levels appear to be elevated. When the patient is dehydrated, potassium levels may, in fact, be reduced.

Decreased Levels (Hypokalemia):

- Deficient dietary intake
- Deficient IV intake

  The kidneys cannot reabsorb potassium to compensate for the reduced potassium intake. Potassium levels decline.

- Trauma, surgery and burns

  The body's response to trauma is mediated, in part by aldosterone, which increases potassium excretion.

- Gastrointestinal (GI) disorders (e.g. diarrhea, vomiting)

  Excessive potassium is lost because of ongoing fluid and electrolyte losses as indicated above.

- Diuretics

  These medications act to increase renal excretion of potassium. This is especially important for cardiac patients who take diuretics and digitalis preparations. Hypokalemia can exacerbate the ectopy that digoxin may instigate.

- Alkalosis

  To maintain physiologic pH during alkalosis, hydrogen ions are driven out of the cell and into the blood. To maintain electrical neutrality, potassium is driven into the cell. Potassium levels fall.

- Insulin administration

  In patients with hyperglycemia, insulin is administered. Glucose and potassium are driven into the cell. Potassium levels drop.

- Ascites

  These patients have a decreased renal blood flow from reduced intravascular volume that results from the collection of fluid. The reduced blood flow stimulates the secretion of aldosterone, which increases potassium excretion. Furthermore, these patients are often taking potassium-wasting diuretics.

Sodium, Blood (Na)

Normal Findings:

Adult: 135-145 mmol/L

Indications:

This test is part of a routine laboratory evaluation of all patients. It is one of the tests automatically performed when "serum electrolytes" are requested. This test is used to evaluate and monitor fluid and electrolyte balance and therapy.

Test Explanation:

Sodium is the major cation in the extracellular space, in which there are serum levels of approximately 140 mEq/L. The concentration of sodium intracellular is only 5 mEq/L. Therefore sodium salts are the major determinants of extracellular osmolality. The sodium content in the blood is a result of a balance between dietary sodium intake and renal excretion. Non-renal (ie: sweat) sodium losses normally are minimal.

Physiologically, water and sodium are closely interrelated. As free body water is increased, serum sodium is diluted and the concentration may decrease. The kidney compensates by conserving sodium and excreting water. If free body water were to decrease, the serum sodium concentration would rise. The kidney would then respond by conserving free water.

The first symptom of ***hyponatremia*** is weakness. When sodium levels fall below normal levels, confusion and lethargy occur. In severe cases stupor and coma can occur. Symptoms of ***hypernatremia*** include dry mucous membranes, thirst, agitation, restlessness, hyperreflexia, mania and convulsions.

Interfering Factors:

- Recent trauma, surgery or shock may cause increased levels because renal blood flow is decreased.
- Drugs that may cause **increased** levels include anabolic steroids, antibiotics, clonidine, corticosteroids, cough medicines, laxatives, estrogens and oral contraceptives.
- Drugs that may cause **decreased** levels include carbamazepine, diuretics, sodium-free IV fluids, angiotensin-converting enzyme (ACE) inhibitors, captopril, haloperidol, heparin, nonsteroidal anti-inflammatory drugs, tricyclic antidepressants and vasopressin.

Test Results and Clinical Significance

Increased Levels (Hypernatremia):

- Increased dietary intake

  If sodium (usually in the form of salt) is ingested at high quantities without adequate free water, hypernatremia will occur.

- Excessive sodium in IV fluids

  If intake of sodium exceeds that amount in a patient without ongoing losses or a prior sodium deficit, sodium levels can be expected to rise.

- Excessive Free Body Water Loss:
  - Gastrointestinal (GI) loss (without dehydration)

    If free water is lost, residual sodium becomes more concentrated.

  - Excessive sweating

    Although sweat does contain some sodium, most is free water. This causes the serum sodium to become more concentrated. If the water loss is replaced without any sodium, sodium dilution and hypernatremia can occur.

  - Extensive thermal burns

    If the burn is extensive, serum and a great amount of free water are lost through the open wounds. Sodium becomes more concentrated.

- Diabetes insipidus

  The deficiency of ADH (antidiuretic hormone) and the inability of the kidney to respond to ADH cause large free water losses. Sodium becomes concentrated.

Decreased Levels (Hyponatremia):

- Deficient dietary intake

  Sodium intestinal absorption is highly efficient. Salt deficiency is rare.

- Deficient sodium in IV fluids

  If IV replacement therapy provides sodium at a level less than minimal physiologic losses or less than ongoing losses, residual sodium will become diluted.

- Increased Sodium Loss:
  - Diarrhea, vomiting or nasogastric aspiration

    Sodium in the GI contents is lost with the fluid. Hyponatremia is magnified if IV fluid replacement does not contain adequate amounts of sodium.

  - Diuretic administration

    Many diuretic works by inhibiting sodium reabsorption by the kidney. Sodium levels can diminish.

  - Chronic renal insufficiency

    The kidney loses its reabsorption capabilities. Large quantities of sodium are lost in the urine.

- Increased Free Body Water:
  - Excessive oral water intake

    Psychogenic polydipsia can dilute sodium.

  - Hyperglycemia

    Each 60 mg/100ml increase of glucose above normal decreases the sodium because the osmotic effect of the glucose pulls in free water from the extracellular space and dilutes sodium.

- Excessive IV water intake:

  When IV therapy provides less sodium than maintenance and ongoing losses, sodium will be diluted. If sodium-free IV therapy is given to a patient who has a significant sodium deficit, sodium dilution will occur with rehydration.

- Congestive heart failure
- Peripheral edema

  These conditions are associated with increased free water retention. Sodium is diluted.

- Ascites

Troponins (Cardiac Specific)

Normal Findings:

Adult: < 0.06 ug/L

Indications:

This test is performed on patients with chest pain to determine if the pain is caused by cardiac ischemia. It is a specific indicator of cardiac muscle injury. Troponin is a cardiac protein. It is a marker of myocardial injury. Except in cases of chronic renal failure, an elevated Troponin is a marker of cardiac injury.

Test Explanation:

Cardiac troponins are the biochemical markers for cardiac disease. This test is used to assist in the evaluation of patients with suspected acute coronary ischemic syndromes. In addition to improving the diagnosis of acute ischemic disorders, troponins are also valuable for early risk stratification in patients with unstable angina.
Troponins are proteins that exist in skeletal and cardiac muscle that regulate the calcium-dependent interaction of myosin with actin for the muscle contractile apparatus.

Because of their extraordinarily high specificity of myocardial cell injury, cardiac troponins are very helpful in the evaluation of patients with chest pain. Cardiac troponins become elevated sooner and remain elevated longer than CPK-MB (see Creatine Kinase pg). This expands the time window of opportunity for diagnosis and thrombolytic treatment of myocardial injury. Finally, Troponins are more sensitive to muscle injury than CPK-MB. This is most important in evaluating patients with chest pain.

Cardiac troponins become elevated as early as 3 hours after myocardial injury. Levels of Trop's may remain elevated for 7 to 10 days after MI, and trop's levels may remain elevated for up to 10 to 14 days. However, if re-infarction is considered, troponins are not helpful because they could be elevated from the first ischemic event. Each cardiac monitor has its specific use depending on the time from onset of chest pain to the time of presentation to the hospital.

Interfering Factors:

Troponins T levels are falsely ***elevated*** in dialysis patients.

Test Results and Clinical Significance

Increased Levels:

- Myocardial injury
- Myocardial infarction

  This myocardial intracellular protein becomes available to the bloodstream after myocardial cell death because of ischemia. Blood levels therefore rise. Normally, no troponins can be detected in the blood.

Hematology Tests

Complete Blood Cell Count & Differential, (CBC, Diff)

The CBC and differential count (diff) are a series of tests of the peripheral blood that provide a tremendous amount of information about the hematological system and many other organ systems. They are inexpensively, easily, and rapidly performed as a screening test. The CBC and diff helps the health professional evaluate symptoms (such as weakness, fatigue, or bruising) and diagnose conditions (such as anemia, infection and many other disorders).

A CBC test usually includes:

- **Red blood cell count:**
  Normal findings: 4.30 - 5.90 X 12^{12}/L

  Red blood cells carry oxygen from the lungs to the rest of the body. They also carry carbon dioxide back to the lungs so it can be exhaled. If the RBC count is low (anemia), the body may not be getting the oxygen it needs. If the count is too high (a condition called polycythemia vera), there is a risk that the red blood cells will clump together and block tiny blood vessels (capillaries).

- **Hemoglobin:**
  Normal findings: Male 135-180 g/L Female: 115-160 g/L

  Hemoglobin is the major substance in a red blood cell. It carries oxygen and gives the blood cell its red color. The hemoglobin test measures the amount of hemoglobin in blood and is a good indication of the blood's ability to carry oxygen throughout the body.

- **Hematocrit or Packed Cell Volume (PCV):**

Normal findings: Male 0.41 - 0.52 Female 0.35- 0.47

The Hematocrit or Packed cell Volume represents the percentage of red blood cells as compared to the total blood volume. The test is usually ordered as part of the CBC and is used to diagnose and monitor anemia, dehydration and to check the severity of ongoing bleeding.

- **White Blood Cell Count:**

Normal findings: 4.0 – 11.0 X 10^9/L

White blood cells protect the body against infection. If an infection develops, white blood cells attack and destroy the bacteria, virus, or other organism causing it. White blood cells are bigger than red blood cells and normally fewer in number. When a person has a bacterial infection, the number of white cells can increase dramatically. The number of white blood cells is sometimes used to identify an infection or monitor the body's response to cancer treatment.WBC can also be elevated in the context of trauma or major stress (anything that causes a major catecholamine release). In these cases, it is not a marker of infection.

- **White Blood Cell Types (WBC differential):**

Normal findings:		
	Neutrophils:	**2 - 8 X 10^9/L**
	Lymphocytes:	**1 – 4 X 10^9/L**
	Monocytes:	**0.1 – 0.8 X 10^9/L**
	Eosinophiols:	**< 0.6 X 10^9/L**
	Basophils:	**< 0.2 X 10^9/L**

The WBC differential is of considerable importance because it is possible for the total WBC count to remain essentially normal despite a marked change in one type of leukocyte. The types of white blood cells include neutrophils, lymphocytes, monocytes, eosinophils, and basophils. Immature neutrophils, called band neutrophils, are also included and counted as part of this test. Each type of cell plays a different role in protecting the body. The numbers of each one of these types of white blood cells give important information about the immune system. An increase or decrease in the numbers of the different types of white blood cells can help identify infection, an allergic or toxic reaction to certain medications or chemicals, and many conditions, such as leukemia.

- **Platelet Count (Thrombocyte Count):**

  Normal findings: 150 - 400 X 10^9/L

  Platelets (thrombocytes) are the smallest type of blood cell. They play a major role in blood clotting. When bleeding occurs, the platelets swell, clump together, and form a sticky plug that helps stop the bleeding. If there are too few platelets, uncontrolled bleeding may be a problem. If there are too many platelets, there is a risk of a blood clot forming in a blood vessel. Also, platelets may be involved in hardening of the arteries (atherosclerosis).

Why It Is Done?

A complete blood count may be done to:

- Evaluate the cause of certain symptoms such as fatigue, weakness, fever, bruising, or weight loss
- Detect anemia
- Determine the severity of blood loss
- Diagnose polycythemia vera
- Diagnose an infection
- Diagnose diseases of the blood, such as leukemia
- Monitor the response to some types of drug or radiation treatment
- Evaluate abnormal bleeding
- Screen for abnormal values before surgery

A complete blood count may be done as part of a routine physical examination. A blood count can provide valuable information about the general state of your health.

Age-Related Concerns:

The WBC values tend to be age related. It is not uncommon for the elderly to fail to respond to infection by the absence of Leukocytes. The elderly may not develop an increased WBC count even in the presence of a severe bacterial infection.

Test Results and Clinical Significance

Increased Levels:

Red blood cell (RBC):

- Conditions that increase RBC values include smoking, exposure to carbon monoxide, long-term lung disease, kidney disease, certain forms of heart disease, alcoholism, liver disease, or a rare disorder of the bone marrow (polycythemia vera).
- Conditions that affect the body's water content can increase RBC values. These conditions include dehydration, diarrhea or vomiting, excessive sweating, severe burns, and the use of diuretics.

White blood cell (WBC):

- Conditions that increase WBC values include infection, inflammation, damage to body tissues (such as a heart attack), severe physical or emotional stress (such as a major trauma, fever, injury, or surgery), burns, kidney failure, lupus, tuberculosis (TB), rheumatoid arthritis, malnutrition, leukemia, and diseases such as cancer.
- The use of corticosteroids, under active adrenal glands, thyroid gland problems, or removal of the spleen can increase WBC values.

Decreased Levels:

Red blood cell (RBC):

- Anemia reduces RBC values. Anemia can be caused by severe menstrual bleeding, stomach ulcers, colon cancer, inflammatory bowel disease, tumors, Addison's disease, thalassemia, lead poisoning, sickle cell disease, or reactions to some chemicals and medications.
- A lack of folic acid or vitamin B_{12} can also cause anemia, such as pernicious anemia.

White blood cell (WBC):

- Conditions that can decrease WBC values include chemotherapy, aplastic anemia, viral infections, malaria, alcoholism, AIDS, lupus, or Cushing's syndrome.

Platelets:

- Low platelet values can occur in pregnancy or idiopathic thrombocytopenic purpura.

What Affects the Test?

Factors that can interfere with the test and the accuracy of the results include:

- Prolonged use of a tourniquet while drawing the blood sample.
- Medications that can cause low platelet levels. These include steroids, some antibiotics, thiazide diuretics, chemotherapy medications, and quinidine.
- A very high white blood cell count or high levels of a type of fat (triglycerides) that can cause falsely high hemoglobin values.
- An enlarged spleen, which may cause a low platelet count (thrombocytopenia). An enlarged spleen may be caused by certain types of cancer.
- Pregnancy, which normally causes a low value RBC value and an increase in WBCs.

- Clumping of platelets in the test tube. This can result in a decreased platelet count and occurs because of the substance used in the test tube.

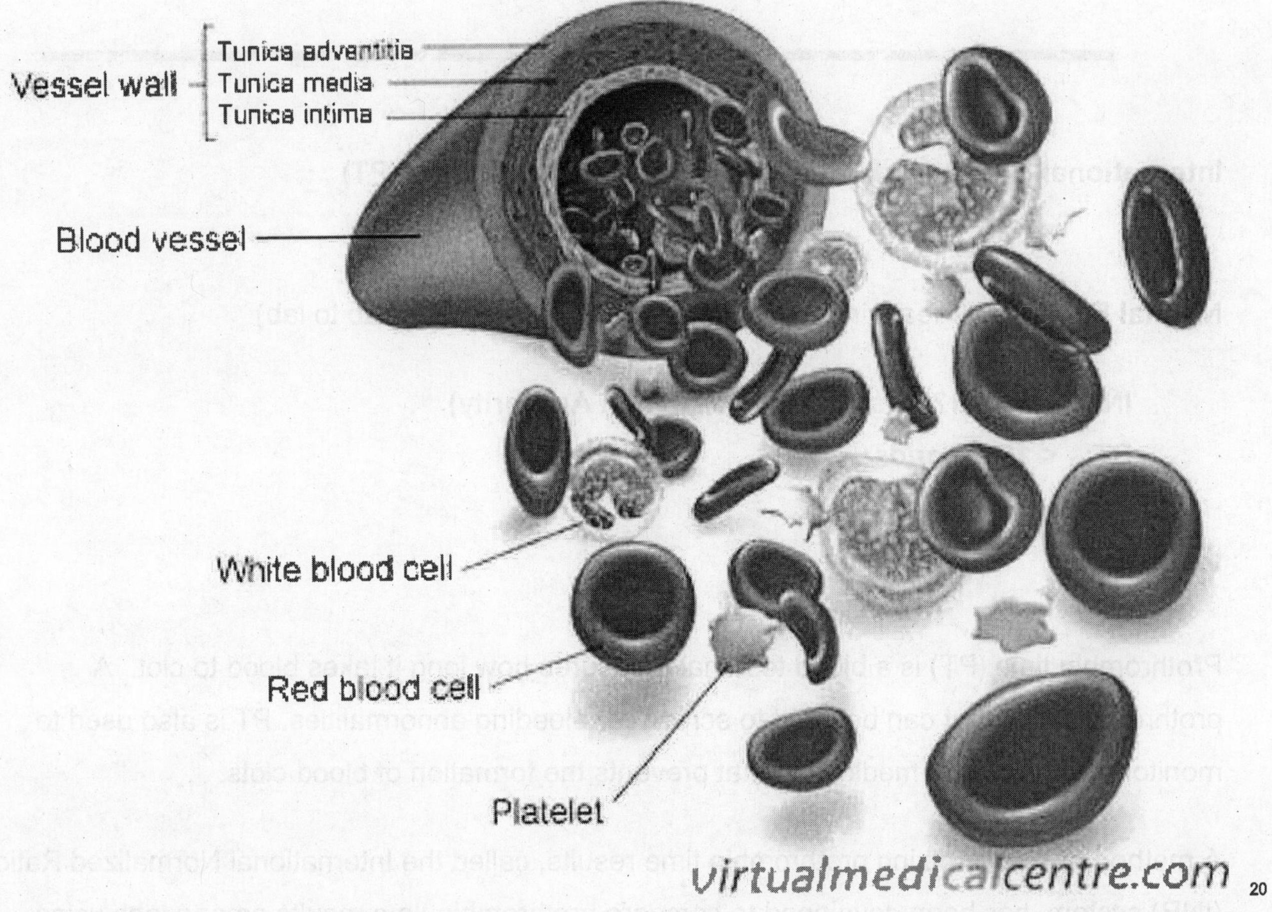

[20]

[20] Reproduced with or without permission from virtual medical centre.com

Coagulation Tests

- **International Normalized Ratio (INR) and Prothrombin Time (PT)**
- **Activated Partial Thromboplastin time (aPTT)**

International Normalized Ratio (INR) or Prothrombin Time (PT)

Normal Findings: (Please note: Normal values may vary from lab to lab)

INR: 0.8 – 1.12 (used at Fraser Health Authority)
PT: < 15 seconds

Indications:

Prothrombin time (PT) is a blood test that measures how long it takes blood to clot. A prothrombin time test can be used to screen for bleeding abnormalities. PT is also used to monitor treatment with medication that prevents the formation of blood clots.

A method of standardizing prothrombin time results, called the International Normalized Ratio (INR) system, has been developed to compare prothrombin time results among labs using different test methods. *Here at RCH we measure and report the prothrombin result as a ratio using the INR system.*

Test Explanation:

Prothrombin time (PT) is a blood test that measures how long it takes blood to clot. PT is used to monitor treatment with medication that prevents the formation of blood clots. The hemostasis and coagulation system is a balance between coagulation factors that encourage clotting and coagulation factors that encourage clot dissolution. The first reaction of the body to active bleeding is blood vessel constriction. In small vessel injury this may be enough to stop bleeding.

In large vessel injury, hemostasis is required to form a clot that will plug the hole until healing can occur.

At least a dozen blood proteins, or blood clotting factors, are needed to clot blood and stop bleeding (coagulation). Prothrombin, or factor II, is one of several clotting factors produced by the liver. Adequate amounts of vitamin K are needed to produce prothrombin. Prothrombin time is an important coagulation test because it measures the presence and activity of five different blood clotting factors (factors I, II, V, VII, and X).

The prothrombin time is lengthened by:

- Low levels of blood proteins (blood clotting factors)
- A decrease in activity of any of the factors
- The absence of any of the factors
- The presence of a substance that blocks the activity of any of the factors

An abnormal prothrombin time is often caused by liver disease or injury or by treatment with the medication warfarin (coumadin), which is used to prevent the formation of blood clots.

The warfarin (coumadin) dosage for people being treated to prevent the formation of blood clots is usually adjusted so that the prothrombin time is about 1.5 to 2.5 times the normal value (or INR values 2 to 3). Prothrombin times are also kept at higher levels for people with artificial heart valves, for the same reason.

Coumadin derivatives are slow acting, but their action may persist for 7 to 14 days after discontinuation of the drug. The action of a coumadin drug can be reversed in 12 to 24 hours by slow parenteral administration of vitamin K. The administration of plasma will even more rapidly reverse the coumadin effect. The action of coumadin drugs can be enhanced by drugs such as aspirin, quinidine, sulfa and indomethacin.

To provide uniform PT results for physician in different parts of the country and the world, the World Health Organization has recommended that PT results now include the use of the international normalized ration (INR) value. Using the INR system, treatment to prevent blood clots (anticoagulant therapy) remains consistent even if a person has the test done at different labs. In some situations, only the INR is reported and the PT is not reported.

Interfering Factors:

- Alcohol intake can prolong PT times. Alcohol diminishes liver function. Many factors are made in the liver. Lesser quantities of coagulation factors result in prolonged PT times.
- A diet high in fat or leafy vegetables may shorten PT times. Absorption of vitamin K is enhanced. Vitamin K-dependent factors are made at increased levels, thereby shortening PT times.
- Diarrhea or malabsorption syndromes can prolong PT times. Vitamin K is mal absorbed, and as a result, factors II, VII, IX, and X are not made.
- Because of drug interactions, instruct the patient not to take any medications unless specifically ordered by the physician.

Test Results and Clinical Significance

- **Increased Levels (Prolonged PT):**
  - Liver disease (egg: cirrhosis, hepatitis): Coagulation factors are made in the liver. With liver disease, synthesis is inadequate and the PT is increased.
  - Hereditary factor deficiency: A genetic defect causes a decrease in a coagulation factor the PT is increased. Factors II, V, VII, or X could be similarly affected.
  - Vitamin K deficiency: Vitamin K-dependent factors (II, VII, IX, X) are not made. The PT is increased.
  - Bile duct obstruction: Fat-soluble vitamins, including vitamin K are not absorbed.
  - Coumadin ingestion: Synthesis of the vitamin K-dependent coagulation factors is inhibited.
  - Massive blood transfusion: Coagulation is inhibited by the anticoagulant in the banked blood. Furthermore, with massive bleeding, the factors are diluted out by the "factor-poor" banked blood.

Why It Is Done?

Prothrombin time (PT) is measured to:

- Determine a possible cause for abnormal bleeding or bruising.
- Monitor the effects of the medication warfarin (Coumadin), which is used to prevent blood clots. If the test is done for this purpose, it may be repeated daily at first and then less often when the correct medication dose is determined.
- Screen for deficiencies of certain blood clotting factors. The lack of some clotting factors can cause bleeding disorders similar to hemophilia.
- Screen for a vitamin K deficiency. Adequate amounts of vitamin K are needed to produce prothrombin.
- Monitor liver function. Prothrombin levels are monitored along with other tests (such as aspartate aminotransferase and alanine aminotransferase) to help evaluate liver function. For more information, see the medical tests Aspartate Aminotransferase (AST) and Alanine Aminotransferase (ALT).

Activated Partial Thromboplastin time (aPTT)

Normal Findings: (Please note: Normal values may vary from lab to lab)

aPTT: 24-35 seconds

Indications:

The activated partial thromboplastin time (aPTT) test is used to determine the most effective dosage of some medications, such as heparin, that prevent blood clots. If the test is done for this purpose, an aPTT may initially be repeated every few hours. When the correct dosage is found, the frequency of testing is decreased. Apart from detecting abnormalities in blood clotting, it is also used to monitor the treatment effects with heparin, a major anticoagulant. Partial thromboplastin time is often measured along with prothrombin time to evaluate bleeding abnormalities.

Test Explanation:

Blood is collected in a tube containing oxalate which halts coagulation by binding with calcium. In order to activate the intrinsic pathway, elements such as calcium are mixed into the plasma sample. The time is measured until a thrombus (clot) forms. Values below 25 seconds and over 35 (depending on local normal ranges) are generally abnormal. Shortening of the PTT has little clinical relevance.

Prolonged aPTT may indicate:

- Use of heparin (or contamination of the sample)
- Antiphospholipid antibody (especially lupus anticoagulant, which paradoxically increases propensity to thrombosis)
- Coagulation factor deficiency (e.g. hemophilia)

The heparin dosage for people being treated to prevent the formation of blood clots is usually adjusted so that the PTT or aPTT is about 1.5 to 2.5 times the normal value.

Abnormal Values:

- A longer-than-normal PTT or aPTT can indicate a deficiency or abnormality of one of the blood clotting factors or another substance needed to clot blood. A deficiency of one or more of these factors results in a bleeding disorder (such as hemophilia or von Willebrand's disease).
- A long PTT or aPTT can be caused by liver disease, kidney disease (such as nephrotic syndrome), or treatment with medications such as heparin or warfarin (Coumadin) that are used to prevent the formation of blood clots.
- A long PTT may be caused by conditions such as antiphospholipid antibody syndrome and lupus anticoagulant syndrome that can cause abnormal clotting or blood clot formation. These syndromes are a complication of lupus in which the immune system produces antibodies that attack certain blood clotting factors, causing the blood to clot easily in veins and arteries.
- PTT can be increased when aspirin is used during heparin therapy, so the PTT value needs to be closely monitored.

What Affects the Test?

Factors that can interfere with your test and the accuracy of the results include:

- Some herbal products or natural remedies
- Some medications, such as antihistamines

URINE Tests

Urinalysis (UA)

Normal findings:

Appearance: Clear

Color: Amber yellow

Odor: Aromatic

Leukocyte: Negative

Nitrites: None

Ketones: None

Indications:

Urinalysis (UA) is part of routine diagnostic and screening evaluations. It can reveal a significant amount of preliminary information about the kidneys and other metabolic processes. UA is routinely done in all patients admitted to the hospital, pregnant women and pre-surgical patients. It is done diagnostically in patients with abdominal or back pain, dysuria, hematuria, or urinary frequency. It is part of routine monitoring in patients with chronic renal disease and some metabolic diseases. It is the most frequently ordered urine test.

Laboratory Examination:

- Appearance and colour:

  Appearance and colour are noted as part of routine urinalysis. A normal urine specimen should be clear. Cloudy urine may be caused by the presence of pus (necrotic WBC's), RBC's or bacteria. However, normal urine also may be cloudy because of ingestion of certain foods (ie: large amounts of fat, urates, phosphates). Urine ranges from pale yellow to amber because of the pigment urochrome (product of cilirubin metabolism). The color indicates the concentration of the urine. Dilute urine is straw colour and concentrated urine is deep amber.

- Odor:

  Determination of urine odor is part of routine urinalysis. The aromatic odor of fresh, normal urine is caused by the presence of volatile acids. Urine of patients with diabetic ketoacidosis has the strong, sweet smell of acetone. In patients with a UTI, the urine may have a foul odor.

- Protein:

  Protein is a sensitive indicator of kidney function. Normally protein is not present in the urine. If significant protein is noted at urinalysis, a 24-hour urine specimen should be collected so that the quantity of protein can be measured. This test can be repeated as a method of monitoring renal disease and its treatment.

- Leukocyte:

  Leukocyte is a screening test used to detect leukocytes in the urine. Positive results indicate UTI. Some patients have no symptoms of UTI (ie: pain or burning on urination). Leukocyte esterase is nearly 90% accurate in detecting WBC's in urine.

- Nitrite:

  Like the leukocyte esterase screen, the nitrite test is a screening test for identification of UTI's. This test is based on the principle that many bacteria produce an enzyme called reductase, which can reduce urinary nitrates to nitrites. Chemical testing is done with a dipstick containing a reagent that reacts with nitrites to produce a pink color, thus indirectly suggesting the presence of bacteria. A positive test result indicates the need for a urine culture. Nitrite screening enhances the sensitivity of the leukocyte esterase test to detect UTI's.

- Ketones:

  Normally, no ketones are present in the urine. However a patient with poorly controlled diabetes and hyperglycemia may have massive fatty acid catabolism. The purpose of this catabolism is to provide an energy source when glucose cannot be transferred into the cell because of insulin insufficiency. Ketones are the end products of this fatty acid break down. As with glucose, ketones spill over into the urine when blood levels in diabetic patients are elevated. Ketonuria may occur with acute febrile illness, especially in infants and children.

Abbreviations for Common Laboratory Tests

ABG	Arterial Blood Gases
BUN	Blood Urea Nitrogen
Ca	Calcium
CK	Creatine Kinase
Cl	Chloride
CSF	Cerebrospinal fluid
Hb	Hemoglobin
INR	International normalization ratio
K	Potassium
LFT	Liver function tests
LP	Lumbar puncture
Mg	Magnesium
Na	Sodium
PT	Prothrombin Time
PTT	Partial Thromboplastin time
RBC	Red blood cell
Trop	Troponin
UA	Urinalysis
WBC	White blood cell

ABG ANALYSIS

Normal ABG Values	
pH	7.35-7.45
PaCO2	35-45 mmHg
HCO3-	22-26 mEq/L
PaO2	80-100 mmHg

DISORDER	CAUSES	ASSESSMENT FINDINGS	TREATMENTS
Respiratory Acidosis pH < 7.35; PaCO2 > 45	Hypoventilation -CNS depression -Pulmonary edema -Respiratory arrest -Airway obstruction	-Bradycardia -Hypotension -Confusion -Somnolence	-Increase RR -Reposition patient -Maintain patent airway -Mechanical ventilation -↑ Rate -↑ Vt
Respiratory Alkalosis pH > 7.45; PaCO2 < 35	Hyperventilation -Excessive mechanical ventilation -Anxiety -Fever -Pneumothorax	-Tachycardia -Palpitations -Anxiety -Seizures -Perspiration/ diaphoresis	-Decrease RR -Administer sedatives -Rebreather mask -Mechanical ventilation -↓ RR - Sedation -↓ Vt
Metabolic Acidosis pH < 7.35; HCO3 < 22	Acid Gain -Shock -Ketoacidosis -Renal failure Bicarbonate loss -Diarrhea -Bile drainage	-Nausea/vomiting -Malaise -Tachypnea -Hypotension -Confusion	-Improve oxygenation -Treat Cause -DKA -Diarrhea -Renal failure
Metabolic Alkalosis pH > 7.45; HCO3 > 26	Acid Loss -Vomiting -Potassium loss (diuretic use) -Hyperaldosteronism - Cushing's - Steroids - Bicarbonate	- Nausea/vomiting/ diarrhea -Confusion -Seizures -Tetany	-Administer buffer -Treat cause

NORMAL BLOOD GAS VALUES

	Arterial	Venous
pH	7.35-7.45	7.31-7.41
PaCO2/PCO2	35-45 mmHg	41-51 mmHg
HCO3	22-28 meq/L	23-29 meq/L
pO2	80-100 mmHg	30-40 mmHg
O2 Sat	>95%	60-80%

INTERPRETING ABNORMAL BLOOD GAS RESULTS

	pH	HCO3	CO2	Possible Causes
Metabolic Acidosis	↓	↓	↓	Diabetes/DKA, Addison's, Liver/Renal Failure, Diarrhea, Toxins/Drugs, Ethylene Glycol
Metabolic Alkalosis	↑	↑	↑	Vomiting, Diuretics, Antacids Use, Cushing's, Administering Alkaline Solutions, Continuous Suctioning of Gastric Contents
Respiratory Acidosis	↓	↑	↑	Obstruction, Pneumonia, Over Sedation, Paralysis, Increased Metabolism, CNS Depression
Respiratory Alkalosis	↑	↓	↓	Anemia, CHF, Over Mechanical Ventilation, Increased Respiratory Rate/Depth, Fever

SHOCK

	BP	HR	CO	Pulse Pressure	SVR	CAP Refill	CVP	UOP	Assessment
Hypovolemia	↓	↑	↓	Narrow	↑	Poor	↓	↓	Weak thready pulse, cool, pale
Cardiogenic	↓	↑	↓	Narrow	↑	Poor	Nml/↑	↓	Weak thready pulse, cool, pale, tachypnea, crackles
Neurogenic	↓	Nml/↓	↓	Nml to Wide	↓↓	Nml	↓	↓	Warm dry skin, vasodilation, loss of sympathetic tone
Anaphylactic	↓	↑	↑	Narrow	↓	Nml	↓	↓	Skin reactions, throat swelling, Dyspnea, pruritus, urticarial, restlessness, decreased LOC, bounding pulses
Early Sepsis	Nml/↑	↑	Nml/↑	Nml to Wide	↓	Nml	Varies	Nml	Bounding pluses, tachypnea, flushed skin, fever, alkalosis
Late Sepsis	↓	↑	↓	Narrow	↑	Poor	↓	↓	Weak pulse, cool, difficulty breathing, acidosis, decreased LOC

BLOOD PRODUCT TRANSFUSIONS - ADULTS

Product	Suggested flow rate		Considerations
PRBC's	1st 15 min: 60-120 ml/hr Active hemorrhage: infuse as rapidly as possible	After 15 min: 240 ml/hr For pt's at risk for fluid overload, 1ml/kg/hr	Infusions must not exceed 4hrs Use filter in line – 170-260 microns
Platelets	1st 5 min: 120-300 ml/hr Active hemorrhage: infuse as rapidly as possible	After 1st 5 min: 300 ml/hr	Generally given over 1 hr. Do not exceed 4 hrs. Use filter in line – 170-260 microns
Plasma	1st 5 min: 120-300 ml/hr Active hemorrhage: infuse as rapidly as possible	After 1st 5 min: 300 ml/hr	Use filter in line – 170-260 microns
Cryoprecipitate	As rapidly as tolerated	Use filter in line – 170-260 microns	
All products	Monitor closely for VS/assessment changes in the first 5-15 minutes of infusion. Normal Vital sign changes Temp +/- 0.5 C RR +/- 5 bpm HR +/- 10 bpm BP +/- 20 mmHg	If reaction is suspected: **Stop** the transfusion **Keep** line open with saline **Call** the physician and blood bank **Document** pt's symptoms **Send** patient's labs and return blood product to the lab	

BASIC ASSESSMENT

Neuro:	Pupils, Orientation, Speech,
Cardiac:	Vein distention, auscultate heart, assess pulses and perfusion.
Respiratory:	Ears, Nose, Throat, auscultate lung sounds, inspect chest rise/rate.
GI/GU:	Inspect, auscultate, palpate 4 quadrants. Palpate/percuss liver. Palpate stomach/bladder. Assess bowel/bladder elimination. Nutritional status.
Skin/ Musculoskeletal:	Color/appearance, intact w/o wounds, rashes, lesions, erythema. ROM. Turn and reposition.

MEDICATION MATH MADE SIMPLE

$$\frac{\text{Desired Dose}}{\text{Available Dose}} * \text{Quantity or Concentration} = \text{Dose}$$

PRESSURE ULCER CLASSIFICATION

Staging	Description
1	Non-blanchable erythema/purple hue of skin changes in temperature and sensation
2	Partial-thickness skin loss (i.e. blister or shallow crater)
3	Full-thickness skin loss involving necrosis of subcutaneous tissue
4	Full-thickness skin loss with extensive necrosis to tendon, muscle, bone, or joint
Unstageable	Ulcer with eschar. Wound base cannot be assessed
DTI	Purple non-blanchable area of intact skin that demarcates between 24-48 hours due to deep tissue destruction

Stages: 1, 2, 3, 4

Skin
Fat
Muscle
Bones

GLASGOW COMA SCALE

Behavior	Response	Score
Eye opening response	Spontaneously To speech To pain No response	4 3 2 1
Best verbal response	Oriented to time, place, and person Confused Inappropriate words Incomprehensible sounds No response	5 4 3 2 1
Best motor response	Obeys commands Moves to localized pain Flexion withdrawal from pain Abnormal flexion (decorticate) Abnormal extension (decerebrate) No response	6 5 4 3 2 1
Total score:	Best response Comatose patient Totally unresponsive	15 8 or less 3

Time	HR	RR	BP	Temp	Sat O2	I	O	✓ Tubes

NCLEX: Fluid and Electrolyte and Acid/Base Balance

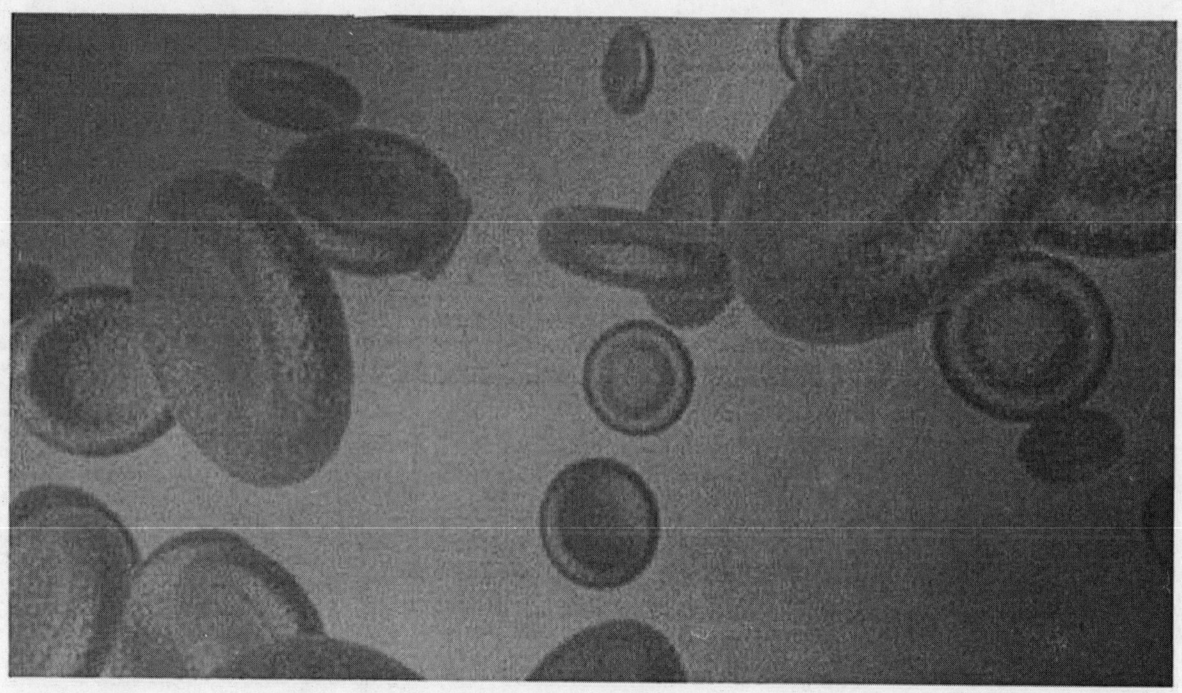

Focus topic: Fluid and Electrolyte and Acid/Base Balance

Cells maintain a balance, or homeostasis, by transference of fluid and electrolytes in and out of the cell. This fluid constantly bathes the cell. Although fluid and electrolyte balance and acid/base balance are separate entities, they directly relate to one another.

For example, dehydration results in a decrease in the pH or metabolic acidosis, whereas overhydration results in an increase in the pH or metabolic alkalosis. To understand how this happens, let's review the basics of fluid movement across the cell membrane.

Water and small particles constantly move in and out of the semipermeable membrane in the cell through active transport and osmosis. This process transports nutrients, hormones, proteins, and other molecules into the cell. It also aids in the movement of waste products out of the cell for excretion from the body.

Along with other functions, fluid also assists with body temperature regulation. When the client has an infection resulting in an elevated temperature, he tends to perspire. This loss of body fluid can lead to dehydration. Dehydration occurs when there is more fluid output than fluid intake.

Other body fluids exist in the form of pericardial fluid, pleural fluid, and spinal fluid. These fluids are compartmentalized into two types:

- Intracellular fluid (fluid that is within the cell): Two-thirds of the body's fluid is intracellular.
- Extracellular fluid (fluid that is outside the cell): One-third of the body's fluid is extracellular. These fluids are divided between the intravascular and interstitial spaces.

NOTE

Intravasular fluid (fluid that is within the vascular space) is composed of blood products, water, and electrolytes.

Interstitial fluid (fluid that is within the interstitial space) is fluid found in organs or tissues.

Contents [show]

Fluid and Electrolyte and Acid/Base Balance: Total Body Water Calculation

Focus topic: Fluid and Electrolyte and Acid/Base Balance

The distribution of body fluid is dependent on age and muscle mass. Total body water in an adult equals approximately 60% of total body weight in kilograms. Infants and the elderly have a higher percentage of body fluid averaging 70%–80%. Fatty tissue contains less water than muscle. For that reason, the elderly and infants lose fluid more quickly than adults and become dehydrated at a more rapid rate, as noted below:

Total body water (TBW) = Extracellular space + Intracellular fluid space (ICF = 2/3 TBW)

Interstitial fluid space + Intravascular fluid space

TBW =

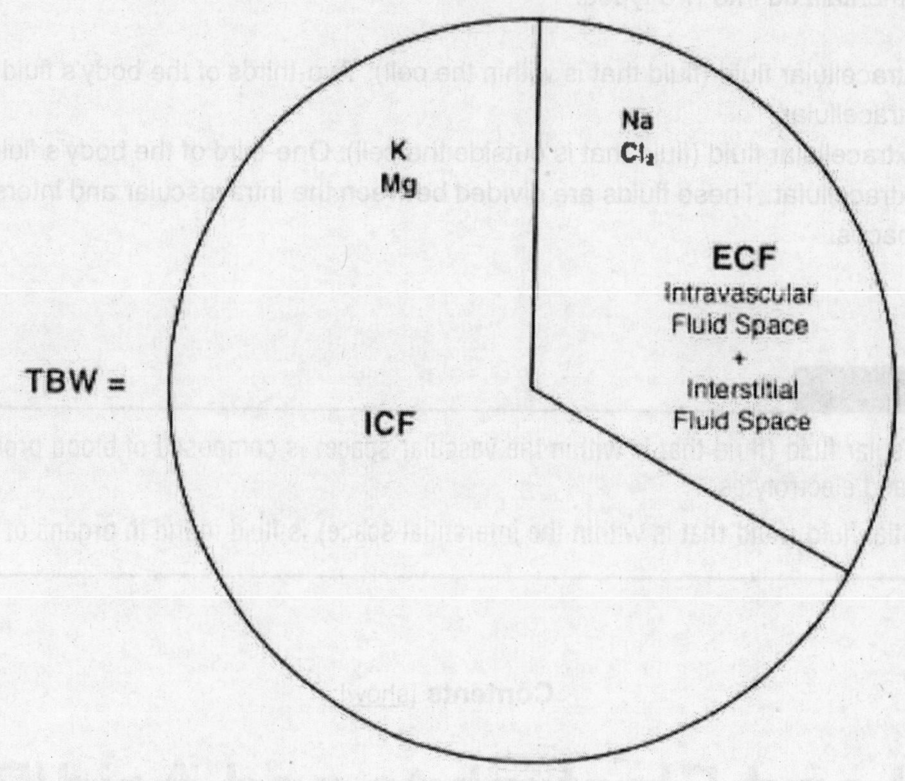

Note: K = potassium
Mg = magnesium
Na = sodium
Cl_2 = chloride

Diffusion is the process whereby molecules move from an area of higher concentration to an area of lower concentration. Diffusion is affected by the amount and type of molecular particles.

These molecular particles are removed from body fluid as they pass through semipermeable membranes in a process known as filtration.

Molecular particles can also pass from an area of lower concentration to one of higher concentration by a process known as active transport. Diffusion and active transport allow positively charged particles, called cations, and negatively charged particles, called anions, to pass in and out of the cell. These particles are also known as electrolytes because they are positively or negatively charged. As cations and anions concentrate, they result in changes in the pH. Some examples of anions are bicarb (HCO3–), chloride (Cl–), proteins, phosphates, and sulfates. Examples of cations are sodium (Na+), potassium (K+), magnesium (Mg++), and calcium (Ca++).

Positive and negatively charged particles are either acidic or alkaline in nature. An acid is a substance that releases a hydrogen (H+) ion when dissolved in water, and a base is a substance that binds with a hydrogen ion when released in water. Therefore, when there is a decrease in bicarbonate hydrogen ions (HCO3–) or an accumulation of carbonic acid, acidosis exists; when there is an increase in bicarbonate hydrogen ions (HCO3–) or a loss of carbonic acid, alkalosis exists.

This chapter discusses how these factors affect acid/base balance (pH) and the regulation of fluid and electrolytes. You will also discover the disease processes that contribute to these alterations.

The sections that follow cover the alteration in acid/base balance as it affects electrolytes and pH.

Fluid and Electrolyte and Acid/Base Balance: Management of the Client with Imbalances in Fluid and Electrolytes

Focus topic: Fluid and Electrolyte and Acid/Base Balance

All body fluid compartments contain water and solutes or electrolytes. The concentra- tion of electrolytes depends on the fluid volume and the body's ability to regulate the fluid:solvent ratio. The electrolytes are as follows:

- Sodium (Na+)
- Potassium (K+)
- Chloride (Cl–)
- Calcium (Ca+)
- Magnesium (Mg+)
- Phosphorus (P–)
- Hydrogen (H+)
- Bicarbonate (HCO3–

The major intracellular electrolytes are potassium and magnesium. The major extracel- lular electrolytes are sodium and chloride. The majority of these electrolytes come from our food and fluid intake. Other sources that can affect electrolytes are medications, blood administration, hyperalimentation, and intravenous fluids.

Fluid and Electrolyte and Acid/Base Balance: Types of Intravenous Fluids

Focus topic: Fluid and Electrolyte and Acid/Base Balance

Intravenous fluid replacement changes the serum by adding electrolytes and/or fluid. There are several indications for the use of intravenous fluid replacement. When the client is unable to maintain a state of fluid and electrolytes within normal limits, the physician might need to institute fluid and electrolyte replacement.

Some of the reasons that the physician might choose to use intravenous fluid replacement are surgery, trauma, gastrointestinal loss of fluid, nothing-by-mouth status, burn injuries, and bleeding. Intravenous fluids are categorized by their composition. Types of IV fluids include isotonic, hypotonic, hypertonic, and colloid.

Intravenous Fluid Solutions

Type of Solution	Uses for These Solutions	Examples
Isotonic solutions: same osmolality as the plasma.	Used to treat isotonic dehydration, burns, mild acidosis, diarrhea	0.9 sodium chloride (normal saline) Lactated Ringer's solution
Hypotonic solutions: more dilute than the plasma; contains more water than particles.	Used to treat the client with edema and kidney disease	5% dextrose and water (D5W) 0.45 sodium chloride (1/2 normal saline) 0.33 sodium chloride
*Hypertonic solutions: higher concentration of particles in solution compared to the plasma.	Used to balance the concentration of fluid and particles across fluid compartments	3% sodium chloride Protein solutions **Hyperalimentation solution 10% dextrose, 50% dextrose, 70% dextrose
Colloid solutions: contain solutes of a higher molecular weight than the serum. These include proteins and are hypertonic. They pull water from the interstitial space.	Used to mobilize third-space fluid; correct hypotension; replenish protein loss during multisystem organ failure, glomerulonephritis, renal failure, or liver disease	Plasmanate Dextran Hespan Salt-poor albumin

*Hypertonic solutions are used only to treat severe hyponatremia and negative nitrogen balance. Hyperalmentation can lead to hyperglycemia, so the client must be monitored for hyperglycemia and might need to have insulin added to the solution or given subcutaneously during the therapy.

**If the infusion is completed and there is no additional hyperalimentation on hand, the nurse should hang a bag of dextrose to prevent a hypoglycemic reaction.

Fluid and Electrolyte and Acid/Base Balance: How the Body Regulates Electrolytes

Focus topic: Fluid and Electrolyte and Acid/Base Balance

The body's electrolytes are regulated by

- The kidneys: The kidneys regulate several electrolytes either directly or indi- rectly. In the kidneys, the glomeruli filter the small particles and water but retain the large particles. Therefore, the waste as well as potassium and sodium are filtered out as needed and the protein—a large particle—is retained.
- The endocrine system: The endocrine system helps by stimulation of an antidi- uretic hormone that helps keep sodium and potassium within a normal range.

- The gastrointestinal system: The gastrointestinal system helps by regulating gastric juices in the stomach and across the small bowel.
- The vascular system: The heart transports electrolytes in the blood.

Fluid and Electrolytes Values

Test	Normal Values
Serum sodium	135–145 mEq/L
Serum potassium	3.5–5.5 mEq/L
Total serum calcium	8.5–10.5 mg/dl or 3.5–4.5 mEq/L
Serum magnesium	1.3–2.1 mEq/L
Serum phosphorus	2.5–4.5 mg/dl
Serum chloride	95–108 mEq/L
Carbon dioxide content	35–45 mEq/L
Serum osmolality	280–295 mOsm/kg
Blood urea nitrogen (BUN)	7–22 mg/dl
Serum creatinine	.6–1.35 mg/dl
Hematocrit	Male: 44–52% Females: 39–47%
Serum glucose	70–110 mg/dl
Serum albumin	3.5–5.5 g/dl
Urinary pH	4.5–8.0 mOsm/L

mEq/L (miliequivalents/liter)
mg/dl (milligram/deciliter)
mOsm/kg (milliosmoles/kilogram)
g/dl (gram/liter)
mOsm/L (milliosmoles/liter)

NOTE

Lab values vary by age and gender, and some laboratory books might have different reference values.

If there is an alteration in electrolytes, the client experiences a state of disequilibrium. The following sections discuss alterations in electrolytes.

Fluid and Electrolyte and Acid/Base Balance: Potassium

Focus topic: Fluid and Electrolyte and Acid/Base Balance

Potassium is the most abundant cation in the body. If damage occurs to the cell, potas- sium leaves the cell. This can result in hyperkalemia or hypokalemia, depending on renal function.

Hypokalemia and Hyperkalemia: Causes, Symptoms, and Treatments

Condition	Causes	Symptoms	Treatment
Hypokalemia	Medications such as diuretics, steroids, and digoxin	Weak pulse, lethargy, confusion, nausea, vomiting, decreased specific gravity of the urine, EKG changes such as depressed S-T segment, inverted T waves	Assess vital signs. Diet (foods high in potassium such as melons, bananas, dried fruits, and baked potatoes with the peel). IV KCl on an IV pump or IV controller. Potassium supplements with juice. Switch to potassium-sparing diuretics. Evaluate the client's intake and output. Check Mg, Cl, and protein when replacing K.
Hyperkalemia	Use of salt substitutes, Addison's disease, renal failure, potassium-sparing diuretics	Muscle twitching, cramps, diarrhea, muscle weakness, paresthesia, slow pulse rate, EKG changes (tall T waves, wide QRS complexes, or prolonged P-R intervals)	Assess vital signs. Dialysis. Measure the intake and output. Calcium gluconate might be given to decrease antagonistic effects of hyperkalemia on the heart. EKG evaluation. Glucose/insulin. Na Bicarb. Polystyrene sulfonate (Kayexalate) PO or enema. Because Kayexalate is constipating, sorbitol is given to induce diarrhea. Monitor lab values. Monitor digitalis levels. Sodium (sodium and chloride go together).

CAUTION

The nurse should assess renal function prior to administering potassium. She should also administer oral liquid potassium with juice because potassium is bitter to taste. If administering with juice, remember that the more acidic juices such as orange or tomato juice are excellent choices because they mask the taste and the ascorbic acid in the juice helps with absorption of the potassium. If the nurse is administering a potassium IV, always infuse using a controller because hyperkalemia can result in cardiac arrhythmias and death (see Figures 2.2 and 2.3). Because potassium can burn the vein and cause discomfort for the client, the nurse should dilute the medication and be sure that the IV is patent.

Fluid and Electrolyte and Acid/Base Balance: Sodium

Focus topic: Fluid and Electrolyte and Acid/Base Balance

Sodium is the major extracellular fluid cation. The major source of sodium is dietary with a minimum sodium requirement for adults of 2 grams per day. Most adults consume more than the necessary amount. Sodium along with potassium facilitates impulse transmission in nerves and muscle fibers.

Hyponatremia and Hypernatremia: Causes, Symptoms and Treatments

Condition	Causes	Symptoms	Treatment
Hyponatremia	Diuretics, wound drainage (particularly GI wounds), renal disease, hyperglycemia, congestive heart failure	Rapid pulse, generalized muscle weakness, lethargy, decreased sensorium, headache, polyuria, decreased specific gravity, dry skin and mucous membranes, anorexia, oliguria	Assess vital signs, replace Na (diet, measure IV therapy), intake and output, foods high in sodium, check complete blood count (will see increased hematocrit), check specific gravity
Hypernatremia	Renal failure, corticosteroids, Cushing's disease, excessive ingestion of sodium, fever	Decreased myocardial control, diminished cardiac output, agitation and confusion, dry and flaky skin	Assess vital signs, correct water balance, administer diuretics, measure intake and output, dialysis, treat fever, decrease sodium intake

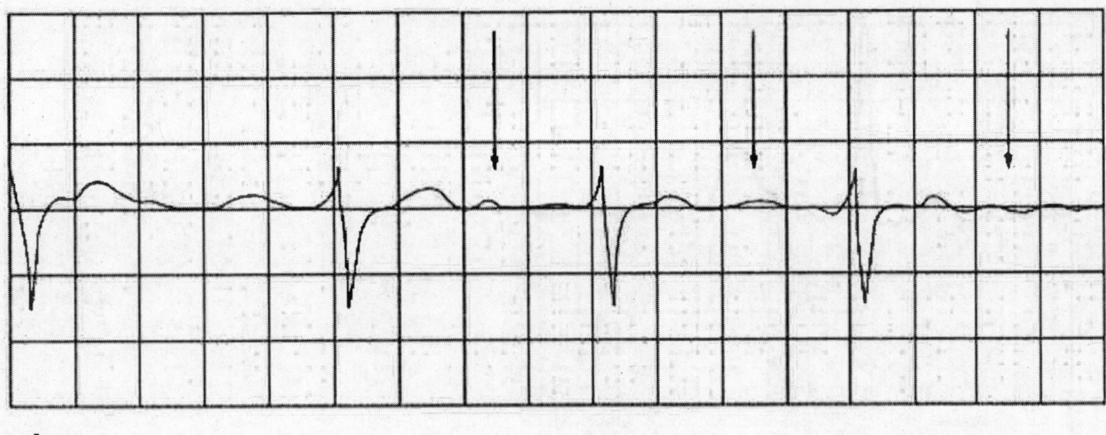

A

B

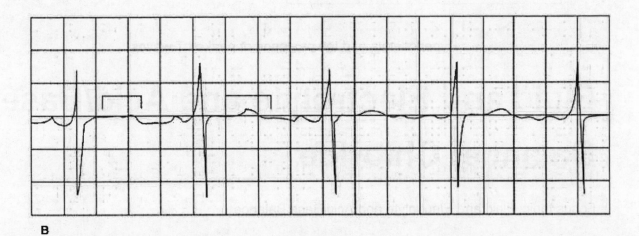

A: Presence of U waves (hypokalemia); B: Fusion of T and U waves with hypokalemia.

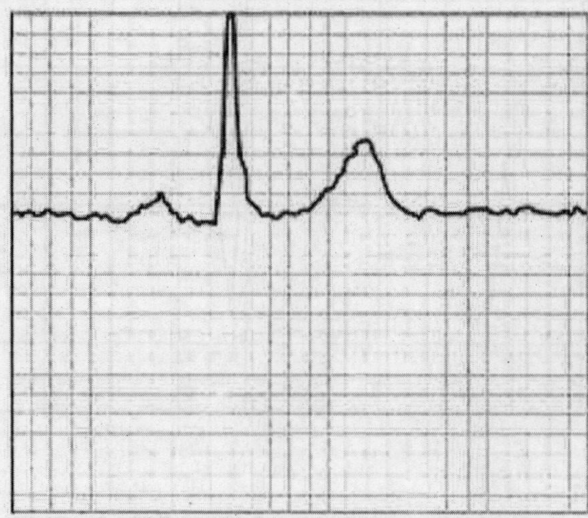

Hyperkalemia and the presence of peaked T waves.

Fluid and Electrolyte and Acid/Base Balance: Chloride

Focus topic: Fluid and Electrolyte and Acid/Base Balance

Chloride is taken in through the diet, especially from foods rich in salt. It is found in combination with sodium in the blood as sodium chloride (NaCl) and is found in the stomach as a hydrogen chloride ion. The function of chloride is to assist sodium with maintaining serum osmolarity. Chloride is regulated primarily by the kidneys and the gastrointestinal system.

Condition	Causes	Symptoms	Treatment
Hypochloremia	Excessive loss in vomitus, nasogastric suction, sodium deficits, losses through the renal system, excessive water within the body due to overinfusion of hypotonic solutions	Accompany loss of sodium, but are nonspecific to chloride.	Replace sodium and chloride, monitor for signs of acidosis
Hyperchloremia	Increased salt intake	No specific symptoms are associated with hyperchloremia, but symptoms usually accompany an excess of sodium.	Monitor electrolytes, monitor intake and output, decrease intake of salt

Most of the total body calcium is found in bone. Calcium not found in the bone is bound to plasma protein. Most of the calcium found and used by the body is taken in through the diet with a recommended daily calcium intake of 800mg. For calcium to be used, vitamin D must be present.

Several systems help in the regulation of calcium. The gastrointestinal system absorbs calcium, and the renal system filters calcium in the glomerulus and absorbs it in the tubules. Calcitonin (a thyroid hormone) helps to regulate calcium by moving it from plasma to bone. The parathyroid gland responds to low plasma levels by releasing parathyroid hormone.

Hypocalcemia and Hypercalcemia: Causes, Symptoms, and Treatments

Condition	Causes	Symptoms	Treatment
Hypocalcemia	Lactose intolerance, celiac disease, Crohn's disease, end-stage renal disease, immobility, acute pancreatitis, thyroidectomy	Increased heart rate, pro longed S-T and Q-T intervals, anxiety, psychosis, hyperactive deep tendon reflexes, positive Trousseau's sign, positive Chvostek's sign, thin hair, dental caries (see Figure 2.4 and Figure 2.5 for diagrams of Trousseau's sign and Chvostek's sign), prolonged Q-T intervals if calcium levels drop below 5.4 mg/dl (see Figure 2.6), osteoporosis, fatigue, dull skin	Assess vital signs, administer calcium supplements, administer vitamin D replacement, check EKG, seizure precautions, place tracheostomy set at bedside in case client experiences laryngeal spasms, monitor for metabolic acidosis
Hypercalcemia	Excessive intake of calcium and vitamin D, thiazide diuretics, hyperparathyroidism, glucocorticoids	Decreased clotting, tachycardia, shortened Q-T intervals (see Figure 2.7), hypertension, disorientation, muscle weakness, increased urinary output and renal calculi, hypotonic bowel sounds	Assess vital signs, advise client to decrease intake of calcium and vitamin D, maintain hydration, monitor for renal calculi, watch for digitalis intoxication, monitor for metabolic alkalosis

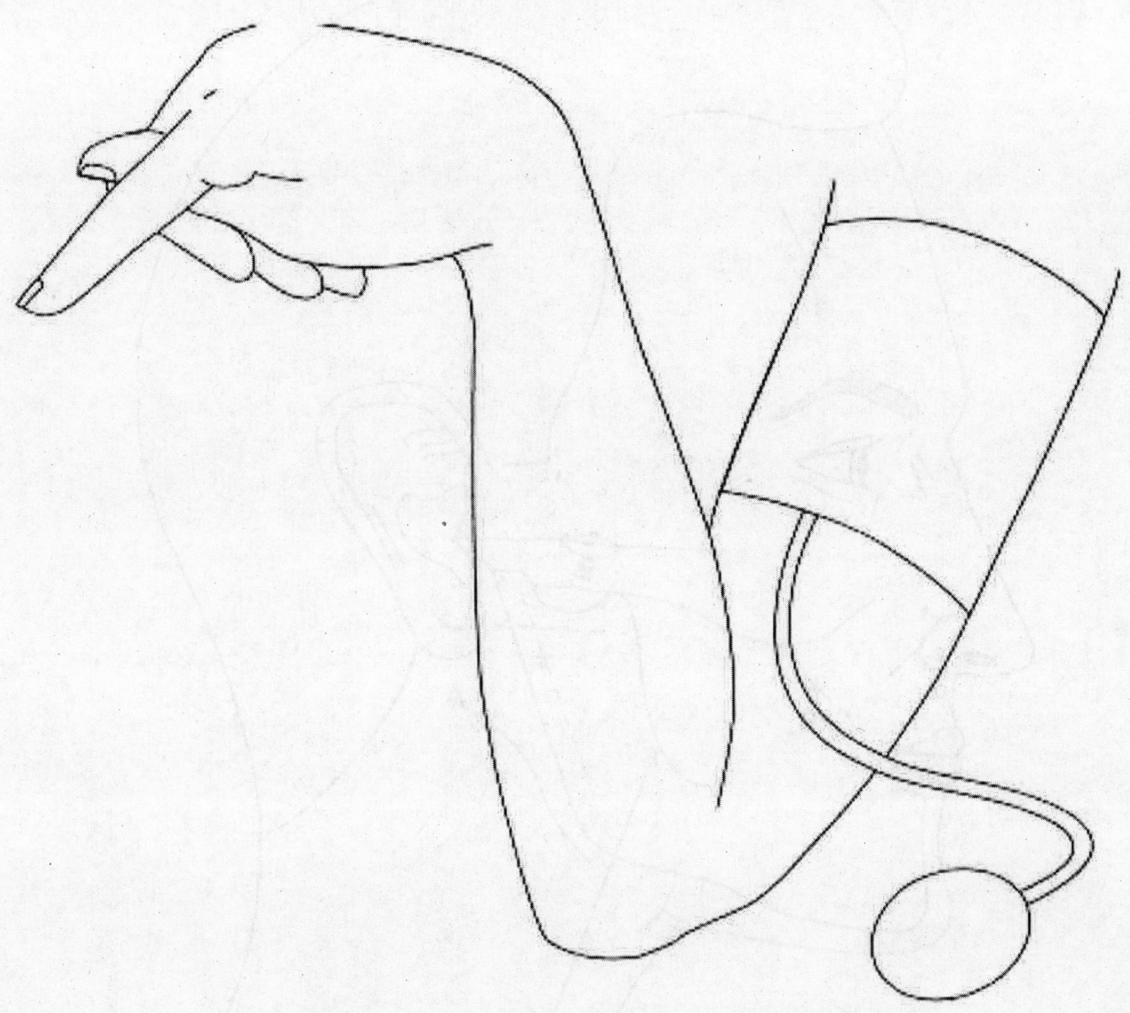

Trousseau's sign.

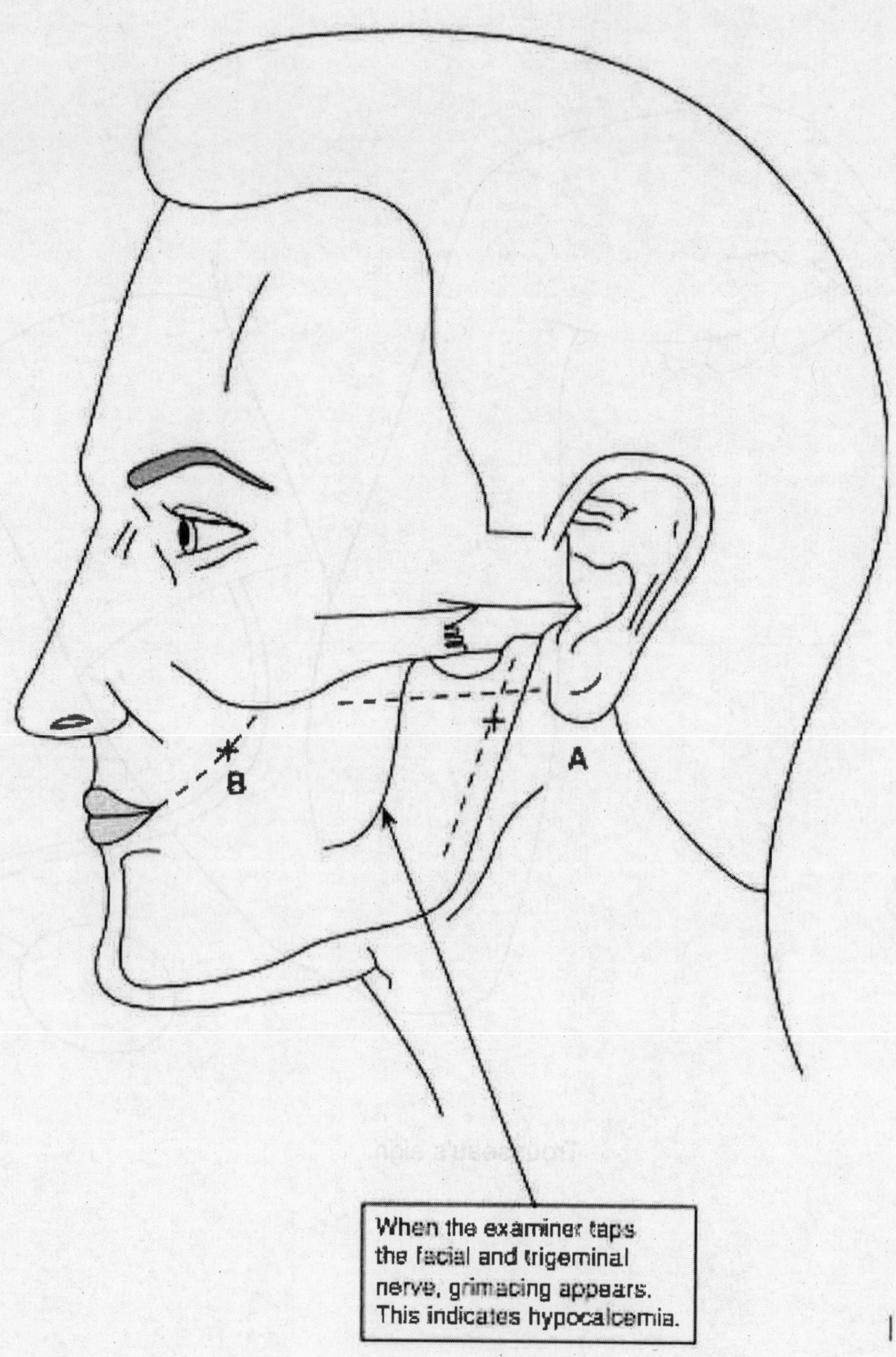
A
B
When the examiner taps the facial and trigeminal nerve, grimacing appears. This indicates hypocalcemia.

Chvostek's sign.

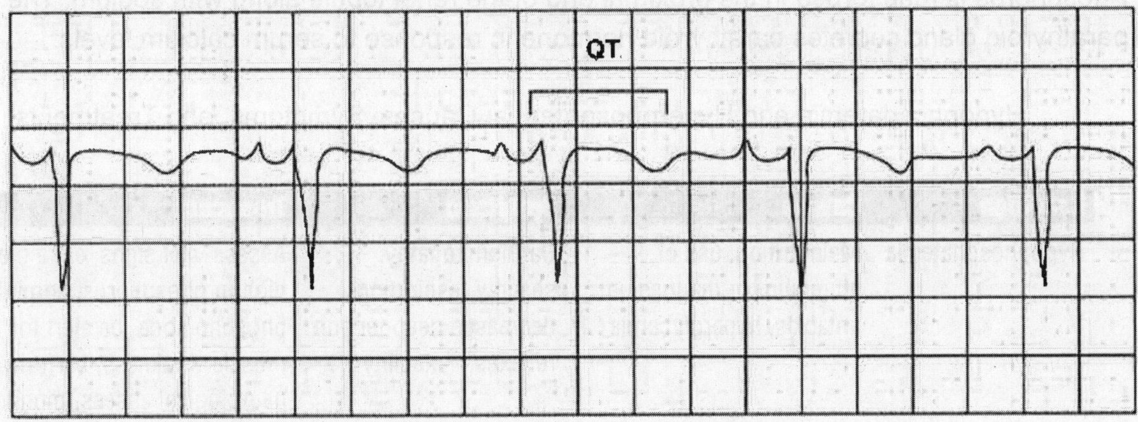

Prolonged Q-T intervals if calcium levels drop below 5.4 mg/dl.

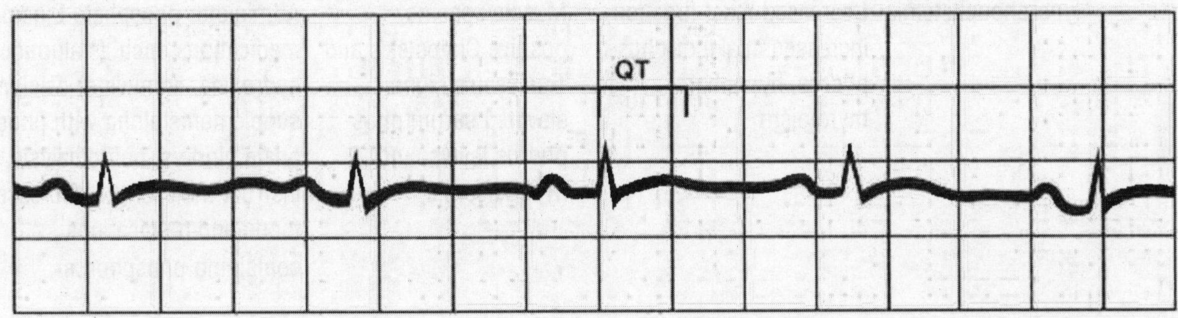

Shortened Q-T intervals.

Fluid and Electrolyte and Acid/Base Balance: Phosphorus

Focus topic: Fluid and Electrolyte and Acid/Base Balance

Phosphorus is the major anion in the intracellular fluid. Its concentration inside the cell is approximately 100 mEq/L. Normal sources of phosphorus intake include almost all foods, especially dairy products. When the phosphorus level is elevated, the calcium level is low, and vice versa. Phosphorus acts as the critical component of the phosphate buffer system that aids renal regulation of acids and bases.

Phosphorus is also a major factor in bone and teeth development; cell integrity; and the function of red blood cells, muscles, and the neurologic system. It is also a component of DNA and RNA.

Phosphorus is reabsorbed in the proximal end of the renal tubule along with sodium. The parathyroid gland secretes parathyroid hormone in response to serum calcium levels.

Hypophospatemia and Hyperphospatemia: Causes, Symptoms, and Treatments

Condition	Causes	Symptoms	Treatment
Hypophosphatemia	Malnutrition, use of aluminum or magnesium antacids, hyperglycemia	Cardiomyopathy, shallow respirations, decreased deep tendon reflexes, irritability	Assess vital signs, eat a diet high in phosphorus, administer phospho soda, be alert for muscle weakness, perform neurological assess, monitor EKG, check calcium levels

Condition	Causes	Symptoms	Treatment
Hyperphosphatemia	Decreased renal function, increased intake of phosphorus, hypopharathyroidism	Muscle spasms, positive Chvostek's and Tousseau's signs, elevated serum phosphorus levels, and hypocalcemia	Administer phosphate-binding medications such as aluminum hydroxide, administer calcium supplements along with phosphate binders, hemodialysis, instruct the client to decrease foods and medications containing phosphorus

Fluid and Electrolyte and Acid/Base Balance: Magnesium

Focus topic: Fluid and Electrolyte and Acid/Base Balance

Magnesium is taken in through the diet and eliminated through the kidneys and gastrointestinal system. It exerts effects on the myoneural junction affecting neuromuscular irritability. Magnesium assists with cardiac and skeletal muscle cells and contributes to vasodilation. Magnesium also activates intracellular enzymes in carbohy- drate and protein synthesis.

Hypomagnesemia and Hypermagnesemia: Causes, Symptoms, and Treatments

Condition	Causes	Symptoms	Treatment
Hypomagnesemia	Malnutrition, diarrhea, celiac disease, Crohn's disease, foods containing citrate, alcoholism	Dysrhythmias, increased blood pressure, positive Trousseau's sign, positive Chvostek's sign, hyper-reflexia, confusion	PO, IV, IM magnesium. (If IV magnesium is administered, always infuse with an IV controller.) Check renal function prior to administration of Mg (insert a Foley catheter for hourly intake and output). Oliguria indicates toxicity to magnesium. Tell the client to expect flushing, sweating, and headache. Monitor magnesium levels and vital signs hourly (decreased respiration is a sign of toxicity to magnesium). Monitor deep tendon reflexes (absence of deep tendon reflexes indicates toxicity to magnesium).
Hypermagnesemia	Increased intake of magnesium, renal failure	Bradycardia, hypotension, drowsiness, lethargy, diminished deep tendon reflexes, respiratory depression	Calcium gluconate. Ventilator support. Dialysis. Monitor hourly intake and output and hourly vital signs. Check DTRs (the absence of patella reflex is the first sign of toxicity). Check LOC. Do not assign the nursing assistant to monitor vital signs or intake and output with this client.

Fluid and Electrolyte and Acid/Base Balance: How the Body Regulates pH

Focus topic: Fluid and Electrolyte and Acid/Base Balance

Many organs are involved in maintaining homeostasis. They are

- Lungs
- Heart
- Pituitary
- Adrenal
- Kidneys
- Blood vessels
- Parathyroids

The body maintains its pH by keeping the ratio of HCO3 (bicarb) to H2CO3 (carbonic acid) at a proportion of 20:1. HCO3, or bicarbonate, is a base, whereas carbonic acid is acidic. This relationship constantly changes and is compensated for by the kidneys and lungs. The normal pH is 7.35–7.45, with the ideal pH being 7.40. If the carbonic acid concentration increases, acidosis occurs and the client's pH falls below 7.40. A pH below 7.35 is considered uncompensated acidosis. If the HCO3 concentration increases, alkalosis occurs and the client's pH rises above 7.40. A pH above 7.45 is considered uncompensated alkalosis.

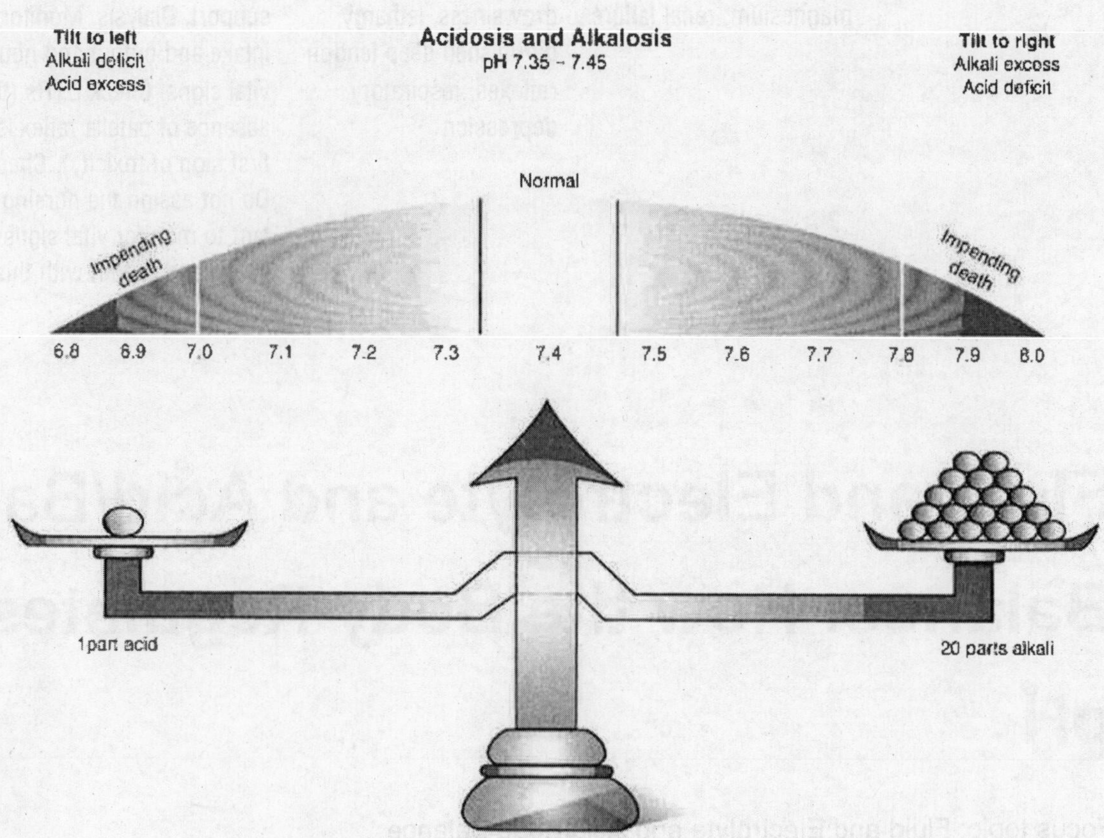

Although several systems assist with the regulation of pH, there are primarily two buffer systems of the body:

- Kidneys: By retaining or excreting $NaHCO_3$ (sodium bicarb) or by excreting acidic urine or alkaline urine. They also help by reabsorbing $NaHCO_3^-$ and secreting free H^+ ions.
- Lungs: By retaining carbonic acid in the form of CO_2 (carbon dioxide) or by rapid respirations excreting CO_2.When there is a problem with the capability of either the lungs or the kidneys to compensate, an alteration in this balance results.

Fluid and Electrolyte and Acid/Base Balance: Metabolic Acidosis

Focus topic: Fluid and Electrolyte and Acid/Base Balance

Metabolic acidosis results from a primary gain of carbonic acid or a loss of bicarbonate HCO_3 with a pH below 7.40.

Causes of Metabolic Acidosis
The following is a list of some causes of metabolic acidosis:

- Certain disease states: Disease states that create excessive metabolism of fats in the absence of usable carbohydrates, leading to the accumulation of ketoacids.
- Diabetes mellitus: Lack of usable insulin, leading to hyperglycemia and ketoacidosis.
- Anorexia: Leads to cell starvation.
- Lactic acidosis: Due to muscle and cell trauma, such as myocardial infarction.
- Renal failure: Leading to waste accumulation in the body and elevated levels of creatinine, BUN, uric acid, and ammonia. All these substances are acidic.
- Diarrhea: With a loss of HCO_3. This loss of HCO_3 and fluid leads to dehydration. When the client is dehydrated, acidosis is likely.
- Excessive ingestion: Ingestion of aspirin or other acids.
- Overuse of diuretics: Particularly non–potassium-sparing diuretics.
- Overwhelming systemic infections: Also called sepsis. Overwhelming infections lead to cell death and nitrogenous waste accumulation.
- Terminal stages of Addison's disease: Adrenal insufficiency results in a loss of sodium and water. This leads to a decrease in blood pressure and hypovolemic shock.

Fluid and Electrolyte and Acid/Base Balance: Symptoms of Metabolic Acidosis

Focus topic: Fluid and Electrolyte and Acid/Base Balance

The following list highlights symptoms of metabolic acidosis that a nurse needs to be aware of for both the NCLEX and for on-the-job observations:

- Lab values: Decreased pH, decreased PaCO2, decreased serum CO2, often increased potassium
- Renal: Polyuria and increased acid in the urine
- Respiratory: Hyperventilation (due to stimulation of the hypothalamus)
- Gastrointestinal: Anorexia, nausea, vomiting, diarrhea, fruity breath
- Neurological: Headache, lethargy, drowsiness, loss of consciousness, coma, death

Fluid and Electrolyte and Acid/Base Balance: Management of the Client with Metabolic Acidosis

Focus topic: Fluid and Electrolyte and Acid/Base Balance

Metabolic acidosis is rarely present without an underlying disease process. Treatment involves early diagnosis and treatment of the causative factors:

- Monitor the potassium level (K+) and treat accordingly: Because potassium (K+) is an intracellular cation, changes in potassium levels commonly occur with metabolic acidosis. The symptoms of hyperkalemia are malaise, generalized weakness, muscle irritability, flaccid paralysis, nausea, and diarrhea. If the potassium is excreted through the kidneys, hypokalemia can result. The symptoms of hypokalemia are diminished reflexes, weak pulse, depressed U waves on the ECG exam, shallow respirations, shortness of breath, and vomiting.

CAUTION

If administering potassium, always check renal function prior to administration. The kidney assists in regulating potassium. If the client has renal disease, life-threatening hyperkalemia can result. Because potassium is bitter to taste, it should be administered with juice. Ascorbic acid also helps with absorption of the potassium. If administering an IV, always control infusion by using an IV pump or controller. An infusion that is too rapid can result in cardiac arrythymias. If giving an IV, dilute the potassium with IV fluids to prevent hyperkalemia and burning of the vein.

- Treat diabetes: Treat with insulin for hyperglycemia; treat with glucose for hypoglycemic.
- Treat hypovolemia: Treat with a volume expander and blood transfusions, and treat shock.
- Treat renal failure: Treatment includes dialysis or transplant. The diet for renal failure clients should control protein, sodium, and fluid. Supplemental with calories and carbohydrates is suggested.
- Treat lactic acidosis: Treatment includes oxygen and NaHCO3.
- Treat Addison's disease: Treatment includes cortisone preparations, a high sodium diet, and fluids for shock.

Nursing care of the client with metabolic acidosis includes frequent monitoring of vital signs and attention to the quality of pulses, intake and output, and oral hygiene. Clients with vomiting should be positioned on their side, with a nasogastric tube to Levin suction. Those with diabetes should be taught the importance of frequent finger sticks and urine checks for hyperglycemia.

Fluid and Electrolyte and Acid/Base Balance: Respiratory Acidosis

Focus topic: Fluid and Electrolyte and Acid/Base Balance

Respiratory acidosis occurs when there is a decrease in the rate of ventilation to the amount of carbonic acid production. Hypoventilation leads to CO2 accumulation and a pH value less than 7.35. Loss of the lungs as a buffer system causes the kidneys to compensate. In chronic respiratory acidosis, the kidneys attempt to compensate by retaining HCO3.

Fluid and Electrolyte and Acid/Base Balance: Causes of Respiratory Acidosis

Focus topic: Fluid and Electrolyte and Acid/Base Balance

The following list highlights causes of respiratory acidosis you need to know. All these involve accumulation of carbonic acid (CO2) and/or a lack of oxygenation:

- Oversedation or anesthesia.
- Head injury (particularly those affecting the respiratory center). This type of head injury leads to an increase in intracranial pressure and suppression of the respirations.
- Paralysis of the respiratory muscles (for example, Guillian-Barrè, myasthenia gravis, or spinal cord injury).
- Upper airway obstruction.
- Acute lung conditions (such as pulmonary emboli, pulmonary edema, pneumonia, or atelectasis).
- Chronic obstructive lung disease.
- Prolonged overbreathing of CO2.

CAUTION

When the client has been given general anesthesia followed by narcotic administration, there is a risk of narcotic overdose. The nurse should keep naloxone hydrochloride (Narcan) available as the antidote for narcotic overdose. Flumazenil (Romazicon) is the antidote for the client who is admitted with an overdose of benzodiazepines such as diazepam (Valium).

Fluid and Electrolyte and Acid/Base Balance: Symptoms of Respiratory Acidosis

Focus topic: Fluid and Electrolyte and Acid/Base Balance

The following list gives the symptoms of respiratory acidosis you need to know:

- Neurological: Dull sensorium, restlessness, apprehension, hypersomnolence, coma
- Respiratory: Initially increased respiratory rate, perspiration, increased heart rate; later, slow respirations and periods of apnea or Cheyne-Stokes respirations (breathing marked by periods of apnea lasting 10–60 seconds followed gradually by hyperventilation) with resulting cyanosis
-

NOTE

Cyanosis is a late sign of hypoxia. Early signs are tachycardia and tachypnea.

Fluid and Electrolyte and Acid/Base Balance: Caring for the Client with Respiratory Acidosis

Focus topic: Fluid and Electrolyte and Acid/Base Balance

Care of the client with respiratory acidosis includes attention to signs of respiratory distress, maintaining a patent airway, encouraging fluids to thin secretions, and chest physiotherapy.

NOTE

Percussion, vibration, and drainage should be done on arising, before meals, and prior to bedtime. Mouth care should be offered after percussion, vibration, and drainage. Cupped hands should be used to prevent trauma to the skin and bruising.

Asthma and cystic fibrosis are common disorders that result in spasms of the airway and accumulation of mucous. These disorders are discussed at length in Chapter 16, "Care of the Pediatric Client." Because these illnesses are common in childhood, the nurse should be aware of the use of play therapy. Effective toys for children with asthma or cystic fibrosis are toys such as horns, pinwheels, and whistles. These toys prolong the expiratory phase of respirations and help with CO_2 exhalation. The best sport is swimming.

Fluid and Electrolyte and Acid/Base Balance: Metabolic Alkalosis

Focus topic: Fluid and Electrolyte and Acid/Base Balance

Metabolic alkalosis results from a primary gain in HCO_3 or a loss of acid that results in a pH level above 7.45.

Fluid and Electrolyte and Acid/Base Balance: Causes of Metabolic Alkalosis

Focus topic: Fluid and Electrolyte and Acid/Base Balance

The following list highlights causes of metabolic alkalosis that you need to be aware of:

- Vomiting or nasogastric suction that might lead to loss of hydrochloric acid
- Fistulas high in the gastrointestinal tract that might lead to a loss of hydrochloric acid
- Steroid therapy or Cushing's syndrome (hypersecretion of cortisol) that might lead to sodium, hydrogen (H^+) ions, and fluid retention
- Ingestion or retention of a base (for example, calcium antacids or $NaHCO_3$)

Fluid and Electrolyte and Acid/Base Balance: Symptoms of Metabolic

Focus topic: Fluid and Electrolyte and Acid/Base Balance

Symptoms of metabolic alkalosis include

- Neurological: Fidgeting and twitching tremors related to hypokalemia or hyperkalemia
- Respiratory: Slow, shallow respirations in an attempt to retain CO_2
- Cardiac: Atrial tachycardia and depressed T waves related to hypokalemia
- Gastrointestinal: Nausea, vomiting, and diarrhea, causing loss of hydrochloric acid
- Lab changes: pH levels above 7.45, normal or increased CO_2, increased $NaHCO_3$

Fluid and Electrolyte and Acid/Base Balance: Caring for the Client with Metabolic Alkalosis

Focus topic: Fluid and Electrolyte and Acid/Base Balance

The following items are necessary care items a nurse should know for treating clients with metabolic alkalosis:

- Administering potassium replacements
- Observing for dysrhythmias
- Observing intake and output
- Assessing for neurological changes

Fluid and Electrolyte and Acid/Base Balance: Respiratory Alkalosis

Focus topic: Fluid and Electrolyte and Acid/Base Balance

Respiratory alkalosis relates primarily to the excessive blowing off of CO2 through hyperventilation. Causes of respiratory alkalosis include

- Hypoxia
- Anxiety
- High altitudes

Fluid and Electrolyte and Acid/Base Balance: Symptoms of Respiratory Alkalosis

Focus topic: Fluid and Electrolyte and Acid/Base Balance

The following list details symptoms of respiratory alkalosis that you will need to know as a nurse and for the exam:

- Neurological: Numbness and tingling of hands and feet, tetany, seizures, and fainting
- Respiratory: Deep, rapid respirations
- Psychological: Anxiety, fear, and hysteria

- Lab changes: Increased pH, decreased PaCO2, decreased K levels, and normal or decreased CO2 levels

To correct respiratory alkalosis, the nurse must determine the cause for hyperventilation. Some causes for hyperventilation are stress and high altitudes. Treatments include

- Stress reduction
- Sedation
- Breathing in a paper bag to facilitate retaining CO2 or using a re-breathing bag
- Decreasing the tidal volume and rate of ventilator settings

EXAM ALERT

Use the following acronym to help you with respiratory and metabolic questions on the exam:

ROME: Respiratory Opposite, Metabolic Equal

This means in respiratory disorders, the pH is opposite to the CO_2 and HCO_3; in metabolic disorders, the pH is equal to or moves in the same direction as the CO_2 and HCO_3. Here's an explanation:

- **Respiratory acidosis:** pH down, CO_2 up, HCO_3 up
- **Metabolic acidosis:** pH down, CO2 down, HCO3 down
- **Respiratory alkalosis:** pH up, CO2 down, HCO3 down
- **Metabolic alkalosis:** pH up, CO_2 up, HCO_3 up

It is important for you to understand the normal blood gas values as they relate to respiratory alkalosis and acidosis. Table 2.9 will help you to determine whether the client is in respiratory or metabolic acidosis or alkalosis.

Blood Gas Values	Acidosis	Alkalosis
pH	pH less than 7.35 (n. 7.35–7.45)	pH less than 7.35 (n. 7.35–7.45)
$PaCO_2$ abnormal with a normal HCO_3 indicates that the disorder is respiratory	$PaCO_2$ greater than 45 is respiratory (n. 35–45 mm Hg)	$PaCO_2$ less than 35 mm Hg is respiratory
An abnormal HCO_3 with a normal $PaCO_2$ indicates a metabolic disorder	HCO_3 less than 22 mEq/L is metabolic (n. 22–26 mEq/L)	HCO_3 greater than 26 mEq/L is metabolic

Blood Transfusion

In this section of the NCLEX-RN examination, you will be expected to demonstrate your knowledge and skills of blood and blood products in order to:

- Identify the client according to facility/agency policy prior to administration of red blood cells/ blood products (e.g., prescription for administration, correct type, correct client, cross matching complete, consent obtained)
- Check the client for appropriate venous access for red blood cell/blood product administration (e.g., correct gauge needle, integrity of access site)
- Document necessary information on the administration of red blood cells/blood products
- Administer blood products and evaluate client response

Blood transfusions are indicated for the client who has hypovolemia secondary to hemorrhage, anemia or another disease process that is associated with a deficiency in terms the client's clotting or another component of blood, for example. Although hypovolemia can be treated with fluid replacement, this fluid does not provide the client with the oxygen carrying components that only blood has. In addition to blood's components in terms of oxygen transporting red blood cells, blood also transports carbon dioxide, and it contains white blood cells to combat infection, clotting factors and essential blood proteins.

There are four blood types each of which has its antigen in its red blood cells. These blood types are A with A antigens, B with B antigens, AB with both A and B antigens, and O which has neither A nor B antigens. People with O type blood are universal donors but they are universal suckers because type O blood can be given to clients with A, B, AB and O blood type clients but the type O blood type client can only receive type O blood. Each blood type also has antibodies, which are referred to as agglutinins. Type A blood has B agglutinins; type B blood has A agglutinins, type AB blood has no antibodies, or agglutinins, and type O blood has both A and B agglutinins.

People also have a rhesus, or Rh, factor antigen or the lack of it. Clients with an Rh positive blood, which is the vast majority of people, have Rh positive blood and people without the Rh factor antigen have Rh negative blood.

Members of the Christian Science religion do not typically accept blood transfusions and members of Jehovah's Witness religion are prohibited from receiving blood. Plasma expanders without any blood or blood products, however, are acceptable to members of both of these religions.

Most clients get blood and blood products that are donate by others through the blood bank, however, some clients can choose to donate their own blood prior to an elective surgery, for example, and then use this blood rather than the blood of a blood donor. This type of blood transfusion is referred to as an autologous blood donation.

Blood and blood components are selected and given as based on the client's specific needs. The different blood products and their components are described below.

- **Packed red blood cells**: Packed red blood cells are used when the client is in need of increased oxygen transporting red blood cells as may occur post operatively and with an acute hemorrhage.

- **Platelets**: Platelets are administered to clients who are adversely affected with a platelet deficiency or a serious bleeding disorder, such as thrombocytopenia or platelet dysfunction that requires the clotting factors that are in platelets.

- **Fresh frozen plasma**: Fresh frozen plasma, which does not contain any red blood cells, is administered to clients who are in need of clotting factors or are in need of increased blood volume as occurs with hypovolemia and hypovolemic shock. Fresh frozen plasma does not have to be typed and cross matched to the client's blood type because plasma does not contain antigen carrying red blood cells.

- **Albumin**: Albumin is administered to clients who need expanded blood volume and/or plasma proteins.

- **Clotting factors and cryoprecipitate**: Clotting factors and cryoprecipitate are administered to clients affected with a clotting disorder including the lack of fibrinogen.

- **Whole blood**: Whole blood is typically reserved for only cases of severe hemorrhage. Whole blood contains clotting factors, red blood cells, white blood cells, plasma, platelets, and plasma proteins.

Identifying the Client According to the Facility or Agency Policy Prior to the Administration of Red Blood Cells and Blood Products

Some blood transfusion reactions and blood transfusion errors occur as the result of inaccurate client identification. Simply stated, client misidentification can be prevented by matching the client to the order, insuring that the blood is accurately matched to the client and the order and by using the two person verification technique that involves two nurses checking the blood, the order and the client's identity using at least two unique identifiers.

The two nurses will check the blood against the order, check the client's identity, check the client's blood type against the type of blood that will be infused, check the expiration of the blood or blood component, and check the client's number against the blood product number. The nurses will also visually inspect the blood for any unusual color, precipitate, clumping and any other unusual signs.

The order for the blood or blood component must be a complete order that specifies exactly what will be administered. The client will also give consent for the transfusion.

The gauge of the intravenous catheter should be 18 gauge and the blood should be administered with normal saline using a Y infusion set that is specifically used for the administration of blood and blood products. Normal saline is compatible with blood; ringer's lactate, dextrose, hyperalimentation and other intravenous solutions with incompatible medications are not compatible with blood and blood products. If a blood filter is used, the filter must be inspected to insure that it is suitable for the specific blood product that the client will be getting.

Blood should not remain in the client care area for more than 30 minutes so it is important that the nurse is prepared to begin the transfusion shortly after the blood is delivered to the patient care area. The nurse must take baseline vital signs just prior to the infusion of blood or a blood product and then the nurse should remain with and monitor the client for at least 15 minutes after the transfusion begins at a slow rate since most serious blood reactions and complications occur shortly after the transfusion begins. All blood and blood products must be administered completely in less than 4 hours.

Only registered nurses and licensed practical nurses can initiate, monitor and maintain blood transfusions. These aspects of care can NOT be delegated to an unlicensed assistive nursing staff member. Additionally, some facilities restrict blood transfusions to only registered nurses, so it is important to check the facility specific policies and procedures relating to the administration of blood and blood products.

Checking the Client for Appropriate Venous Access for Red Blood Cells and Blood Product Administration

The nurse must insure that the intravenous line is patent and they must insure that a 18 or 20 gauge catheter is being used and patent.

Documenting the Necessary Information on the Administration of Red Blood Cells and Blood Products

All aspects of the administration of red blood cells and blood products are documented. This documentation must minimally include:

- The date and time that the blood transfusion began
- The name of the second nurse who did the two person verification process
- The name and amount of the specific type of transfusion such as 1 unit of packed red cells
- The number of the blood product
- Where the IV site was
- Size of the angiocath that was used
- The duration of the transfusion
- The vital signs that were taken and when they were taken
- The fact that the client was informed about when and why to contact the nurse after the initial 15 minute monitoring period

Administering Blood Products and Evaluating the Client's Responses

Whenever blood or a blood product is being administered, the nurse must closely monitor the client for the signs and symptoms of a possible complication. The first thing that the nurse must do when a reaction or a complication is possible is to discontinue the administration of the blood or blood product.

The complications associated with the administration of blood and blood components are discussed below:

Febrile Reactions

Febrile reactions are the most commonly occurring reaction to blood and blood products administration. Although a febrile reaction can occur with all blood transfusions, it is most frequently associated with packed red blood cells and this reaction is not accompanied with hemolysis. The signs and symptoms of this transfusion reaction include fever, nausea, anxiety, chilling and warm flushed skin.

Hemolysis

Hemolysis occurs as the result of an incompatibility of the donor's and recipient's blood which is referred to as an ABO incompatibility. This incompatibility can occur as the result of a laboratory error in terms of typing and cross matching and a practitioner error in terms of checking the blood and matching it to the client's blood type. This complication is signaled when the client has flank pain, chest pain, restlessness, oliguria or anuria, respiratory distress, brown urinary output, hypotension, fever, low blood pressure and tachycardia. The treatment of hemolysis includes the administration of normal saline after the transfusion is stopped and all the tubing is changed to prevent kidney failure and circulatory collapse. Although rare, a delayed, rather than an acute and immediate, hemolytic reaction can occur up to about 4 weeks after the transfusion. This delayed reaction is not as severe as an acute hemolytic reaction and it is characterized with jaundice, discolored urine and anemia.

The intravenous tubing, the blood filter, the blood bag with its remaining contents are retained and sent to the laboratory. A sample of the client's blood and urine are also taken and sent for diagnostic testing.

Allergic Reactions

Allergic reactions to a blood transfusion can range from mild to severe. A mild allergic reaction typically occurs as the result of an allergy to the plasma proteins in the blood, and severe allergic reactions occur from a severe antibody - antigen reaction. Mild allergic reactions are accompanied with possible itching, pruritic erythema, swelling of the lips, tongue or pharynx and eyelids, and flushing of the skin; severe allergic reactions can manifest with chest pain, decreased oxygen saturation, loss of consciousness, flushing, shortness of breath and respiratory stridor. Mild allergic responses are treated with the administration of a corticosteroid and/or antihistamine medication; severe allergic reactions are treated with the administration of supplemental oxygen and medications. At times, a serious allergic reaction can be life threatening.

Sepsis

Sepsis is characterized with fever, hypotension, oliguria, chilling, nausea and vomiting This transfusion reaction occurs as the result of some contaminate in the blood. This complication is treated with intravenous fluids and antibiotics. The intravenous tubing, the blood filter, the blood bag with its remaining contents are retained and sent to the laboratory. A sample of the client's blood and urine are also taken and sent for diagnostic testing as is also done when the client has a hemolytic reaction.

Blood Typing

Blood Type	Donate Blood To	Receive Blood From
A	A AB	A O
O	O A B AB Universal Donor	O
B	B AB	B O
AB	AB	Universal Recipient

Blood and Blood Product Transfusion

- Whole blood or components of whole blood can be transfused for a client who requires replacement of blood loss or blood disease
- Blood Components
  - Packed RBCs
  - Plasma
  - Albumin
  - Prothrombin complex
  - Platelets
  - Clotting factor
  - Cryoprecipitate
- Transfusion Types
  - Homologous -blood from donors not used
  - Autologous- clients own blood
    - Intraoperative blood salvage- cell-saver, collects blood intraoperatively and transfused back to client
- Indications
  - Excessive blood loss- Hgb 6-10g/dl- Whole blood
  - Anemia- Hgb 6-10g/dl- **Packed RBCs**
  - CRF- **Packed RBCs**
  - Coagulation factor deficiencies such as hemophelia- **Fresh frozen plasma**
  - Thrombocytopenia/platelet dysfunction (platelets less than 200,000 or greater than 80,000 and active bleeding) **Platelets**

- Follow facility protocol for transfusion of blood or blood products
- Procedure for Administration:
  - Check lab values Hgb + Hct
  - Verify order
  - Blood samples should be obtained for cross match
  - Check for Hx of transfusion reactions
  - Obtain blood products from blood bank
  - Check for discoloration, air bubbles, or cloudiness
  - Confirm identity, blood compatibility, expiration date
  - Large bore IV cannula, 20 gauge for standard admin
  - Ascertain if filter is to be used
  - Ensure 0.9% NaCl to prime tubing and to hang with blood
  - A Y-tubing is to be used
  - Baseline vital sings before administration
- Nursing Actions:
  - Remain with client for the first 15-30 min of transfusion as reaction can occur most often during this time
  - Monitor V/S q hour
  - Rate of infusion
  - Resp. status
  - Sudden increase in anxiety
  - Breath sounds
  - Neck vein distention
  - Notify provider is any reaction signs occur

- Complete transfusion within 2-4 hours

Types of Reactions	Onset	S&S/ Nursing Interventions
Acute Hemolytic	Immediate	Reaction may be mild or life-threatening CV collapse, ARF, DIC, shock death Chills, fever, low back pain, tachycardia, flushing hypotension, chest pain, tachypnea, nausea, anxiety hemoglobinuria
Febrile	30min- 6 hours after infusion	S&S/Chills , fever, flushing, H/Ache. Use WBC filter Admin and antipyretic- Tylenol
Mild Allergic	During or up to 24 hours after transfusion	S&S- itching uticaria, flushing Admin antihistamine-Benadryl
Anaphylactic	Immediate	S&S- wheezing, dyspnea, chest

		tightness, cyanosis, hypotension. Assist with emerg. care- Maintain airway, admin O2, IV fluids, antihistamines, corticosteroids, epinephrine

- STOP transfusion is a reaction is noted
    - Maintain patent IV with 0.9% NaCl
    - Save blood and bag and tubing for lab testing as per facility protocol
- Circulatory overload
    - Clients who have impaired cardiac function can have overload
        - S&S- Dyspnea, chest tightness, tachycardia, tachypnea, H/A, HTN, JVD, peripheral edema, orthopnea, sudden anxiety, Crackles in lungs
        - AdminO2, monitor V/S, slow infusion rate, admin prescribed diuretic

Cardiovascular

The four concepts related to oxygenation and perfusion are:

1. Hypoxemia: Decreased oxygen concentration of arterial blood
2. Hypoxia: Oxygen deficiency in body tissues
3. Ischemia: Tissue not getting enough oxygen
4. Necrosis: The tissue dies

Overview

CV disease is the leading cause of death in the US. One death occurs every 33 seconds, and 25% of the population has CV disease. It's bad.

Technology

Various diagnostic procedures are used to detect disease and various procedures/surgery are used to treat disease:

- *Ultrasound* (ECHO) is used to evaluate the structure and function of the heart. It's not really do-able in pts with COPD (due to a lot of air between heart and chest cavity) and pts who are obese.
- *EKG* uses monitoring electrodes to create a graphic representation of the electrical impulses that the heart generates during the cardiac cycle. Interfering factors are electrolyte imbalances and certain drugs such as digitalis, quinidine and barbiturates.
- *Angiography* is cardiac catherization, and it is used to visualize the heart chambers, arteries and great vessels. It is used most often to evaluate pts with chest pain. Pts with a positive stress test also undergo this test to locate the region of coronary occlusion. It is also used to determine the effects of valvular heart disease. Right heart catheterization is used to calculate cardiac output and measure right heart pressures (also used to identify pulmonary emboli).
- *Radioisotope studies* (couldn't find anything about this online that was understandable)
- *Clot prevention drugs and lysis drugs*
- *Angioplasty* involves placing a balloon is placed at the stenotic area to widen a narrowed or obstructed blood vessel.
- *Endarterectomy* is a surgical procedure to remove plaque material or blockage in the lining of an artery.
- *Stent placement* holds an artery open
- *CABG and Peripheral Bypass* are surgical procedures. CABG is coronary artery bypass, in which arteries or veins from elsewhere in the body are grafted to the coronary arteries to bypass artherosclerotic narrowings and improve the blood supply to the heart. Peripheral arterial bypass refers to treating blockages in the legs.
- *Amputation* is often for a vascular reason (if not for diabetes or trauma).

Arterial Disorders

These are disorders that affect arteries…not veins! Try to keep that straight! Examples are:

- Artherosclerosis (CAD and Peripheral): thickening and hardening of arterial walls.
- Hypertension: BP over 140/90
- Aneurysm: localized abnormal dilation of a blood vessel (usually artery)

- Raynaud's: A primary vasospsastic disease of small arteries, presents as an exaggerated response of vasomotor controls to cold or emotion.
- Buerger's: a chronic, recurring, inflammatory, vascular occlusive disease, chiefly of the peripheral arteries and veins of the extremeties.

<u>Venous Disorders (ex)</u>
- Thrombophlebitis: inflammation of a vein in conjunction with the formation of a thrombus.
- Emboli: masses of undissolved matter present in a blood or lymphatic vessel and brought there by the blood or lymph.
- Venous Stasis Ulcers: ulcers in the lower leg (usually inner part of leg just above ankle). Common in pts who have a history of leg swelling, varicose veins or blood clots.
- Lymphedema: an abnormal accumulation of tissue fluid in the interstitial spaces.

<u>CV Disease</u>
Though CV disease is the leading cause of death in the U.S. the really sad thing is that there are many risk factors associated with this disease that are modifiable:
- Hypertension
- Obesity
- Smoking
- Hyperlipidemia
- Stress
- Lack of Exercise
- Diabetes
- Na Intake
- Alcohol

<u>Hypertension</u> affects about 25% of the US population (50 million folks), and represents any BP above 140/90. However, it is important to note that ANYTHING above 120/80 is considered risky b/c there is a direct relationship to CV…so it's not like if you're 138/84 that you're a-ok.

HTN damages the intima of the vessel wall. This attracts macrophages which come in and cause an increase in inflammation. This creates more work for the heart to pump against (afterload), and can lead to CHF and cardiovascular "events" such as heart attack and stroke. Note that elderly people can have an increase in systolic pressure only…this is b/c artherosclerosis causes a loss of elasticity in the large arteries and diastolic pressure does not increase as well.

Pathophysiology of HTN:
Kidnesys relase renin into the bloodstream, which travels to the liver where it converts aniotensinogen to ang I. Ang I goes to the lungs where it is converted to ang II. Ang II then goes to the kidneys which cause aldosterone to be released. Aldosterone causes sodium and water retention. This retained sodium and water increase blood volume. Arteriolar constriction increases peripheral vascular resistance (remember that ang II is a potent vasoconstrictor). Increased blood volume and vascular resistance cause hypertension.

> Studies show that the incidence of MI increases proportionately with increases in systolic pressure over 120.
>
> Studies also show that diabetics are less at risk of "CV events" when diastolic pressure is <80.

Treating HTN:
Lifestyle modifications are fantastic, but they won't fix everyone's HTN. Most people need to be on more than one drug (for example, a diuretic would lower BP, as would a beta-blocker and an Ace-inhibitor or vasodilator…lots of ways to drop BP!) If someone is going to implement lifestyle changes, they can drop their BP 5-20 mmHg for every 10kg they lose…this is great IF they can stick to it!

Pre-hypertension:	the plan is lifestyle modification (diet, stop smoking, be more active, cut back on Na).
Stage I:	thiazide diuretic +/- beta blocker (also for pre-hypertension diabetic…the treatment is more aggressive)
Stage II:	thiazide diuretic + ACEi/ARB/BB/CCB

Obesity
Obesity is associated with increased risk of CV disease. This is especially true for "central obesity". Obesity is also associated with other risk factors…Type 2 DM, HTN, Inactivity and Hyperlipidemia. Note that obesity is an INDEPENDENT risk factor, but it is often combined with others. The dangers are very real…one study followed 1 million Americans for 14 years and found the risk of CV death to be 2x higher in obese individuals. Get off the couch!!!

Some scary statistics:
- 60% of adults are overweight or obese
- the % of young people who are overweight has more than doubled in the past 30 years
- between 10-15% of Americans age 6-17 are overweight
- The annual cost for the US is $100 billion. Get off the couch!!!

Smoking
24% of adults in the US continue to smoke, but this is down from 42% in 1965. We're doing better, but we're not there yet! Smoking is the strongest promoter for artherosclerosis…a truly horrible disease. How does this happen: Well, smoking increases PVR, increases LDL ("lethal" cholesterol) and decreases HDL ("healthy" cholesterol). The arterial endothelium is damaged, and platelets (which have increased aggregation due to smoking), are thought to adhere to subendothelial connective tissue exposed by endothelial denutation, initiating the smooth muscle proliferation that leads to artherosclerotic plaque formation. What's more, as many as 30% of CHD deaths in the US each year are attributed to smoking and the risk is strongly dose-related. It also nearly doubles the risk of ischemic stroke because the carbon monoxide more readily binds to hemoglobin than does oxygen and tissues suffer from lack of oxygen.

Environmental smoke has about 34% of the impact on artherosclerotic progression that occurs with active smoking.

Smokers who have had an MI:
- If you quit smoking, there is a 50% reduction in the risk of reinfarction, sudden cardiac death and total mortality
- This group is highly receptive to teaching, so teach!
- When MI pts are given information about quitting, there is a 50% long-term cessation rate…this is awesome!
- Modest telephone-based counseling can increase this percentage to 70% and is cheap!

Quitting:

- ~1.3 million quit each year
- After 1 year off cigarettes, the excess risk of heart disease is reduced by half.
- After 15 years of abstinence, the risk is similar to that of people who never smoked.
- In 5-15 years, the risk of stroke returns to the level of those who've never smoked.
- Only 50% of smokers seen in primary care were spoken to about smoking.
- It is better to have a "quit day" than to taper.
- Hypnosis is not supported by sufficient evidence
- There is a vaccine in clinical trials
- Counseling works!
- Drugs work! Nicotine patch or gum, bupropion, varenicline
- Chart all smoking cessation teaching!
- Smoking is the cause of more than 10% of CV deaths
- Smoking costs the US $90 billion year

<u>Lipids</u>

LDL = lethal. Each 1% drop in LDL confers to a 2% reduction in CV events. Yay for oatmeal!
HDL = healthy

Treatment for hyperlipidemia depends on lipid profile/levels, other CV risks and the cost of therapy. Generally, pts should change their diet (low-fat, low cholesterol), adopt lifestyle changes, and take drugs (statins, resins, fibrates, niacin).

<u>Stress</u>

Perceived high stress DOUBLES the risk of CV morbidity. So RELAX!

<u>Lack of Exercise</u>

Sadly, 60% of Americans are sedentary! Physical inactivity is another one of those independent risk factors for CVD. Improving activity reduces weight, improves lipid profiles and reduces BP... yay for exercise!

A 1996 statement from the NIH recommends that adults accumulate at least 30 mins of moderate activity on most days (and yes, walking to class counts so park far far away!), and more vigorous activity 3-4x a week for 30-60 minutes. Your heart and lungs will thank you!

<u>Diabetes</u>

The more I learn about diabetes the more I am convinced it is a truly horrible disease. Interestingly, the goal is not to keep pts at "the right level" for their blood glucose...this is because there were too many incidents of hypoglycemia. Instead, the goal is to keep pts within a healthy range and all I know about that is that <200 is the goal for wound healing so maybe that's it? One of the problems diabetics have is with arterial perfusion, which leads to necrotic tissues in the periphery. And yes, there is a definite parallel between obesity and diabetes. Once more folks, "get off the couch!"

<u>Na intake</u>

In obesity, each 2g increase in sodium intake is associated with a 61% increase in CV mortality.

Alcohol Intake

And now for some good news! Moderate alcohol consumption (identified as 1 glass of wine for women and 2 glasses for men) increases HDL, may decrease coagulation and lower BP! Yippeee! However, moderation is the key. Large alcohol intake increases BP, risk of stroke, cardiomyopathy and non-cardiac disorders. So, do the benefits outweigh the risks? In the US, 100k excess deaths can be attributed to alcohol-related deaths each year. On the other hand, if current alcohol consumers abstained from drinking, approximately 80,000 of them would die from CV disease.

Binge drinking is a real problem, especially among college aged males.

Homocysteine, Folic Acid and CVD

Homocysteine is an amino acid, and high levels of this are associated with CAD, CVA and PVD in epidemiological studies. However, folic acid and other B vitamins break down this amino acid in the body. Note that there have been no controlled studies supporting whether taking these vitamins decreases the risk so the AHA does not currently recommend. However, it is important to get lots of fruit and green leafy veggies.

Pathophysiology of Artherosclerosis
Look up the pathophys..what causes it. The consequences of artherosclerosis are decreased blood flow and decreased elasticity. The difference between chronic and acute artherosclerosis relates to the time it takes to develop collateral vessels and the amount of ischemia, pain and necrosis.

Congestive Heart Failure
The definition of CHF is "The situation when the heart is incapable of maintaining a cardiac output adequate to accommodate metabolic requirements and the venous return." (E. Braunwald) It affects 4.6 million Americans, with 400,000 new cases each year. 260,000 people die each year from this disease, and many of these pts died without ACEi.

Right vs. Left
The two things that basically occur with CHF is that 1) the heart is not pumping enough blood, so you get decreased BP, decreased cardiac output and fatigue; and 2) blood backs up!

Most common symptoms of CHF are dyspnea and fatigue.

In left heart failure, blood backs up to the lungs causing pulmonary edema. Because fluid gets into the alveoli and reacts with the surfactant, you get foamy sputum…the foam is basically the detergent (surfactant) mixed with fluid. If the right heart fails, you get peripheral edema and a tender/enlarged liver.

CHF Etiology and Risk Factors
Heart failure may result from a primary abnormality of the heart muscle (like an infarction) that impairs ventricular fxn and prevents the heart from pumping enough blood. It can also be caused by other problems:

- Mechanical disturbances in ventricular filling during diastole (due to blood volume that's too low for the ventricle to pump) occur in mitral stenosis secondary to rheumatic heart disease or constrictive pericarditis and in a-fibb.
- Systolic hemodyamic disturbances (excessive cardiac workload caused by volume overload or pressure overload) limit the heart's pumping ability. This can result from mitral or aortic insufficiency, which leads to volume overload. It can also result from aortic stenosis or systemic hypertension, which causes increased resistance to ventricular emptying and decreased cardiac output.

Factors Favorable to Failure

arrhythmias
bradycardia
pregnancy
thyrotoxicosis
pulmonary embolism
infectins
anemia
increased physical activity
increased salt or water intake
emotional stress
failure to comply with heart disease Tx

To sum this up:

- Heart attack
- High BP…the heart is pumping against increased pressure, so the left heart is affected.
- Lung disease decreases O2, the body compensates with vasoconstrinction in the lungs causing a lot of resistance and right heart has trouble pumping.

Determinants of Ventricular Function

- Contractility: How well does the heart contract? This affects stroke volume, which affects cardiac output.
- Preload: How much blood is delivered to the heart (venous return). If you are dehydrated, this will cause low preload, so you need to give that person fluids. Preload also affects stroke volume (and thus cardiac output)
- Afterload: Is the heart pumping against a lot of pressure? If so, stroke volume will go down.
- Heart rate: less time for ventricular filling, so reduced cardiac output.
- LV wall integrity, synergistic LV contraction and valvular competence all related to cardiac output.

Evolution of clinical stages

CHF can range from asymptomatic LV dysfunction all the way to refractory CHF. If we treat it early before symptoms appear, we have a better chance of treating the disease.

- Normal heart has no symptoms, normal exercise and normal LV fxn
- Asymptomatic LV dysfunction has no symptoms, normal exercise and abornmal LV fxn (EF may be down, but you'd only know this if you did an ECHO)
- Compensated CF has no symptoms unless exercising and abnormal LV fxn
- Decompensated CHF has symptoms when not exercising and abnormal LV fxn
- Refractory CHF has symptoms that are not controlled with treatment. This guy needs a heart transplant.

Treatment Objectives

The goals with treating CHF are to increase survival, decrease morbidity (well, duh), increase exercise capacity, increase quality of life, decrease neurohormonal changes, halt progression of the disease (or at least slow it) and decrease symptoms. The reason you want to decrease neurohormonal changes is because when BP is low, the neurohormonal response activates the SNS…this stresses the heart (think about what the SNS does to the heart). So, the heart remodels which means it gets fibrous tissue. Unfortunately, fibrous tissue does not work as well so we will turn off the neurohormonal response with medications to prevent fibrosis in the heart.

Treatments for CHF

The main goal with CHF is to correct aggravating factors:

- Pregnancy
- Arrythmias (AF)
- Infections
- Hyperthyroidism
- Thromboembolism
- Endocarditis
- Obesity
- Hypertension
- Physical activity
- Dietary excess
- MEDICATIONS (note that digoxin causes arrythmias, which are probably never good)

Key Points

Know that CHF used to be managed with the goal to relieve the symptoms…now the progression of the disease can be altered. Yay! The key to this is early interpretation with the appropriate drugs. B-Blockers and ACEi can slow the disease by turning off the neurohormonal pathway.

The disease is classified by the New York Heart Association as Class I-IV, based on the ability of the pt to exercise without symptoms.

The disease is staged as A-D, based on the evolution of the disease.

- A = High Risk. The goal here is to lower the risk and we do this by giving an ACEi.
- B is for anyone who has asymptomatic LV dysfunction, an EF < 40% (class I). This person will get an ACEi and a B-Blocker in an effort to reduce risk.
- C is for symptomatic CHF (class II and III). This person will get an ACEi, a B-Blocker, diuretics and be on a low sodium diet... all in an effort to reduce risk. They may also get angiotensin II RB and digoxin.
- D is for the most at risk person...symptomatic CHF (class IV). This person will get specialized therapy and get in line for a heart translplant.

<u>Common Clinical Features</u>
Fatigue and dyspnea
Cheyne Stokes
Orthostatic Hypotension
Liver tenderness
Peripheral edema
Pulmonary crackles
Weak pulses

Q: A 56 year old tests negative for a heat attack. His BP is 145/84 and he has an ejection fraction of 55%. He denies dyspnea and walks several miles a day. On discharge from the hospital, which meds would you anticipate he should have?

A: A thiazide diuretic...his BP is just too high to ignore. He won't get the other therapies because his EF is ok, and he has never had a heart attack.

<u>Various Drugs for Treating CHF (need to look over the slides, and maybe look these up)</u>

- ACEi
  - ACE inhibitors inhibit the renin-angiotensin-aldosterone system. Recall that this system is activated in response to hypotension, decreased sodium concentration in the distal tubule, decreased blood volume and renal sympathetic nerve stimulation. The kidneys release renin which cleaves angiotensinogen into ang I. Ang I is then converted ingo ang II via the angiotensin converting enzymes (ACE) in the lungs (also in the endothelium of blood vessels in many parts of the body). Ang II causes vasoconstriction and the release of ADH (among other things). Both of these work to increase blood pressure. If this pathway is inhibited, then the increase in blood pressure is thus inhibited. That's what an ACEi does.
  - ACEi drugs end in the word "pril". Quinapril was studied in 1993 and it shows that pts who received quinapril did not require any additional treatment, as compared to the group who took quinapril for a while and then took a placebo.
  - The advantages of ACEi are:
    - Inhibit left ventricular remodeling post myocardial infarction
    - Modify the progression of chronic CHF (increased survival and decreased hospitalizations, also improved quality of life)
    - In contrast to other vasodilators, does not produce neurohormonal activation or reflex tachycardia
    - Tolerance to its effects does not develop!

        - Studies show that the probability of death decreases when taking Enalopril vs a placebo.
    - ACEi indications are:
        - Clinical cardiac insufficiency (all patients)
        - Asymptomatic ventricular dysfunction (LVEF < 35%)
        - High risk for CHF pts (DM, HTN, ASVD, s/p MI)
- Angiotensin II Inhibitors (AKA AT1 receptor blocker, or ARB)
    - These drugs block vasoconstrictor and aldosterone-secreting effects of ang II at various receptor sites including vascular smooth muscle and the adrenal glands. It leads to vasodiation, an antiproliferative action and lowers blood pressure!
    - Some common ARBs are Losartan, Valsartan, Irbersartan and Candersartan.
- Diuretics
    - Thiazides act on the cortex of the kidney. They inhibit active exchange of Cl and Na in the cortical diluting segment of the ascending loop of Henle. They increase the excretion of sodium and water by inhibiting sodium reabsorption.
    - K-sparing diuretics act on the medulla and inhibit resportion of Na in the distal convoluted and collecting tubule…they also save K, so you will want to make sure K not too high! They also save H ions…will this affect pH?
    - Loop diuretics act on the medulla and inhibit the exchange of Cl, Na, K in the thick segment of the ascending loop of Henle.
- Digoxin
    - Digoxin binds to the Na/K/ATPase pump in the membranes of heart cells and decrease its function. This causes an increase in the level of sodium ions in the myocytes which then leads to a rise in the level of calcium ions. This causes an increase in the length of Phase 4 and Phase 0 of the cardiac action potential, which when combined with the effects of Dig on the NS, leads to a decrease in heart rate. Increased amounts of Ca are then stored in the sarcoplasmic reticulum and released by each action potential, which is unchanged by dig. This leads to increased contractility of the heart. Dig also increases vagal activity via its action on the CNS, decreasing the conduction of electrical impulses through the AV node.
    - Increases the force of myocardial contraction
    - Prolongs refractory period of the AV node
    - Decreases conduction through the SA and AV nodes
    - Causes increased cardiac output and slowing of the heart rate.
    - Studies show that when pts are given digoxin (along with a diuretic and ACEi), the CHF does not experience dramatically increased worsening (as compared to pts who received a placebo instead of digoxin).
    - The long term effects of dig are:
        - Survival similar to that of the placebo
        - Fewer hospital admissions
        - More serious arrhythmias
        - More myocardial infarctions
- Vasodilator Drugs
    - Vasodilators affect preload and afterload. There are different kinds of vasodilators:
        - Arterial vasodilators reduce arterial pressure by decreasing systemic vascular resistance. This benefits patients in heart failure by reducing the

afterload on the left ventricle, which enhances stroke volume and cardiac output and leads to secondary decreases in ventricular preload and venous pressure. Anginal pts benefit from arterial dilators because they decrease the oxygen demand of the heart, thereby improving the oxygen supply/demand ratio. Ex: Minoxidil, Hydralazine

- Venous vasodilators reduce venous pressure, which reduces preload on the heart thereby decreasing cardiac output. This also decreases proximal capillary hydrostatic pressure, which reduces capillary fluid filtration and edema formation (which is a result of heart failure).

- Nitrates
  - Have several different affects:
    - Venous Vasodilation (reduce preload leading to reduced pulmonary congestion, reduced ventricular size, reduced ventricular wall stress and reduced MVO2)
    - Coronary Vasodilation increases myocardial perfusion
    - Arterial Vasodilation decreases afterload leading to decreased cardiac output and decreased BP
  - Tolerance
    - Develops with all nitrates
    - Is dose-dependent
    - Disappears in 24 hours after stopping the drug
    - Can be avoided
      - Use the last effective dose
      - Create discontinuous plasma levels
      - Intermittent administration (nitrate-free period)
      - Allow peaks and valleys in plasma levels
  - Hold Nitrates when BP is low…it will drop BP even more!
- Aldosterone Inhibitors
  - The one discussed in class is called Spironolactone…it is a diuretic, but not as potent as Lasix. It is the only diuretic that actually makes people live longer. It is a competitive agonist of the aldosterone receptor in the myocardium, arterial walls and kidney. It BLOCKS aldosterone which decreases the fibrous tissue formation. Note that this drug conserve potassium, so you will hold the drug if the pt becomes hyperkalemic.
- Beta-Blockers
  - The Beta Blocker discussed in class is Carvedilol. It blocks Beta-1 (myocardial) and Beta-2 (pulmonary, vascular, uerine) adrenergic receptor sites. It also has alpha-1 blocking activity which means it may result in orthostatic hypotension. Be careful when getting this pt out of bed!
  - Therapeutic effects are decreased heart rate and BP, improved cardiac output, slowing of the progression of CHF and decreased risk of death. Yay!
  - These drugs have other awesome possible benefits:
    - Increased density of B-1 receptors (not sure what this means)
    - Inhibit cardiotoxicity of catecholamines

Remember This!
Beta Blockers end in "olol"
ACEi end in "pril"
ARB end in "sartan"

- Decreased neurohormonal activation
- Decreased HR
- Antihypertensive and antianginal
- Antiarrhythmic
- Antioxidant
- Antiproliferative (I've got to look this up and see what it means!)

  - Survival of pts on Beta-Blockers is pretty darn good. See the slides to get the details, but basically, if people are on B-Blockers and ACEi, the mortality rate goes down to 13.3% (down from 27.7%)
- Anticoagulants are given for lots of really interesting reasons (interesting if you're a NS!)
  - Previous embolic episode
  - Atrial fibrillation
  - Identified thrombus
  - Left ventricular aneurysm (3-6 months post MI)
  - Class III-IV CHF in the presence of an Ejection Fraction less than 30%, and/or an aneurism or a very dilated left ventricle.
  - Phlebitis (inflammation of a vein)
  - Prolonged bed rest (ok, that one's not interesting)

<u>Nursing Interventions for CHF</u>

Assist with ADLs: this patient is going to be fatigued
Improve SOB: raise HOB up, administer O2, give meds to decrease preload & afterload (ACEi and B-Blockers, plus others discussed above)
Keep an eye on K: Know how the meds affect K levels, keep an eye on I&O.

<u>Peripheral Vascular Disease</u>

Peripheral Vascular Disease can be broken down into arterial and venous diseases. Once again, Dr. Van warned us about getting the arterial diseases all combobulated with the venous ones. Probably the best thing to do would be to look at the table in the book. In general, here's what to look for when determining arterial vs. venous:

- Location
  - Arterial: Can be in aorta, legs? What about arms?
  - Venous: Is this always in extremities?
- Characteristics
  - Arterial: Dependent rubor, pallor with elevation, hypertrophied toenails, cool skin, hairless extremity, tissue atrophy.
  - Venous: Red color to skin, induration, warmth
- Pain
  - Arterial: Typically brought on by exercise and relieved by rest (intermittent claudication); sometimes unremitting pain in foot even at rest.
  - Venous: Tendernes along vein, discomfort may be relieved by applying heat
- Pulses
  - Arterial: Weak or absent
  - Venous: not sure?
- Surrounding tissue
  - Arterial: Gangrene, delayed wound healing

- Venous: Edematous (did I just make up a word?), itchy and scaly skin, thick/ coarse/brownish skin around the ankles

Assessment for PVD is the check for CSM. To manage it, we're going to do a few really fun things:

- Reduce risks
- Clot prevention/dissolution
- Surgery

Aneurysm

- Classification
  - Saccular = a unilateral outpouching
  - Fusiform = a bilateral outpouching
  - Dissecting = a bilateral outpouching in which layers of the vessel wall separate, creating a cavity
  - False = the wall ruptures and a blood clot is retained in an outpouching of tissue… or there is a cnnxn btwn a vein and an artery that does not close
- Pathophysiology.
  - An aneurysm can be venous or arterial. The exact cause is unknown, but recent evidence includes atherosclerosis and hypertension. Genetics can also come into play such as with Marfan syndrome.
  - True aneurysms contain all three layers of the arterial wall; saccular have a neck and mouth; fusiform invole the entire circumference; a dissecting is not a true aneurysm, but is ahematoma in the arterial wall that separates the layers of the wall.
  - Other causes of anueysms include infection, mycotic infections and even trauma (though that last one is rare)
- Clinical Manisfestations
  - AAA
    - Most abdominal ones are asymptomatic, can be palpated once it's at 5 cm (unless obese…see, another reason to go for a run!).
    - Most common clinical manisfestations is the client's awareness of a pulsating mass in the abdomen, followed by abdominal pain and back pain.
    - Groin pain and flank pain
    - Bruits can be heard over the aneurysm…a bruit is an adventitious sound of venous or arterial origin heard on auscultation.
    - Sometimes mottlinf of the extremeties or distal emboli in the feet alert the clinician to a source in the abdomen.
    - Ultrasonography and CT are dx tools
  - Ruptured AAA
    - Pulsating sensation in abdomen
    - Abrubt excruciating pain (ripping or knife-life that radiates)
    - Hypertension (but elsewhere it says hypotension?)
    - Manisfestations of shock (pallor, tachycardia, hypotension, dry skin, excessive thirst)

- Diminished peripheral pulses or unequal pulses
- Abdominal rigidity
- Differing BP in arms
- Paraplegia, hemiplegia
- Decreased urine output or hematuria

Raynaud's Syndrome

An arterial disease in which the small arteries and arterioles constrict in response to various stimuli. This can be caused by cold, nicotine, caffeine and stress. Obstructive Raynaud's often seen with autoimmune diseases.

Buerger's Disease

This is an inflammatory disease of the small and medium-sized arteries and veins of the extremities…it appears to be directly related to smoking (reason #5,673 why smoking is bad for you). The main clinical manisfestation is pain, digital ulcerations and ischemia. Pts may also have cold sensitivity with color changes and pain. Pulsations in the posterior tibial and dorsalis pedis are weak or absent and in advanced cases the extremeties may be abnormally red or cyanotic. Ulceration and gangrene are frequent complications…if pt don't stop smoking they are very likely to lose fingers (or whatever part is affected). This disease is hard to treat…drugs don't work very well.

DVT

This is a very common disease that happens most often in the lower extremities. DVT is often asymptomatic, but you may see unilateral edema, calf pain and fever. The three factors that affect the formation of DVTs are known as **Virchow's Triad**:

- Endothelial injury due to trauma or surgery
- Circulatory stasis due to immobility
- Hypercoagulable state due to birth control pills (may be other things, not sure)

Prevention and Treatment of DVTs

- Heparin
- Warfarin (COUMADIN)
- TEDs/SCDs (prevention only)
- Elevation
- Early ambulation (prevention only)

Mechanism of Action of Antithrombotic Agents (sounds so fancy!)

- Anticoagulants prevent clot formation and extension
- Antiplatelet drugs interfere with platelet activity
- Thrombolytic agents dissolve existing thrombi

Pulmonary Embolism

When thrombi break off and travel to the lungs (where it obstructs the pulmonary arterial bed), this is a very very bad situation. Though it can be so mild as to produce no symptoms, a massive embolism obstructing more than 50% of the circulation) is rapidly fatal.

What to look for:

- First sign is usually dyspnea, may be accompanied by angina or pleuritic chest pain
- Tachycardia
- Air hunger
- Feeling of impending doom
- Productive cough (may have blood)
- Low-grade fever
- Pleural effusion

Less common signs:

- Massive hemoptysis
- Splinting of the chest
- Leg edema
- Cyanosis, syncope, distended neck veins
- Pleural friction rub
- Signs of circulatory collapse
- Hypoxia

Treatment/Management

- Resuscitate as needed
- Give O2
- Give heparin
- If can't tolerate heparin, then surgery

Edema

Lymphedema occurs when lymphatic flow is blocked, but can also occur with low serum protein and high venous pressure. It is treated by elevating the affected body part, compressing the affected body part, providing skin care and infection treatment and administering diuretics.

Aging and the CV system

As we age, the efficiency of the heart's pumping action decreases. This is related to connective tissue changes (decreased compliance), increased fat/sclerosis causing lower cardiac output, arrhythmias and valve incompetence. The vasculature changes as well, with decreased elastin and increased arteriosclerosis.

Nursing Dx (related to???)

- Decreased tissue perfusion
- Health maintenance (risk reduction, medication compliance)
- Knowledge deficit

Labs, labs, labs!

Na < 135 = fluid overload
K < 3.5 = loop diuretics
K > 5.0 = renal insufficiency
BUN > 20 = renal insufficiency
BUN < 7 = malnutrition
Creatinine > 1.2 = renal insufficiency
INR 1 = normal, 2-3 therapeutic warfarin level
aPTT 30 = normal, 60-90 therapuetic heparain
Cholesterol > 200mg/dl = risk; >240 mg/dl = high risk
LDL >130 mg/dl = risk
HDL <37 = male risk; <47 = female risk
Triglycerides >200 mg/dl = risk; > 400 mg/dl = high risk
C-reactive protein = women < 1.5 mg/l; men < 5mg/l

Outcomes
BP < 130/86, No MI, CVA or renal failure

Brain Attack, CVA, Stroke
Most strokes are caused by thromboemboli! The concepts of perfusion/stasis are the same as for CV disease, as are the risk factors. Brain attack is the 3rd leading cause of death in the US and is very expensive for both the government and the individual patient. The good news is, the death rate due to brain attack has declined due to better risk prevention and management, quicker diagnoses and more timely intervention technologies.

Causes & Pathophysiology Brain Attack
Thromboembolic, hemorrhage and aneurysm. The brain has no oxygen reserve, so when an artery is occluded (ischemia) this causes the Na/K pump to no loner work. The Na stays in the cell and since water follows salt, the cell swells. This swelling limits the amount of perfusion that can get to the brain and causes cells to die.

Sadly, people don't often recognize the signs of stroke, but if you can get the pt to the hospital within 3 hours (and it's a thromboembolic stroke), then that person can fare very well with the administration of TPAs (which dissolve clot).

Stages of Brain Attack
- TIA (transcient ischemic something or other)…these symptoms resolve on their own in minutes or hours. They are caused by microemboli from plaque. However, all is not peaches and candy for this person…they are likely to go on to have a bona fide CVA.
- RIND (reversible ischemic neurological disease) symptoms persist for 24-48 hours. There is ischemia, but no necrosis…comlete recovery!
- Stroke in evolution: 20-35% of pts have symptoms that get worse over the course of the week after the CVA.
- Completed stroke causes permanent neuro damage.

Clinical Manifestations of Brain Attack (CVA)
The clinical manifestations have to do with which blood vessel is involved (see book). The most common are the middle cerebral artery and the internal carotid artery.
- Middle Cerebral Artery
  - Contralateral paralysis, paresis, sensory loss
  - Dysphasia, aphasia
  - Spatial perception problems, judgment/behavior
  - Contralateral homonymous hemianopsia
- Internal Carotid Artery
  - Same as above, plus…
  - Ipsilateral visual impairment
  - Ipsilateral Horner's syndrom (ptosis, miosis, no sweating on same side of face)

With both you have decreased LOC, could have seizures and VS changes. Visual problems vary with the site of the stroke...see book for diagram of how the ocular pathways criss-cross. Also, the motor and sensory tracts cross over, so a stroke on the left side of the brain is going to cause right-sided weakness.

Prevention of Brain Attack/CVA/Stroke

- Risk factor modification (ex: stop smoking, lose weight, control HTN)
- Anticoagulants
    - Warfarin for atrial fibrillation
    - Aspirin
    - Aspirin/extended release dipyridamole
    - Not heparain (except for DVT/afib*)
- Surgical revascularization

*Pts with past history of afib are taught to feel radial pulse to evaluate return of irregular heart beat and to self administer LMWH prior to seeking medical care. Several strokes have been prevented!

Treatment: Evolving Stroke

- 911…get the stroke team activated!
    - Stabilize airway, O2, BP, CT scan
    - Give or not to give thrombolytics
- Maintain cerebral perfusion
    - Reduce swelling
        - BP < 200/120 (<185/110 with TPA plans). You might think "WOAH", that BP is high! Well, we want it to be high so the blood can perfuse the brain.
        - Good ventilation
        - Mannitol: osmular agent used in first 72-96 hours (pulls fluid out of cell to decrease edema)
        - Steroids: Not useful except after SAH (subarachnoid hemorrhage)
        - HOB up slightly (though this may get sticky with MD…let them has it out)
        - Glyburide: experimental, reduces swelling
    - Prevent vasospasm: nimodipine (a calcium channel blocker)…used for bleeds but not ischemic strokes.
- Protect brain cells…make sure no fever, use neuroprotectants (experimental drugs)
- Surgery: external decompressions, remove clot with hemorrhagic stroke
- Seizure prevention (not sure how you prevent a seizure)…anti-seizure meds?

> When CO2 goes up, blood vessels in the brain dilate, causing increased pressure in the brain, leading do decreased perfusion.

Rehab/Treatment: Evolving and Completed Stroke

In this stage you will protect your pt from complications of immobility and decreased neuromuscular status. This is a multidisciplinary approach with a lot of people involved.

- No aspiration (HOB up, NPO/PEG or feeding tube, speech therapy, swallow evaluation)
- No pressure sores (turn pt, OOB to chair)
- No contractures (position of max function, ROM)
- Bowel and bladder function support
- Communication
- Interaction with environment when visual field impaired
- Depression

Blood flow through the heart

Oxygen poor blood travels through the inferior or superior vena cava or coronary sinus
ronary blood circulation)
Deoxygenated blood enters the right atrium
Blood passes through the tricuspid valve
Blood enters right ventricle
Blood moves through the pulmonary valve
Blood enters the pulmonary trunk and arteries where the blood is carried to the lungs
Blood loses CO2 and gains O2 in the pulmonary capillaries
The oxygenated blood enters the pulmonary veins
Blood enters the left atrium
Blood travels through the mitral/bicuspid valve
Blood enters the left ventricle
Blood moves through the aortic valve
Blood travels through the aorta and systemic arteries
Blood loses O2 and gains CO2 in the systemic capillaries

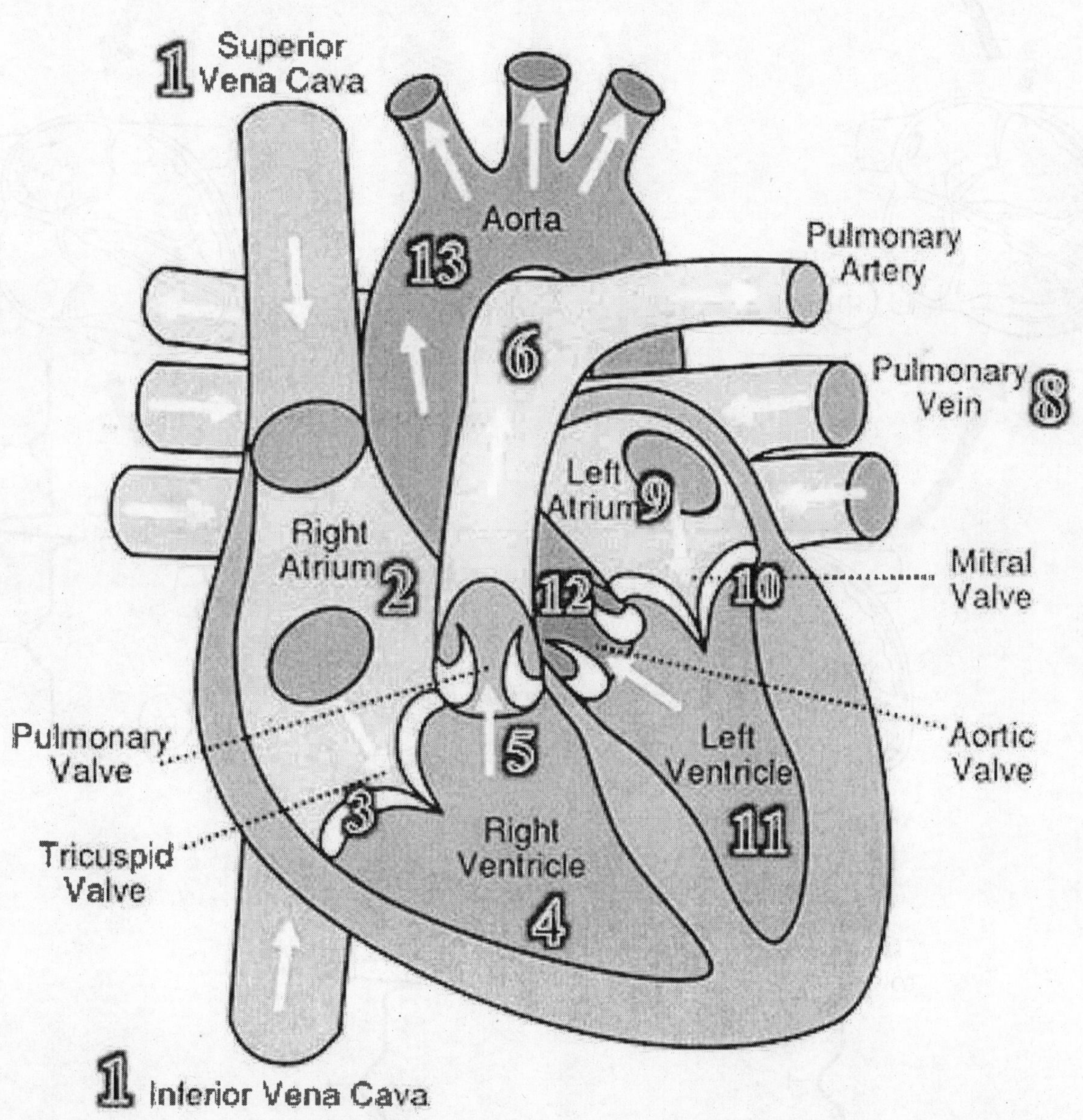

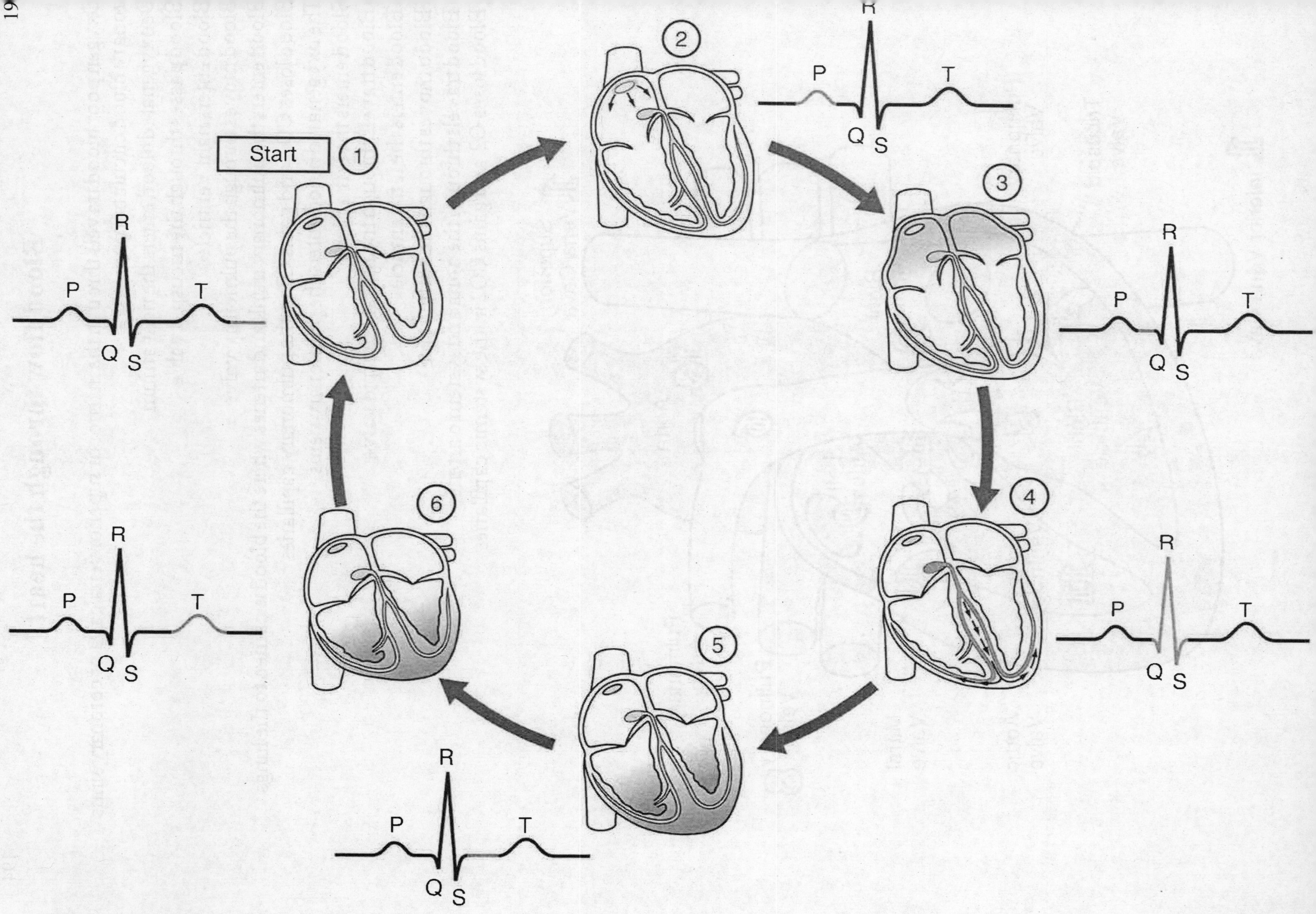

Start

1

2

3

4

5

6

P Q R S T

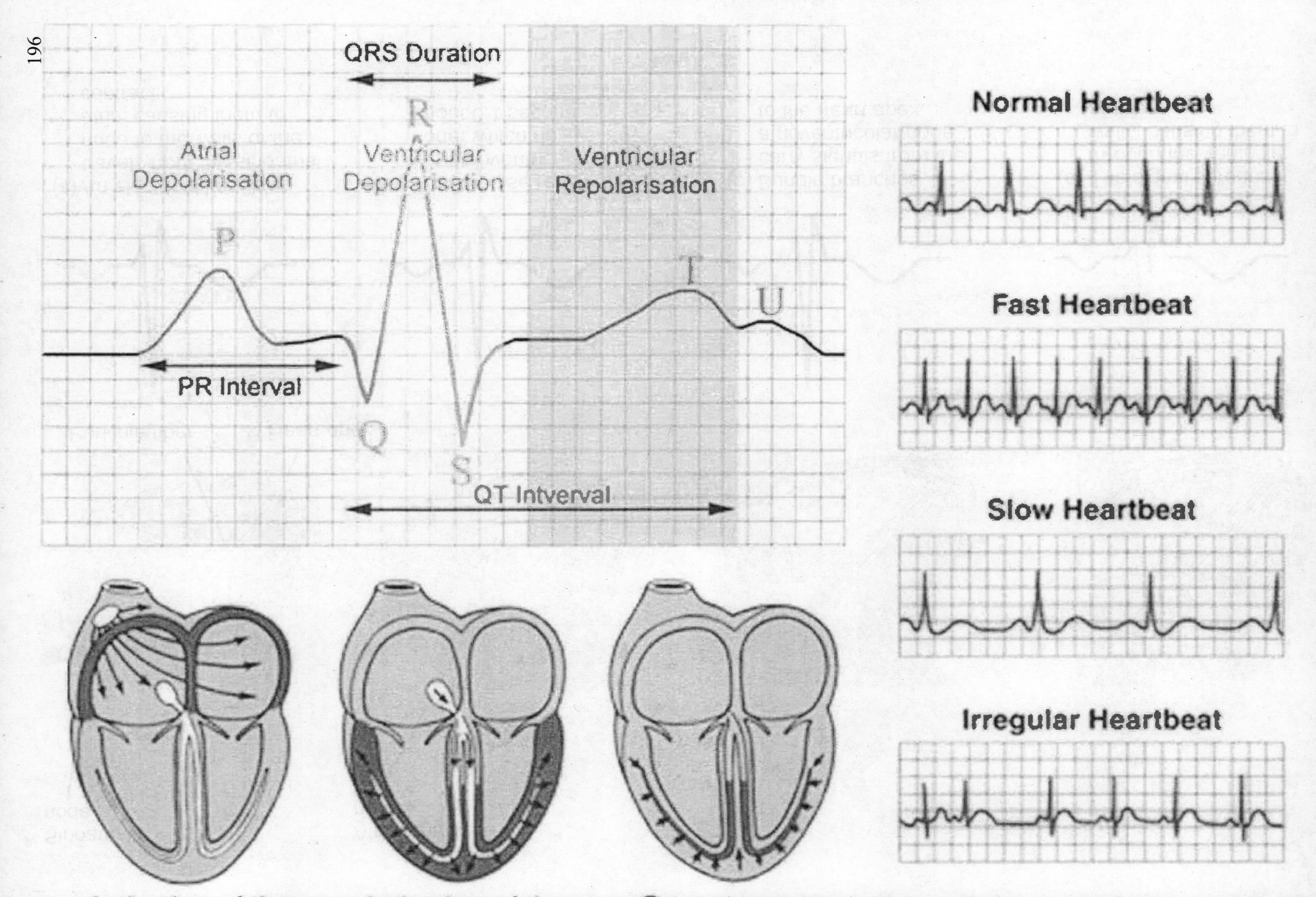
QRS Duration
R
Atrial
Depolarisation
Ventricular
Depolarisation
Ventricular
Repolarisation
P
T
U
PR Interval
Q
S
QT Intverval
Normal Heartbeat
Fast Heartbeat
Slow Heartbeat
Irregular Heartbeat

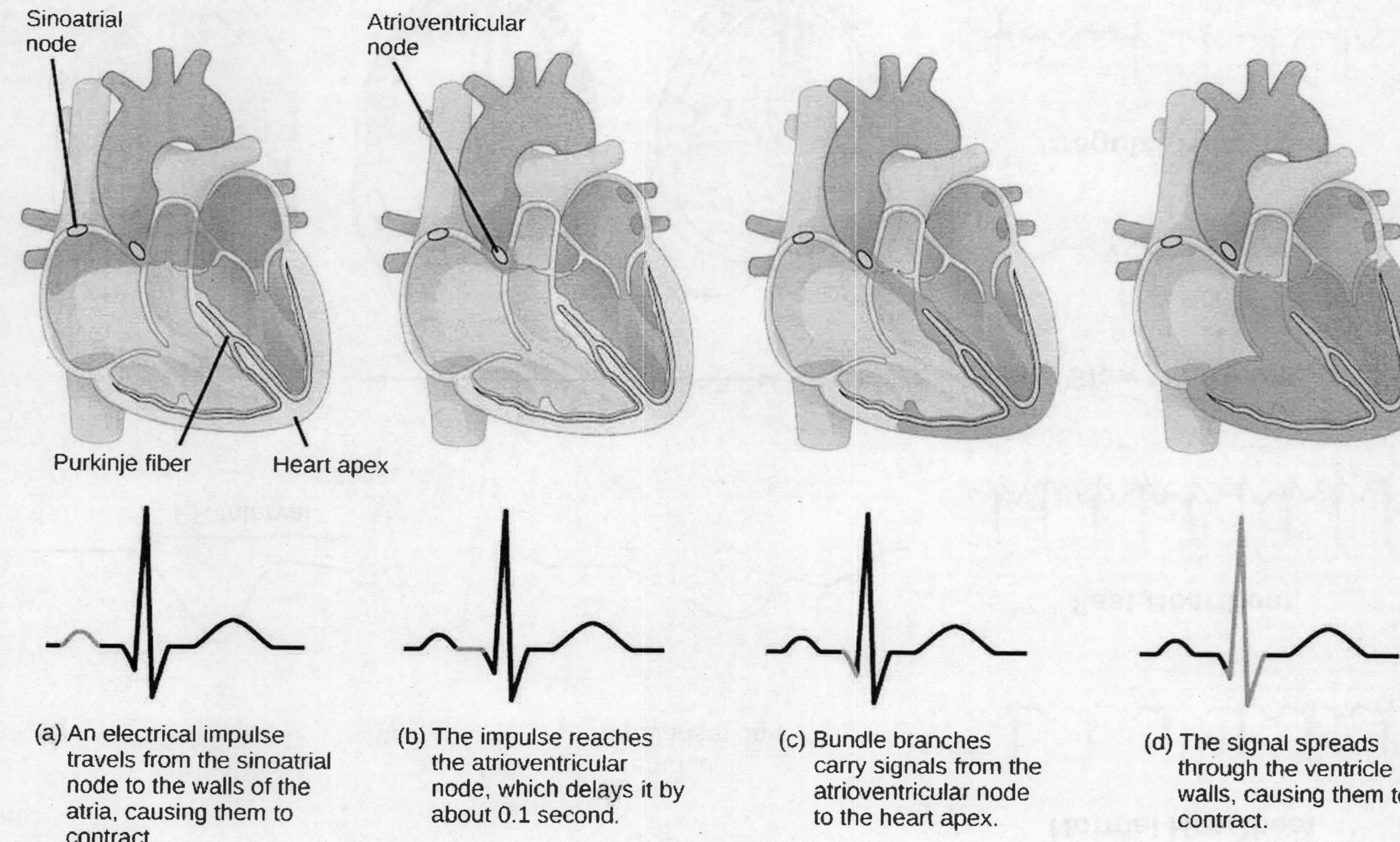

(a) An electrical impulse travels from the sinoatrial node to the walls of the atria, causing them to contract.

(b) The impulse reaches the atrioventricular node, which delays it by about 0.1 second.

(c) Bundle branches carry signals from the atrioventricular node to the heart apex.

(d) The signal spreads through the ventricle walls, causing them to contract.

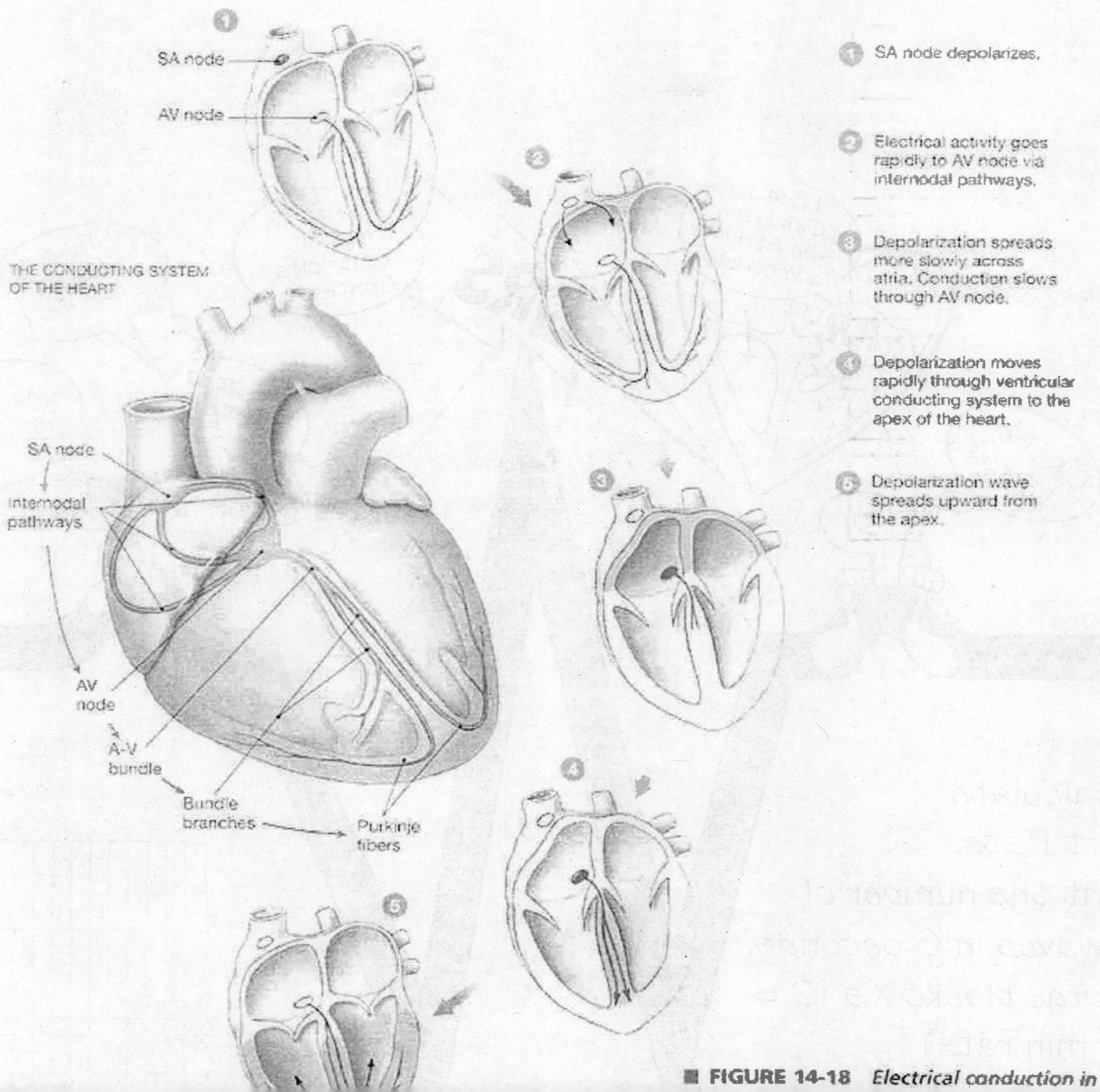

SA node
AV node

THE CONDUCTING SYSTEM OF THE HEART

SA node
Internodal pathways
AV node
A-V bundle
Bundle branches
Purkinje fibers

1. SA node depolarizes.
2. Electrical activity goes rapidly to AV node via internodal pathways.
3. Depolarization spreads more slowly across atria. Conduction slows through AV node.
4. Depolarization moves rapidly through ventricular conducting system to the apex of the heart.
5. Depolarization wave spreads upward from the apex.

■ **FIGURE 14-18** ***Electrical conduction in the***

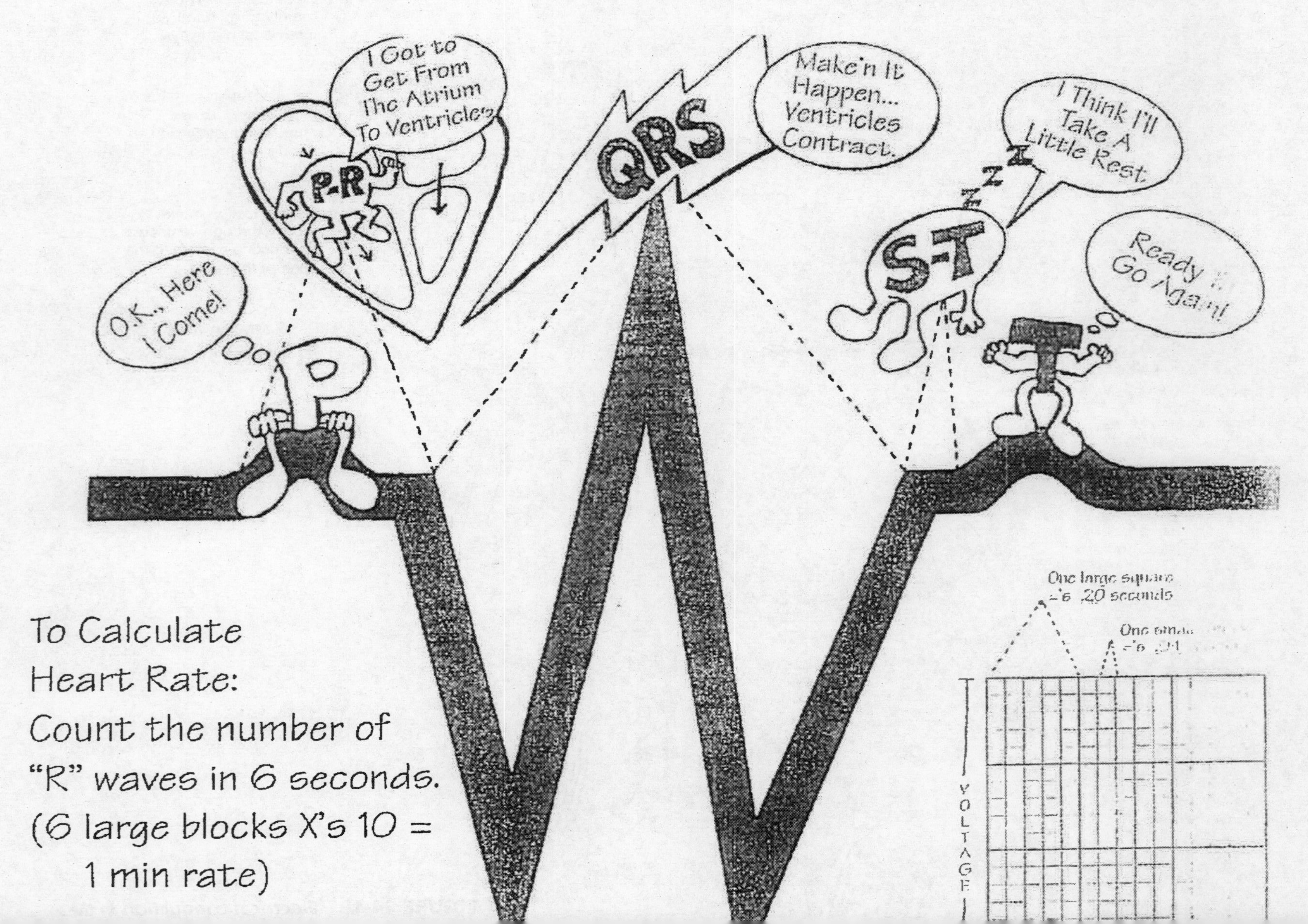

To Calculate
Heart Rate:
Count the number of
"R" waves in 6 seconds.
(6 large blocks X's 10 =
1 min rate)

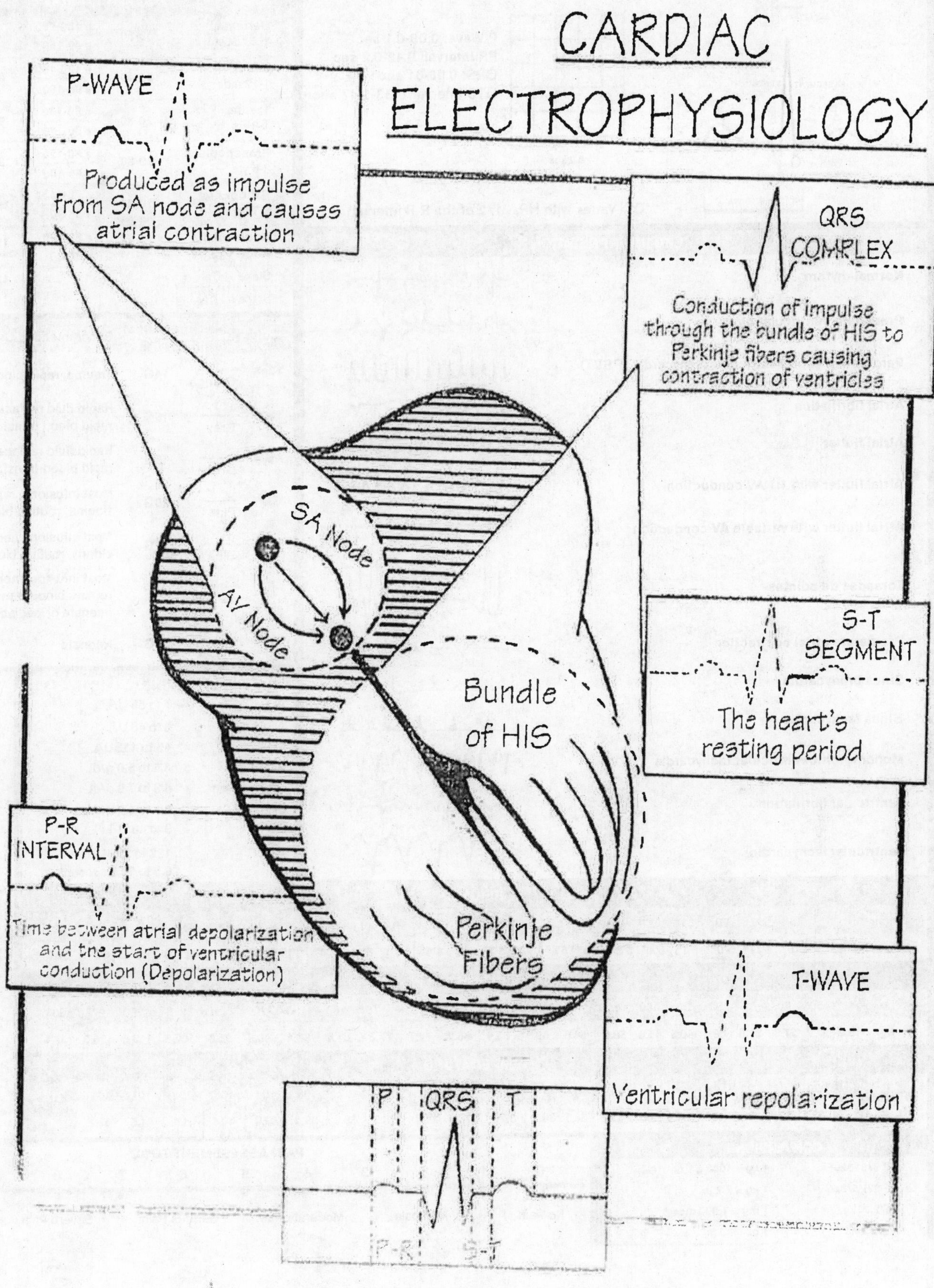
CARDIAC
ELECTROPHYSIOLOGY
P-WAVE
Produced as impulse from SA node and causes atrial contraction
QRS COMPLEX
Conduction of impulse through the bundle of HIS to Perkinje fibers causing contraction of ventricles
SA Node
AV Node
Bundle of HIS
S-T SEGMENT
The heart's resting period
P-R INTERVAL
Time between atrial depolarization and the start of ventricular conduction (Depolarization)
Perkinje Fibers
T-WAVE
Ventricular repolarization
P
QRS
T
P-R
S-T

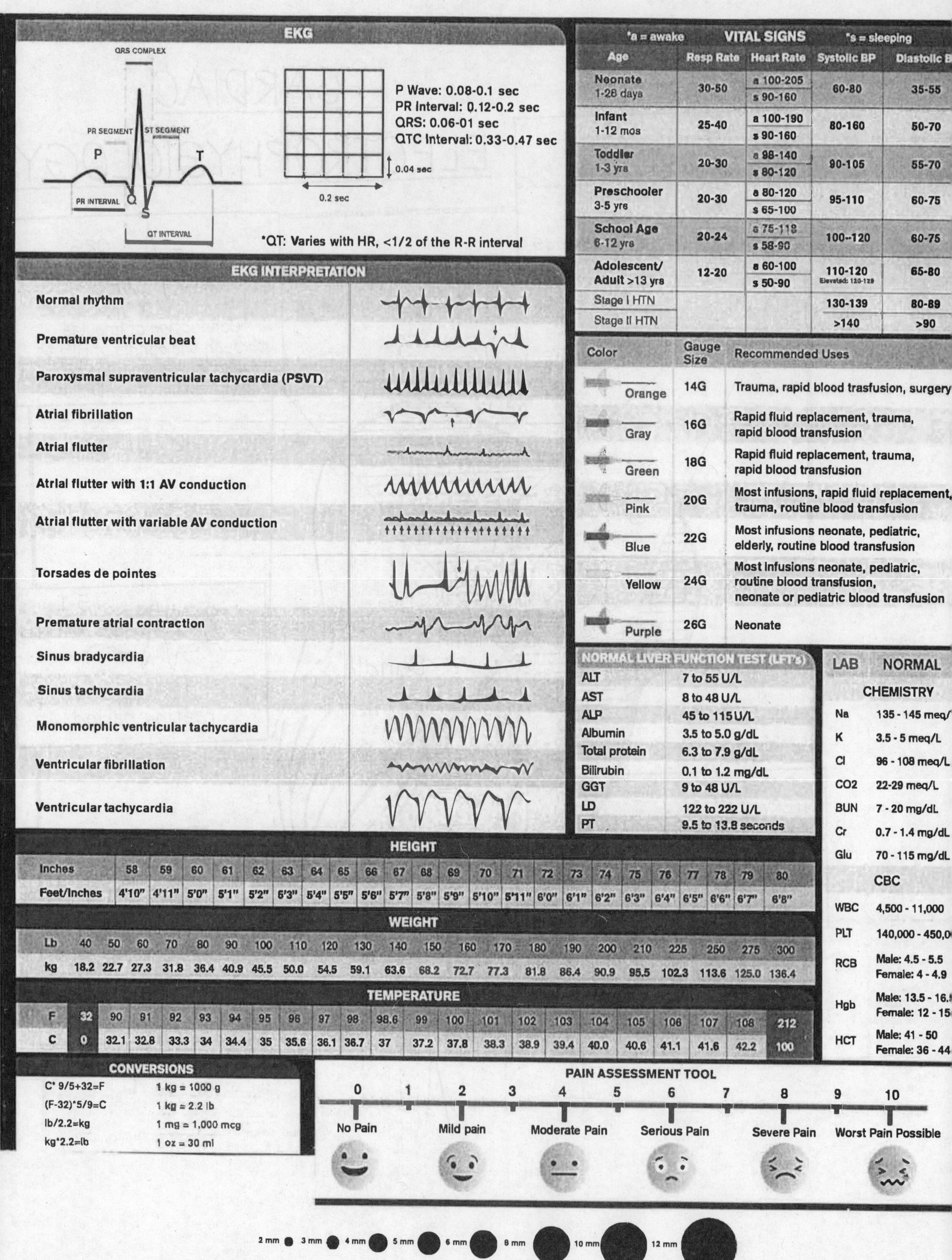

EKG

P Wave: 0.08-0.1 sec
PR Interval: 0.12-0.2 sec
QRS: 0.06-01 sec
QTC Interval: 0.33-0.47 sec

*QT: Varies with HR, <1/2 of the R-R interval

EKG INTERPRETATION

- Normal rhythm
- Premature ventricular beat
- Paroxysmal supraventricular tachycardia (PSVT)
- Atrial fibrillation
- Atrial flutter
- Atrial flutter with 1:1 AV conduction
- Atrial flutter with variable AV conduction
- Torsades de pointes
- Premature atrial contraction
- Sinus bradycardia
- Sinus tachycardia
- Monomorphic ventricular tachycardia
- Ventricular fibrillation
- Ventricular tachycardia

VITAL SIGNS

*a = awake *s = sleeping

Age	Resp Rate	Heart Rate	Systolic BP	Diastolic B
Neonate 1-28 days	30-50	a 100-205 s 90-160	60-80	35-55
Infant 1-12 mos	25-40	a 100-190 s 90-160	80-160	50-70
Toddler 1-3 yrs	20-30	a 98-140 s 80-120	90-105	55-70
Preschooler 3-5 yrs	20-30	a 80-120 s 65-100	95-110	60-75
School Age 6-12 yrs	20-24	a 75-118 s 58-90	100--120	60-75
Adolescent/ Adult >13 yrs	12-20	a 60-100 s 50-90	110-120 Elevated: 120-129	65-80
Stage I HTN			130-139	80-89
Stage II HTN			>140	>90

Color	Gauge Size	Recommended Uses
Orange	14G	Trauma, rapid blood trasfusion, surgery
Gray	16G	Rapid fluid replacement, trauma, rapid blood transfusion
Green	18G	Rapid fluid replacement, trauma, rapid blood transfusion
Pink	20G	Most infusions, rapid fluid replacement, trauma, routine blood transfusion
Blue	22G	Most infusions neonate, pediatric, elderly, routine blood transfusion
Yellow	24G	Most infusions neonate, pediatric, routine blood transfusion, neonate or pediatric blood transfusion
Purple	26G	Neonate

NORMAL LIVER FUNCTION TEST (LFT's)

ALT	7 to 55 U/L
AST	8 to 48 U/L
ALP	45 to 115 U/L
Albumin	3.5 to 5.0 g/dL
Total protein	6.3 to 7.9 g/dL
Bilirubin	0.1 to 1.2 mg/dL
GGT	9 to 48 U/L
LD	122 to 222 U/L
PT	9.5 to 13.8 seconds

LAB NORMAL

LAB	NORMAL
CHEMISTRY	
Na	135 - 145 meq/
K	3.5 - 5 meq/L
Cl	96 - 108 meq/L
CO2	22-29 meq/L
BUN	7 - 20 mg/dL
Cr	0.7 - 1.4 mg/dL
Glu	70 - 115 mg/dL
CBC	
WBC	4,500 - 11,000
PLT	140,000 - 450,0
RCB	Male: 4.5 - 5.5 Female: 4 - 4.9
Hgb	Male: 13.5 - 16. Female: 12 - 15
HCT	Male: 41 - 50 Female: 36 - 44

HEIGHT

Inches	58	59	60	61	62	63	64	65	66	67	68	69	70	71	72	73	74	75	76	77	78	79	80
Feet/Inches	4'10"	4'11"	5'0"	5'1"	5'2"	5'3"	5'4"	5'5"	5'6"	5'7"	5'8"	5'9"	5'10"	5'11"	6'0"	6'1"	6'2"	6'3"	6'4"	6'5"	6'6"	6'7"	6'8"

WEIGHT

Lb	40	50	60	70	80	90	100	110	120	130	140	150	160	170	180	190	200	210	225	250	275	300
kg	18.2	22.7	27.3	31.8	36.4	40.9	45.5	50.0	54.5	59.1	63.6	68.2	72.7	77.3	81.8	86.4	90.9	95.5	102.3	113.6	125.0	136.4

TEMPERATURE

F	32	90	91	92	93	94	95	96	97	98	98.6	99	100	101	102	103	104	105	106	107	108	212
C	0	32.1	32.8	33.3	34	34.4	35	35.6	36.1	36.7	37	37.2	37.8	38.3	38.9	39.4	40.0	40.6	41.1	41.6	42.2	100

CONVERSIONS

C° 9/5+32=F	1 kg = 1000 g
(F-32)*5/9=C	1 kg = 2.2 lb
lb/2.2=kg	1 mg = 1,000 mcg
kg*2.2=lb	1 oz = 30 ml

PAIN ASSESSMENT TOOL

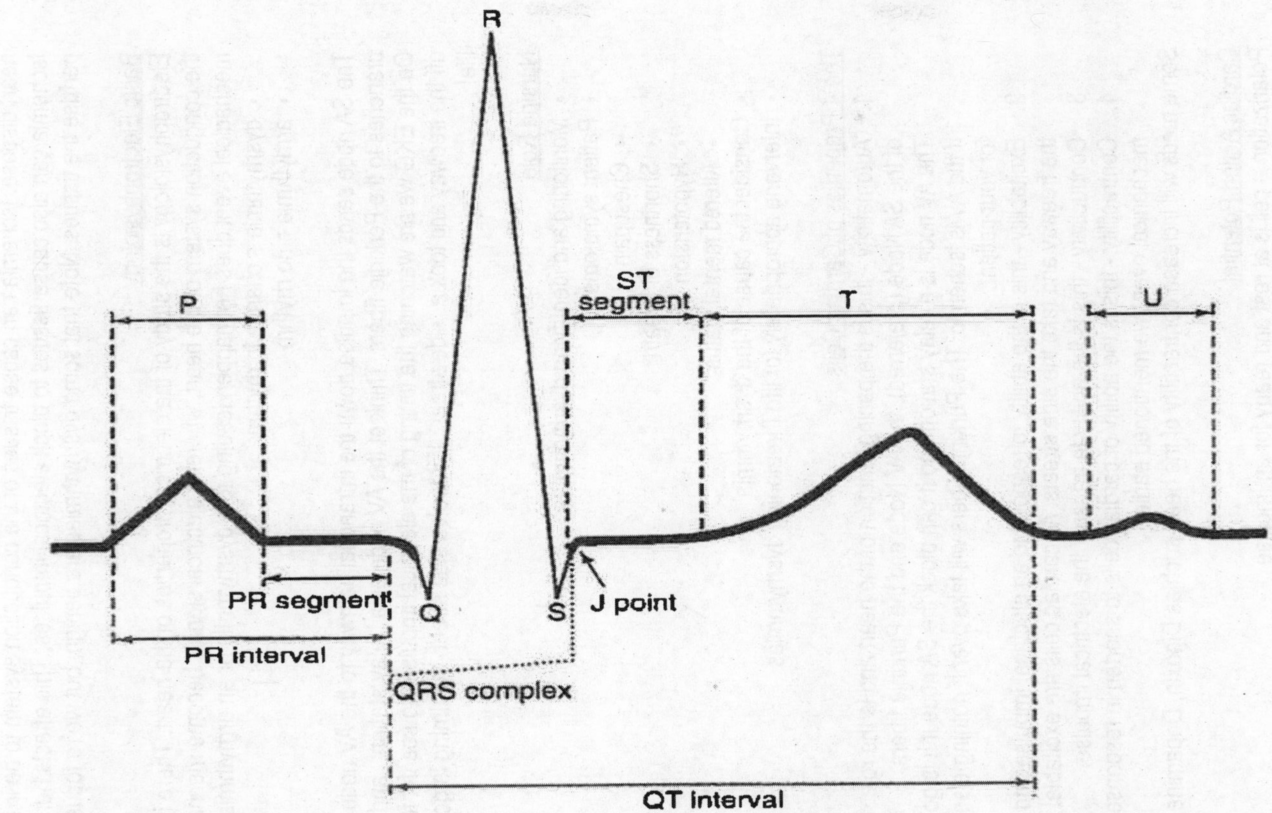

P wave:	Represents atrial depolarization.
PR segment:	Represents the time required for the impulse to travel through the AV node, where it is delayed, and through the bundle of His, bundle branches, and Purkinje fiber network, just before ventricular depolarization.
PR interval:	Represents the time required for atrial depolarization as well as impulse travel through the conduction system and Purkinje fiber network, inclusive of the P wave and PR segment. It is measured from the beginning of the P wave to the end of the PR segment.
QRS complex:	Represents ventricular depolarization and is measured from the beginning of the Q (or R) wave to the end of the S wave.
J point:	Represents the junction where the QRS complex ends and the ST segment begins.
ST segment:	Represents early ventricular repolarization.
T wave:	Represents ventricular repolarization.
U wave:	Represents late ventricular repolarization.
QT interval:	Represents the total time required for ventricular depolarization and repolarization and is measured from the beginning of the QRS complex to the end of the T wave.

EKG Interpretation

Epidemiology of dysrhythmia
In 2003, dysrhythmias caused or contributed to 479,000 deaths. The conduction system is susceptible to damage by heart disease. Ischemia can cause tissues of the conduction system to be irritable or excitable (extra beats). Ischemia can also cause tissues to block electrical impulses. This effects hemodynamics and the hearts ability to perfuse the tissues. Note that some dysrhythmias are benign, but we're focusing today on the lethal ones.

Basic Electrophysiology
Electrophysiology is the study of the electrical properties of the heart. There is a pattern of electrical impulses through the conduction system of the heart, whereby electrical signals become mechanical events. However, sometimes the mechanical event does not happen leading to a dysrhythmia or an arrhythmia.

- dysrhythmia = change in rhythm
- arrhythmia = no rhythm

The SA node sends the impulse down the intranodal pathway to the AV node to the Bundle of His through the bundle branches to the Perkinje fibers. Think of the AV node as a "relay station", and the branches as a "freeway system." On the EKG we are watching the timing of the electrical impulses to see if it follows a pathway (freeway), or if it got off the freeway and took a "side street". If it took a side street, the timing is going to be slooowwwer...just like in real life!

Nursing Role
- Monitoring and identifying dysrhythmias
- Patient symptoms
  - Chest pain
  - Shortness of Breath
  - Hypotension
  - Altered mental status
- Consider the cause of the dysrhythmia
- Intervene appropriately for life threatening dysrhythmias

Intrinsic Rates of the Heart
SA Node: 60-100 beats per minute
AV Node: 40-60 beats per minute
Purkinje: 20-40 beats per minute

The 4 Properties of Cardiac Cells
1. Automaticity - this is the pacing function of the heart and is the role of the SA Node (preferred), the AV Node and the Purkinje fibers.
   The AV node is a relay station and it can block the SA node if it is going too fast, or block the SA completely if the AV is ischemic. The Purkinje fibers will take over if nothing else is working well...this is pretty bad news for your patient.
2. Excitability - this is the ability to respond to an electrical impulse and explains why the impulse can get off the freeway and take the side streets. All cardiac cells are excitable!
3. Conductivity - this is the ability to transmit the electrical impulse
4. Contractility - this is the ability of cardiac cells to shorten in response to an electrical stimulus. This is the mechanical event we mentioned earlier!

Some meds will increase contractility of the heart such as Digoxin, Dopamine, Dobutamine.

Cardiac Action Potential
Polarization = cell is at rest and ready for an impulse
Depolarization = reversal of electrical charge across cell membrane (this is the Na and K changing places)
Repolarization = recovery of the cell to its original polarized state (Na and K returning to their original positions). The cell is refractory during this time period. If a cell receives an impulse during this period, it gets irritable leading to a lethal rhythm and sudden cardiac death. No bueno! More on refractory periods below.

Refractory Periods...3 Stages

- Absolute refractory period: Cardiac cells will NOT respond to a stimulus AT ALL! No way Jose!
- Relative refractory period: This is a vulnerable period. Some cells have repolarized and the tissue may respond with a strong impulse.
- Supernormal period: Weaker than normal stimulus could cause depolarization. The cell is "hyper" during this time and it doesn't take much to set it off. Stimulation at this time often results in very fast, dangerous rhythms.

Cardiac Conduction System

- SA Node is the pacemaker for the heart. It is located on the upper posterior wall of the RA. It generates a stimuli at regular intervals (60-100 bpm), and it corresponds with the P WAVE on the ECG.
- Intranodal pathways (between SA and AV nodes)
- AV Node slows the impulse coming from the SA Node (recall that the AV is the "relay station"). The slowing of the SA node allows the atria time to contract and the ventricles to fill. The ventricles have to be nice and full in order to have optimal cardiac output! The AV can spontaneously generate an impulse btwn 40-60 bpm and this is usually an "escape mechanism" or "rescue mechanism". The AV node's impulse is portrayed as the PR interval on the EKG. We want to keep an eye on the length of this line!
- The Bundle of His is the "freeway system" of the heart. It bifurcates into the left and right branches and travels through the ventricles.
- The Purkinje fibers allow for rapid depolarization of the ventricle. It is seen as the QRS on the ECG. If left to its own devices, Purkinje would fire at 20-40 bpm...not very good!

ECG Waveforms

The full cardiac cycle consists of a P wave, a PR interval, a QRS complex, an ST segment, a T wave and an isoelectric line.

- **P wave** is the start of the cardiac cycle. It results from the electrical firing of the SA node/atrial depolarization. It is rounded and smooth in appearance, and has a positive deflection (it points up like a little hill). All P waves on the EKG should look the same. If they don't something is going on with the AV node.
- **The PR Interval** relates to the depolarization of the right and left atria, and the impulse delay through the AV junction (which is your relay station). This is a period of electrical silence and it establishes the isoelectric line. Your ST segment needs to be at the same level as this line!
  - It is measured from the beginning of the P wave to the beginning of the QRS complex. It's normal length is 0.12 to 0.20 seconds (3-5 little boxes).
  - If the PR interval is long this means there is a blockage in the AV node (most likely d/t ischemia)

> ***The Boxes***
>
> Each little box signifies TIME
> Each LITTLE box = 0.04 seconds
> Each BIG box = 0.20 seconds

- **The QRS Complex** is made up of 3 waveforms and these can vary dramatically depending on the view you are utilizing. It represents the depolarization of the ventricles.
  - Q wave is the FIRST downward deflection after the P wave...it can be pathological indicating damage to the heart muscle. The Q wave is usually not there unless the pt has had an acute MI in the past. Tiny ones are OK though.
  - R wave is the FIRST upward deflection in the QRS. This is always a good thing! On a 12-lead view, we are looking for R-wave progression...it should get taller and taller as time goes on. If pt has had an acute MI, the R wave will not progress normally b/c the Q gets in the way.
  - S wave is the downward deflection AFTER the R wave.
  - The QRS should be no wider than 3 little boxes (0.12 seconds) If it is wider, this means there is a blockage along the bundle and the impulse got off the freeway and took the side street.
- ST segment is an isoelectric line between the QRS and the T-wave. It should be on the same plane as the PR interval.
  - If it is elevated or depressed this is indicative of injury in the myocardium.
  - It begins at the end of the QRS and ends at the beginning of the T wave.
  - It represents early repolarization of the ventricle
- T Wave follows the ST segment and represents ventricular repolarization
  - It is usually rounded and deflected in the same direction as the QRS.
  - A negative T-wave following a positive QRS is suggestive of ischemia

- Tall pointy (tented) T waves can mean hyperkalemia
- An electrical impulse during this time can lead to an "R on T" phenomenon, causing a lethal dysrhythmia.

How does the electrocardiogram work?

The ECG provides a graphic picture of the electrical waves of depolarization and repolarization. These waves are transmitted to the body surface and picked up by conductive gel within the electrode pads. It is transmitted to the ECG monitor via the leads.

- The Leads provide views of the heart, and the standard ECG has 12 leads (12 views). The lead is a graphic picture of electrical current flowing between a positive and negative electrode.
- Monitoring is usually in two leads.
  - Limb leads or precordial leads (V1-V6) These precordial leads go around the chest to view R waves
  - Lead I, II, III (bipolar leads look at the negative to positive. When you look at the upper right to the lower left (lead II), you will have a positive QRS deflection. We like lead II the best!
  - Modified chest lead
- Lead Names
  - Limb leads: Bipolar (I, II, III)
  - Precordial leads: Unipolar (V1-V6)
  - Augmented leads: Bipolar (aVf, aVl, aVr)
- Einthoven's Triangle is defined as an equilateral triangle whose vertices lie at the left and right shoulders and the pubic region, and whose center corresponds to the vector sum of all electric activity occurring in the heart at any given moment, allowing for the determination of the electrical axis. It is approximated by the triangle formed by the axes of the ECG limb leads I, II and III. The center of the triangle offers a reference point for the unipolar ECG leads.
- Lead Placement
  - White on right upper chest
  - Black on left upper chest
  - Brown at 5th ICS, right sternal border
  - Green at right hip
  - Red at left hip
  - An easy way to remember this is: White on right, smoke over fire, poop over grass.
  - Lead wires are often labeled RA, LA, MCL, LL, and RL.
  - Note that you will get a better picture over flat bone.

ECG Paper

Graph paper with little boxes and big boxes.

- Small squares = 0.04 seconds or 1 mm
- Large squares = 0.20 seconds or 5 mm
- 5 large squares = 1 second
- Horizontal axis measures time
- Verticle axis measures amplitude
- ECG monitors all record at a standard speed of 25 mm/sec
- You can speed up the flow of the paper through the machine if you are looking at a really fast rhythm...this will spread the rhythm out a bit so you can see the detail.

Interpreting ECG Strips

- Step 1: Look for regularity or irregularity.
- Step 2: Determine the heart rate
- Step 3: Look for P waves
- Step 4: Measure the PR interval
- Step 5: Examine QRS complex
- Step 6: Check out the T wave

Step 1: Look for regularity or irregularity

- Are the P-R intervals the same?

- Are things generally happening in a consistent manner?
- The faster the rhythm the more difficult to tell if it is irregular

Step 2: Determine the heart rate

- Easy way: count the complexes on a 6-second strip and multiply by 10. This is your heart rate.
- Math way: count the boxes between two consecutive R waves
  - Divide 300 by the number of boxes between R waves (i.e. 300 ÷ 6 = 50 bpm)

Step 3: Look for the P waves

- Are there P waves present?
- Are they consistent...do they fall in the same place relative to the QRS?
- Is there a P wave preceding every QRS?

Step 4: Measure the PR interval

- Normal is 0.12 - 0.20 seconds
- A PR interval of > 2.0 seconds indicates a delay across the AV node
- A PR interval of < 0.12 is considered questionable for conduction (not enough time for impulse to go from SA to AV)
- The PR interval should be consistent from beat to beat

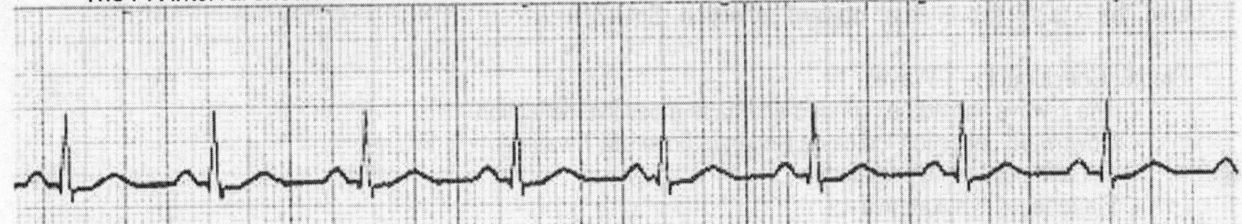

In the above EKG strip, it is REGULAR, the P waves are CONSISTENT, there is a QRS after every P. This is a normal sinus rhythm.

Step 5: Examine the QRS complex

- Determine the polarity (up or down). Both can be normal depending on the lead used.
- Is it a QRS, or just an RS?
- What is the width of the QRS? Should be , 0.12 or 3 little boxes. If it is wider this means there is a block in the Bundle of HIS or bundle branches
- Is it rSR' (RSR prime). This indicates a block somewhere along the bundle branches (looks kind of like an M)
- Is there a QRS following every P wave?

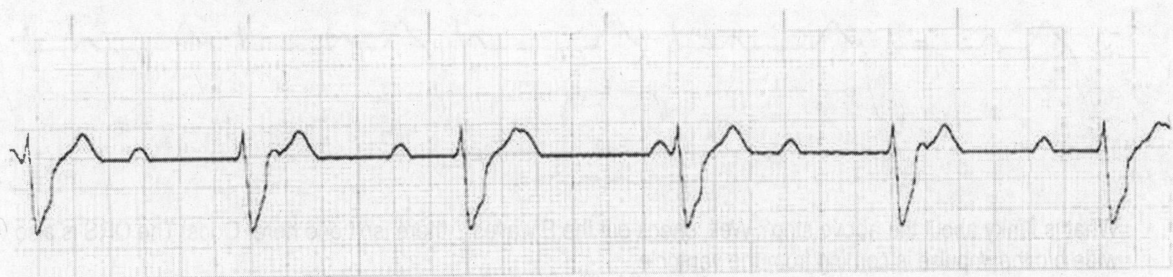

In the above example, the P waves are regular, the QRS are not coordinated, indicating that it is the Purkinje fibers firing. The SA node and the Purkinje fibers are each doing their own thing. The QRS is wide b/c the impulse has taken the side streets. This is called a 3rd Degree Block.

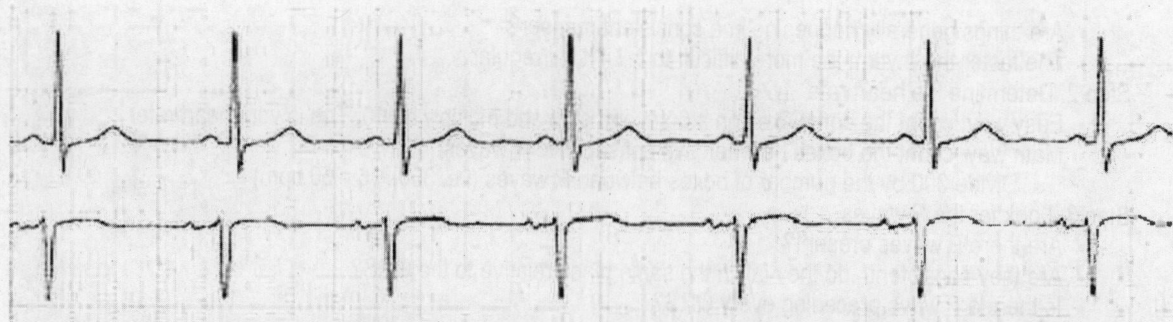

In the above graph, the top line is Lead II, the bottom line is MCL (brown lead). Notice that the QRS points down, this is normal for the MCL lead. See the QRS and that there is no Q (recall that the Q is the first downward deflection after the P wave. There is no downward deflection after the P, so no Q is present. This is OK! If that little upward deflection was not there, then the big downward deflection would actually be the FIRST downward deflection after the P, meaning it would be a GINORMOUS Q wave, which would be super-duper pathological. When looking at the MCL lead, the R is still shown as an upward deflection. Got it? :-)

Step 6: Check out the T-Wave

- The T-wave should be rounded and have a positive deflection
- Downward deflection indicates ischemia (inverted T wave)
- Tall and pointy = hyperkalemia
- Flattened = hypokalemia
- There's lots more than can be determined by the T wave, but we'll just start with that.

Ex: Right bundle branch block (see diagram to right). Remember the rSR' we mentioned earlier? See how it looks kind of like an M?
Also notice how the T wave is inverted? This is ischemia!

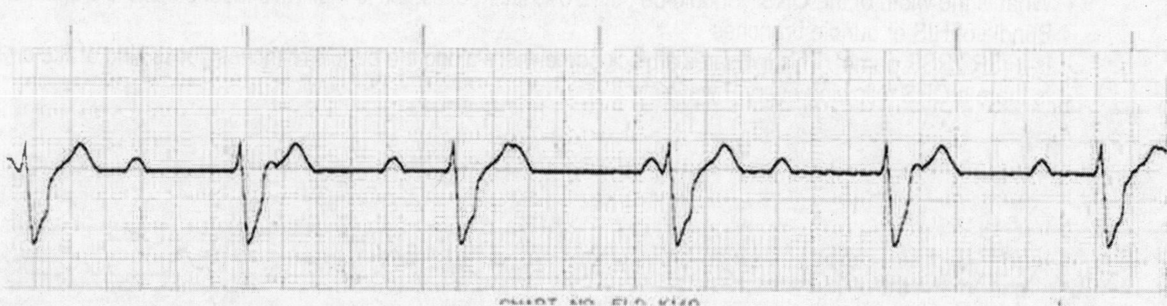

What is funky about the above strip? Well, check out the P waves....there isn't one here! Oops! The QRS is also very wide b/c the impulse is coming from the ventricle.

<u>Types of Rhythms</u>
Sinus rhythms are any rhythms that originate from the SA node.

- Rhythm is regular
- PR interval is normal (0.12 to 0.20 seconds)
- P wave precedes each QRS
- QRS follows each P wave
- QRS width is 0.08 to 0.12 seconds.

Sinus Tachycardia is a rate > 100 bpm. It is important to determine the reason for the tachycardia

- Fever
- Dehydration
- Anxiety or pain
- Hyperthyroid
- Hypoxia (keep this top of mind!)
- CHF
- Shock

Sinus Bradycardia is a rate < 60 bpm. It may or may not be symptomatic (an athlete could have a normal HR of 45)

- Assess these 4 things when you see a change in rhythm
  - Hypotension
  - Altered mental status
  - SOB, tachypnea
  - Chest pain

Sinus Arrhythmia is a variation of a NSR that is also called respiratory sinus arrhythmia.

- This is a normal finding in the young (20 year old)
- Occurs with respiration
- HR increases during inhalation and decreases during expiration
- It is cyclical with "regular irregularity" and is repetitive
- Strip to the right is one strip

Sick Sinus Syndrome is an abnormality of the sinus node (it's a little ischemic)

- Persistent sinus bradycardia
- Sinus arrests or pauses
- Combinations of SA and AV nodal conduction disturbances
- Alternating paroxysms of rapid atrial tachycardias
- Fast, slow, fast, slow
- Shown at right

<u>Sino-Atrial Dysrhythmias</u>

These are problems with transmission from the Sinus node to the AV node. This can occur b/c the impulse from the SA Node is not generated, or the impulse from the SA Node is not conducted. The causes are:

- Conditions that increase vagal tone (vaso-vagal episode: pt starts to pass out, but once they are no longer upright, it corrects itself...when you pass out, you fall down and this makes it "self limiting).
- Coronary artery disease
- Acute MI
- Digitalis and calcium channel blocker toxicity
- Hypertensive disease
- Tissue hypoxia
- Scarring of intra-atrial pathways
- Electrolyte imbalances
- Ischemia

<u>Atrial Dysrhythmias</u>

- Premature atrial contractions: causing an irregularity in rhythm, pretty benign and pretty common
- Paroxysmal atrial tachycardia (PAT): starts and stops abruptly, difficult to see P waves, common in mitral valve prolapse and people experiencing anxiety
- Atrial fibrillation: most common, there are no P waves, atrial rate is 350-700, ventricular rate varies (ventricular rate > 100 is "rapid ventricular response" aka "rapid atrial fib", affects 1-2% of general population, irregular irregularity
- Atrial flutter: saw tooth pattern

Blocks Across the AV Node

- First degree block has a prolonged PR interval (slows down SA conduction)
- Second degree block will block SOME impulses from SA).
    - The PR interval is inconsistent
    - No QRS following a P wave
- Third degree block will block ALL impulses and the ventricle does its own thing
    - No connection between P wave and QRS
    - Lethal rhythm

Ventricular Rhythms

- These are often VERY lethal
- Usually a disturbance in automaticity and excitability
- Premature ventricular contractions. These are more worrisome than AVC, especially if >6 x minute or 'R on T'. These may be prodromal (I suspect we'll learn what AVC is at some point?)
- Ventricular tachycardia (can be lethal)
- Ventricular fibrillation (always lethal)

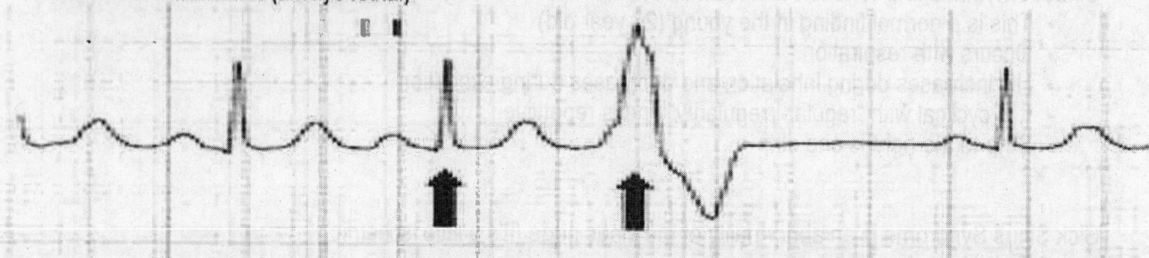

In this strip, you see that there is no P wave, the QRS is wide and "odd looking". This QRS with no P is a premature ventricular contraction...if you feel the pulse as this rhythm is going on, you won't feel this one...does not perfuse.

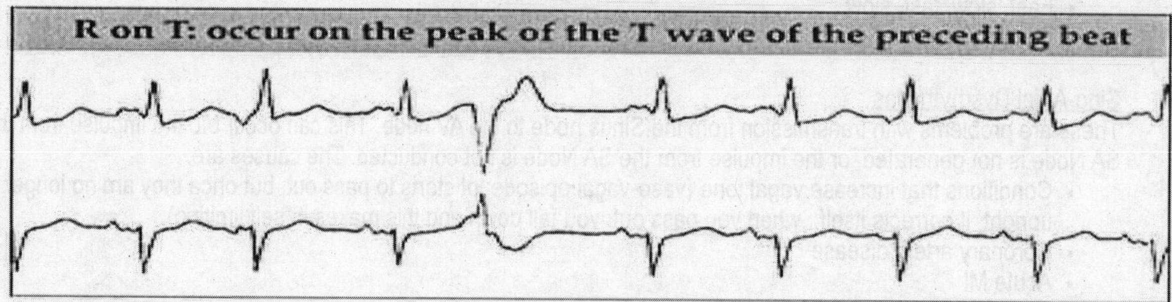

R on T: occur on the peak of the T wave of the preceding beat

The rhythm directly below is V-Tach...will probably lead to V-Fib. V-tach usually does not generate a blood pressure. Pt may lose consciousness and can be VERY symptomatic VERy quickly!
The rhythm directly above is V-Fib...pt will be non responsive with no pulse, cold and pale. This is LETHAL!

To end on a somber note...Sudden Cardiac Death occurs from an abrupt loss of heart function and pt may not even have coronary artery disease...more than 163,000 deaths annually!

- MYOCARDIAL INFARCTION (MI) -

- CORONARY OCCLUSION -

- HEART ATTACK -

- Pain:
  - Sudden Onset
  - Substernal
  - Crushing
  - Tightness
  - Severe
  - Unrelieved by Nitro
  - May Radiate To: Back, Neck, Jaw, Shoulder, Arm
- Dyspnea
- Syncope (↓ BP)
- Nausea
- Vomiting
- Extreme Weakness
- Diaphoresis
- Denial is Common
- ↑ HR

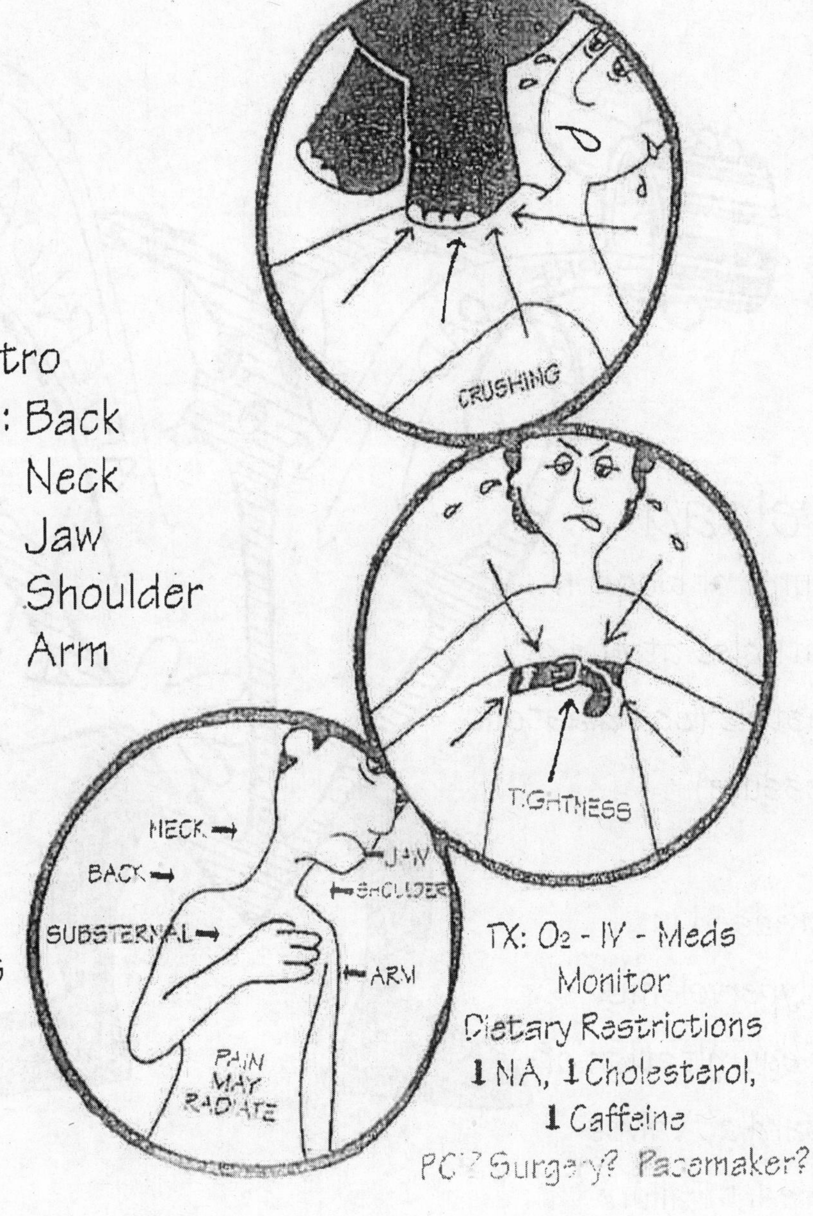

TX: O_2 - IV - Meds
Monitor
Dietary Restrictions
↓ NA, ↓ Cholesterol,
↓ Caffeine
PCI? Surgery? Pacemaker?

PRELOAD AND AFTERLOAD

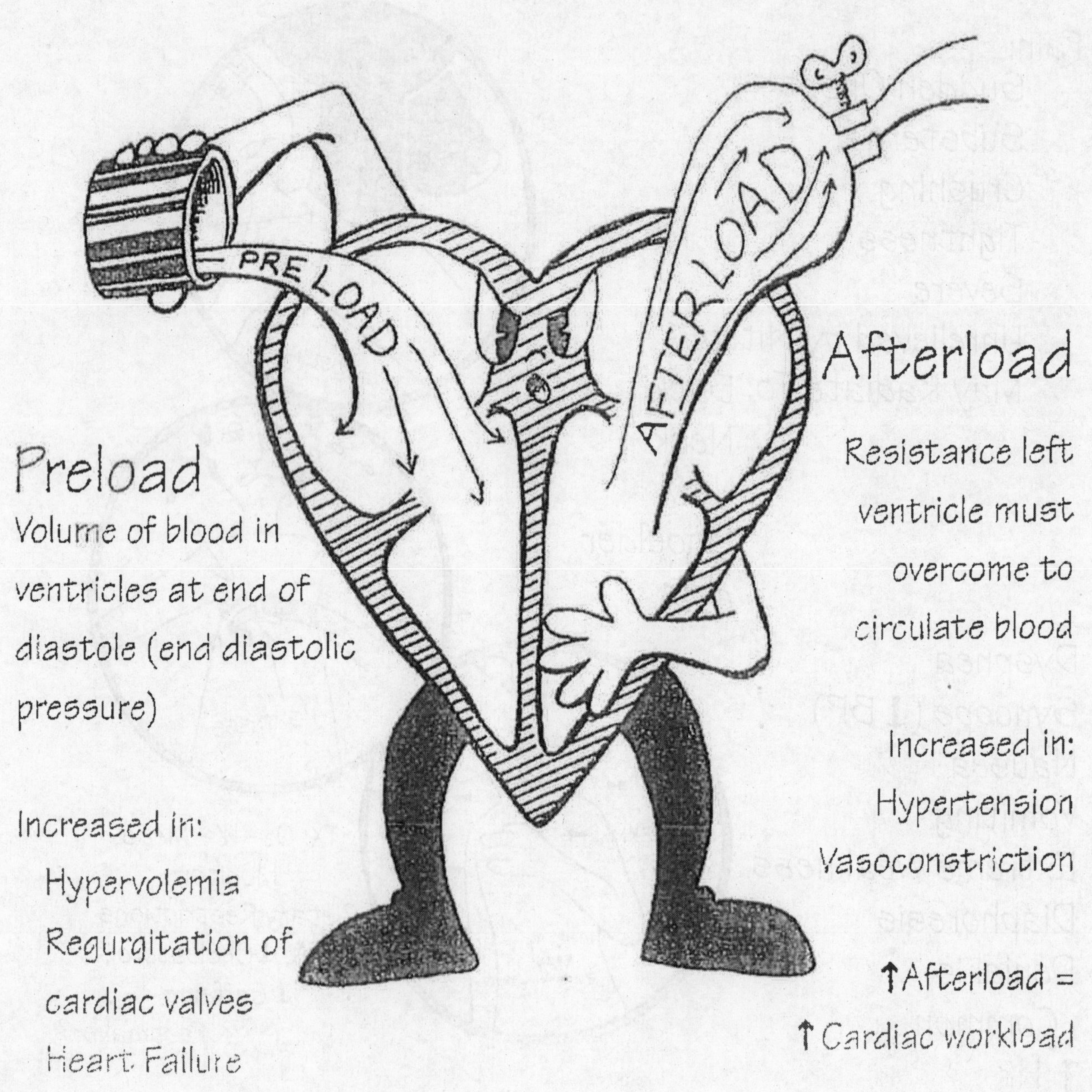

PRELOAD
AFTERLOAD
Preload
Volume of blood in ventricles at end of diastole (end diastolic pressure)
Increased in:
Hypervolemia
Regurgitation of cardiac valves
Heart Failure
Afterload
Resistance left ventricle must overcome to circulate blood
Increased in:
Hypertension
Vasoconstriction
↑Afterload =
↑ Cardiac workload

AUSCULATING HEART SOUNDS

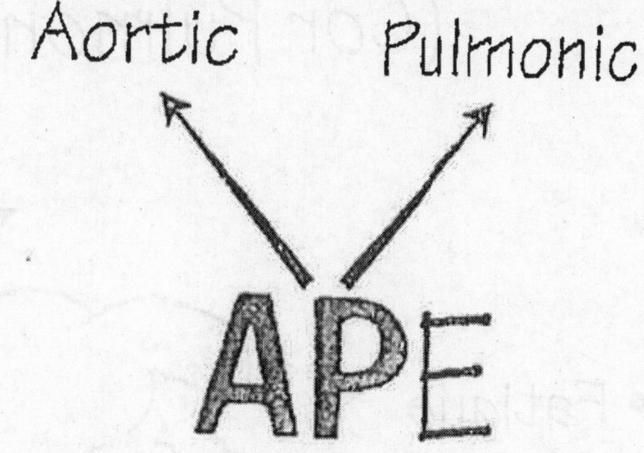

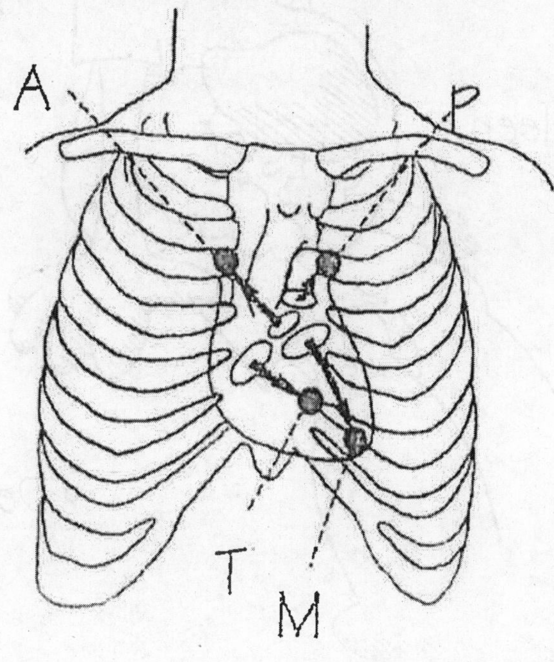

RIGHT SIDED ♥ FAILURE

(Cor Pulmonale)

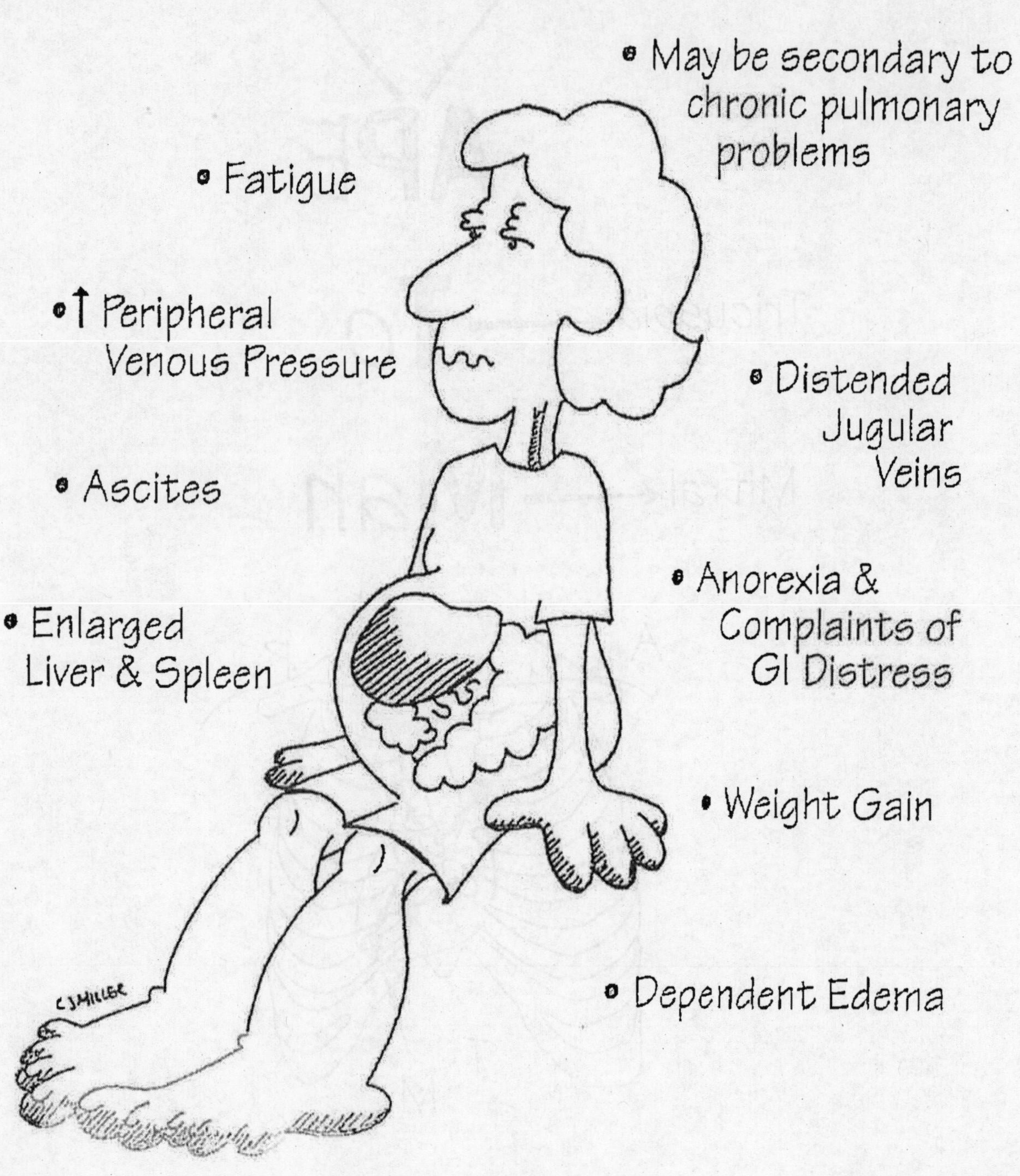

LEFT SIDED ♥ FAILURE

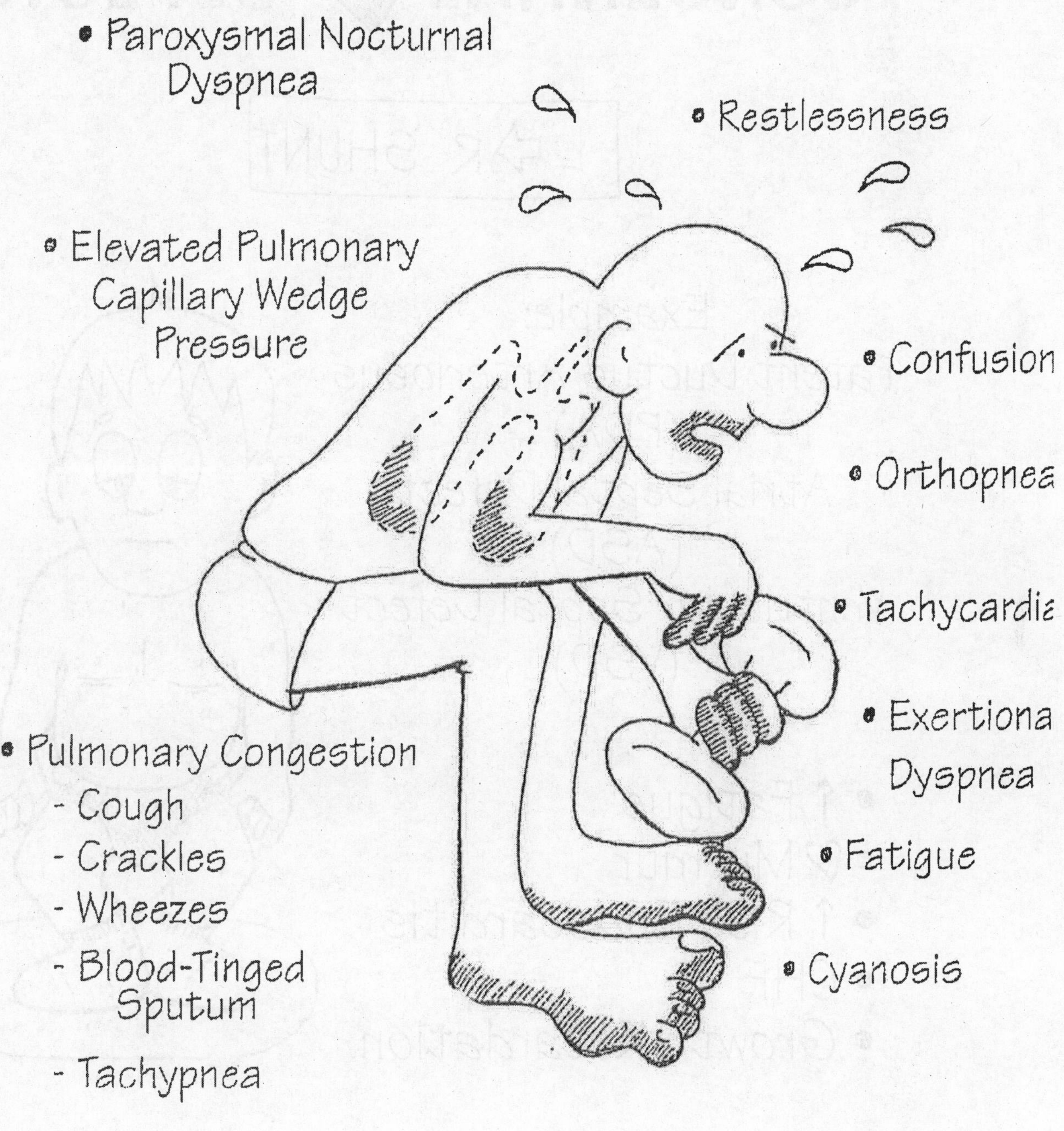
• Paroxysmal Nocturnal Dyspnea
• Restlessness
• Elevated Pulmonary Capillary Wedge Pressure
• Confusion
• Orthopnea
• Tachycardi
• Exertiona Dyspnea
• Pulmonary Congestion
- Cough
- Crackles
- Wheezes
- Blood-Tinged Sputum
- Tachypnea
• Fatigue
• Cyanosis

ACYANOTIC CONGENITAL ♥ DEFECTS

L ⇨ R SHUNT

Example:
Patent Ductus Arteriosus (PDA)
Atrial Septal Defect (ASD)
Ventricular Septal Defect (VSD)

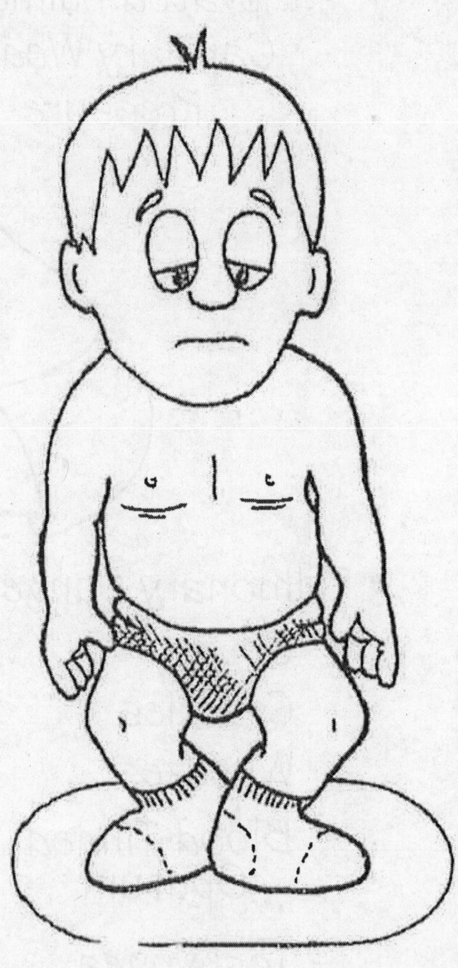

- ↑ Fatigue
- ♡ Murmur
- ↑ Risk Endocarditis
- CHF
- Growth Retardation

CONGENITAL ♥ DEFECT SYMPTOMS

- ♥ ↑ Pulse
- ♥ ↑ Respirations
- ♥ Retarded Growth
- ♥ Dyspnea, Orthopnea
- ♥ Fatigue
- 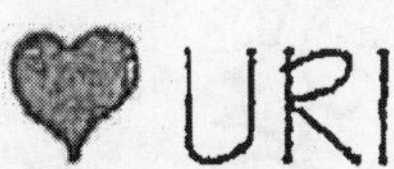 URI

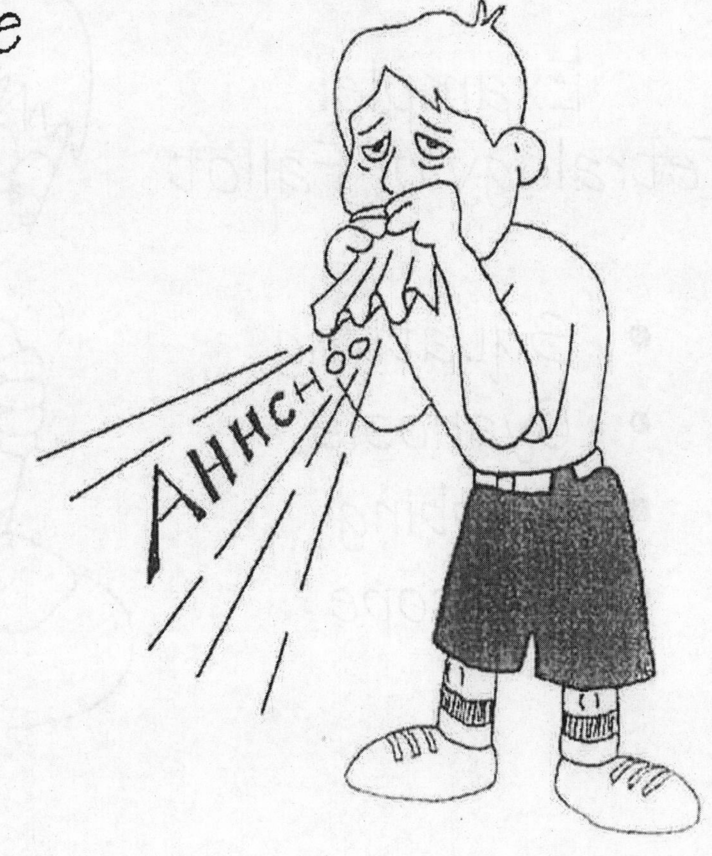

Cyanotic Congenital ♥ Defects

R ⇨ L SHUNT

Example:
Tetralogy of Fallot

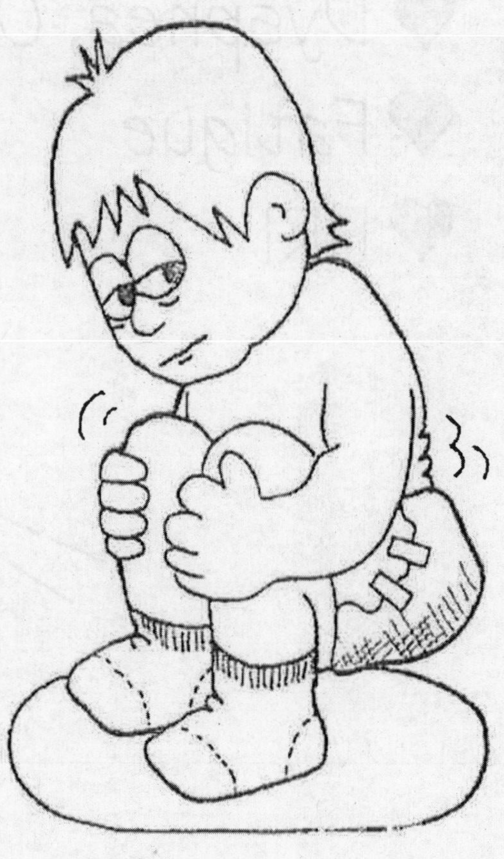

- Squatting
- Cyanosis
- Clubbing
- Syncope

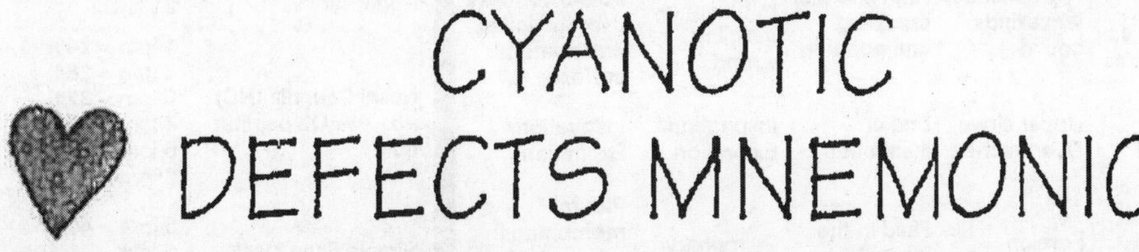

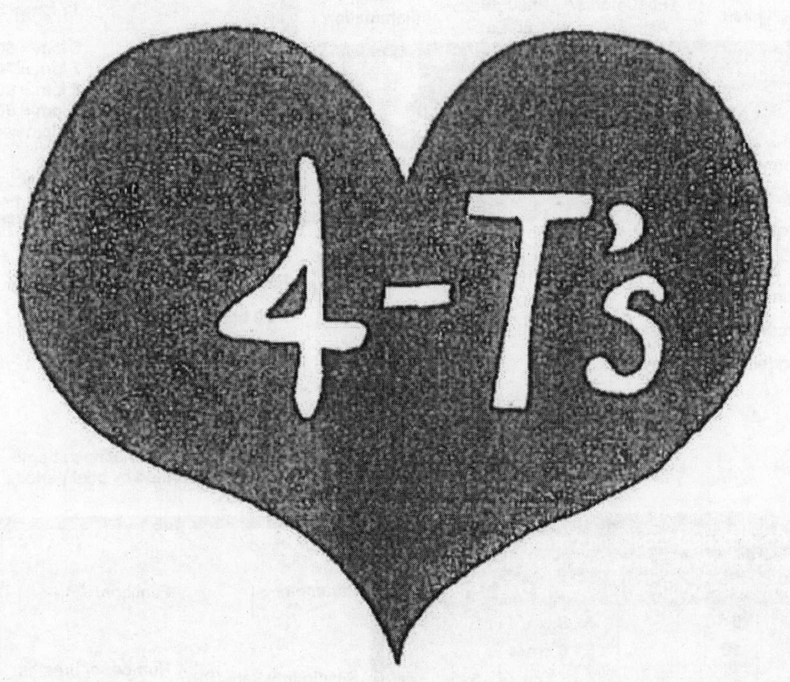

- Tetralogy of Fallot
- Truncus Arteriosus
- Transposition of The Great Vessels
- Tricuspid Atresia

RESPIRATORY

Lung Sounds

Clinical Assessment	Rales	Rhonchi	Wheezing	Stridor	Fine Crackles	Coarse Crackles	Pleural rub
What you hear	Crackles	Coarse rattling sound	Air trying to pass through the bronchioles	High-pitched, wheezing sound	High pitched crackling and popping	Low pitched, bubbling or gurgling sound	Rubbing sound, loudest over the lower anterolateral surface
Where or When	Smaller airways	Medium size airways	Effects Bronchi	Upper airway Over trachea	End of inspiration	Inspiration/ Expiration	Inspiration/ Expiration
Cause of noise	Fluid in alveoli	Obstruction or fluid accumulation in the larger airways	Constriction	Foreign airway obstruction	Fluid in the lungs/Not cleared by cough	Pulmonary Edema/ Fibrosis	Pleural membranes rub against each other/ Not cleared by cough
Commonly heard	CHF/ Pneumonia	COPD/ Pneumonia/ CHF	Asthma/ Bronchitis	Croup in children	CHF/ Pneumonia/ Asthma	CHF/ Pneumonia/ Asthma	Pleural inflammation

Ventilator Alarm Checklist

Paw High (High airway pressure)	Paw Low (Low airway pressure)
☐ Air-trapping	☐ Chest wounds/drains allowing air to escape
☐ Bronchospasm	☐ Disconnect from the circuit
☐ Mucous plug	☐ Esophageal intubation
☐ PEEP set too high	☐ ETT cuff delated
☐ Pmax set too low	☐ Tidal Volume (VT) set too low
☐ Pneumothorax	☐ Loose circuit/tubing connections
☐ PT coughing/biting/gagging	☐ Water condensation in the circuit
☐ PT-Ventilator dyssynchrony	
☐ Tube in R main bronchus	
☐ Pooling of condensation	
☐ Wet filter increasing resistance	

Hierarchy of O2 Delivery

Exact FiO2 will be based on the patient's anatomic reservoir and minute ve

Method of delivery	% O2 delivered	Recommendation Considerations
Room Air	21% O2	Sat 90-100%
Nasal Cannula (NC) ~3 - 4% O2 per liter flow	1 lpm = 24% 2 lpm = 28% 3 lpm = 32% 4 lpm = 36% 5 lpm = 40% 6 lpm = 44%	1-6 lpm via NC FiO2 0.24-0.44 FiO2 decreases a Ve increases
Simple Face Mask ~3- 4% O2 per liter flow	5 lpm = 40% 6 lpm = 45-50% 7 lpm = 50-55% 8 lpm = 55-60%	5-8 lpm FiO2 0.35-0.55 Minimum flow 5 l to flush CO2 fron mask
Venturi Mask	4 lpm = 24-28% 8 lpm = 35-40% 12 lpm = 50%	Variable lpm Flow and FiO2 va manufacture
Non-rebreather	6 lpm = 60% 7 lpm = 70% 8 lpm = 80% 9 lpm = 90% 10 lpm = ~100%	6-10 lpm FiO2 0.6 - 1 Flow must be suf to keep reservoir from deflating up inspiration
Trach Collar	21-70% @ 10 lpm	Ensure humidific is in place

Breathing Patterns

Normal (eupnea)	Regular rate and rhythm 12-20 bpm
Tachypnea	> 20 bpm
Bradypnea	< 12 bpm
Kussmaul's	Raid, deep, and labored – Common in DKA
Cheyne-Stokes	Neurological – alternating patterns of depth separated by brief periods of apnea

Approximate Size and Depth for Placement of Endotracheal Tubes and Central Venous Lines

Ages 1-10 yrs Uncuffed ETT size (mm) = (age in years/4) + 4 - Cuffed ETT size (mm) = (age in years/4) + 3

Age	Uncuffed ETT mm	Cuffed ETT mm	Initial Depth cm	Central Line length/size
Newborn	3 - 3.5	3	9-10	5 - 8 cm/4 Fr
1-5 mons	3.5	3 - 3.5	10	5 - 8 cm/4 Fr
6-11 mons	3.5 - 4	3.5	11	8 - 12 cm/4 - 5 Fr
1 yr	4 - 4.5	4	12	8 - 12 cm/4 - 5 Fr
2-3 yrs	4.5 - 5	4 - 4.5	12-13	8 - 12 cm/4 - 5 Fr
4-5 yrs	5 - 5.5	4.5 - 5	13-15	8 - 12 cm/5.5 - 6 Fr
6-9 yrs	5.5 - 6	5 - 5.5	15	8 - 12 cm/5.5 - 6 Fr
10-12 yrs	6.5 - 7	6 - 6.5	17	12 - 15 cm/6 + Fr
13+ yrs	7 - 7.5	6.5 - 7	19	12 - 15 cm/6 + Fr

Modes of Mechanical Ventilation

Modes	Types of Breaths	Independent Variable	Dependent Variable	Notes
Volume Assist/ Control	Assisted or Controlled	Preset Tidal Volume	PIP & Plateau Pressures	Control tidal volume (protect the lungs) Control minute ventilation (RR & Vt)
Pressure Assist Control	Assisted or Controlled	Preset Pressure	Adequate Tidal Volumes (not too high or low)	Patient comfort (decelerating flow). Control over delivered pressures (avoid barotrauma)
Pressure Support (PS)	Supported	Preset Pressure	Adequate Tidal Volumes (not too high or low)	Patient comfort Allows patient to maintain respiratory work effort
Synchronized Intermittent Mandatory Ventilation (SIMV) + PS	Assisted, Controlled or Supported	PC - SIMV=Preset Pressure VC - SIMV=Preset Tidal Volume	PC-SIMV=Adequate Tidal Volumes (not too high or low) VC-SIMV=PIP & Plateau Pressures	Can get benefits of supported breaths (PS), but still ensure minimum number of mandatory breaths (controlled or assisted)
Pressure Regulated Volume Control (PRVC)	Assisted or Controlled	Preset Tidal Volume	PIP & Plateau Pressures	Control Minute Ventilation Control Vt. Patient comfort (decelerating flow). Can limit high pressures (avoid barotrauma)

Ventilator Management

Parameter	Function	Usual Parameters
Respiratory Rate (RR)	Number of breaths delivered per min	Normal Lungs: 12 - 14 bpm ARDS/ALI: 12 - 14 bpm Asthma/COPD: 8 - 12 bpm Head Injury: 14 - 16 bpm Metabolic Acidosis: 20 - 30 b Severe Obesity: 12 - 14 bpm
Tidal Volume (VT)	- Volume of gas delivered during each breath - Measured in ml/kg based on IBW (ideal body weight)	Normal Lungs: 8 ml/kg ARDS: 6 ml/kg ALI: Monitor Closely Asthma/COPD: 5 - 8 ml/kg Head Injury: 6 - 8 ml/kg Metabolic Acidosis: 8 - 10 m Severe Obesity: 8-10 ml/kg
FiO2	Amount of O2 delivered	21%-100% to keep SaO2 > or pO2>70. Avoid hyperoxia
I:E ratio	Ratio length of inspiration compared to length of expiration	Normal Lungs: 1:2 ARDS: 2:1 ALI: 2 - 4:1 Asthma/COPD: 1:4 - 1:5 Head Injury: 1:2 Metabolic Acidosis: 1:1 - 1:2 Severe Obesity: 1:1-2:1
PEEP (cm H2O)	PEEP increases the volume of gas remaining in the lungs at the end of expiration in order to decrease the shunting of blood through the lungs and improve gas exchange	Normal Lungs: 5 ARDS/ALI: 10 - 15 Asthma: 0 COPD: 5 Head Injury: 5 Metabolic Acidosis: 5 Severe Obesity: 10 - 15
Position	Ensure your patient's HOB is elevated to decrease risk of VAP	30 - 40° unless reduced cere perfusion or hypotension is a concern

Assessing Lung Sounds

(3) Normal Breath Sounds

Bronchial breath sounds: *loud, harsh and high pitched.* Heard over the trachea, bronchi—between clavicles and midsternum, and over main bronchus.

Bronchovesicular breath sounds: *blowing sounds, moderate intensity and pitch* Heard over large airways, either side of sternum, at the Angle of Louis, and between scapulae.

Vesicular breath sounds: *soft breezy quality, low pitched.* Heard over the peripheral lung area, heard best at the base of the lungs.

ADVENTITIOUS LUNG SOUNDS

Sound	Characteristics	Lung Problem
Crackles	Popping, crackling, bubbling, moist sounds on inspiration	Pneumonia, pulmonary edema, pulmonary fibrosis
Rhonchi	Rumbling sound on expiration	Pneumonia, emphysema, bronchitis, bronchiectasis
Wheezes	High-pitched musical sound during both inspiration and expiration (louder)	Emphysema, asthma, foreign bodies
Pleural Friction Rub	Dry, grating sound on both inspiration and expiration	Pleurisy, pneumonia, pleural infarct

Assessing Heart Sounds

These tones are produced by the closing of valves and are best heard over 5 points:

1.) Second intercostals space along the right sternal boarder. AORTIC AREA

2.) Second intercostals space at the left sternal boarder. PULMONIC AREA

3.) Third intercostals space at the left sternal boarder ERB'S POINT

4.) Fifth intercostals space along the left sternal boarder. TRICUSPID AREA

5.) Fifth intercostals space, midclavicular line MITRAL AREA—APEX

This is where the Point of Maximal Impulse (PMI) is found—document location (note: with enlarged hearts mitral area may present at anterior axillary line)

S_1 ("lub") the start of cardiac contraction called systole. Mitral and tricuspid valves are closing and vibration of the ventricle walls due to increased pressure.

S_2 ("dub") end of ventricular systole and beginning of diastole. Aortic and pulmonic valves close.

S_3 ("Kentucky") a ventricular gallop heard after S_2. Normal in children and young adults, pregnancy, and highly trained athletes. In older adults it is heard in heart failure. Use bell of stethoscope and have pt in the left lateral position.

S_4 ("Tennessee") atrial diastolic gallop. Resistance to ventricular filling and heard before S_1. Heard in HTN and left ventricular hypertrophy. Listen at apex in left lateral position.

Grading Murmurs

Grade I	Faint; heard with concentration
Grade II	Faint murmur heard immediately
Grade III	Moderately loud, not associated with thrill
Grade IV	Loud and may be associated with a thrill
Grade V	Very loud; associated with a thrill
Grade VI	Very loud; heard w/stethoscope off chest, associate w/a thrill

EDEMA: Assess by placing thumb over dorsum of the foot or tibia for 5 seconds	
0	No edema
1+	Barely discernible depression
2+	A deeper depression (< 5 mm) w/ normal foot & leg contours
3+	Deep depression (5-10 mm) w/ foot & leg swelling
4+	Deeper depression (> 1 cm) w/ severe foot and leg swelling

Normal B/P for all <120/<80; Prehypertension 120-139/80-89

Guidelines and education site for adult B/P.

http://www.nhlbi.nih.gov/hbp/index.html

For children & adolescents:

http://www.nhlbi.nih.gov/health/prof/heart/hbp/hbp_ped.htm

Routine & Advanced Techniques Respiratory		Normal	Common Abnormal
Inspection	*General Appearance, posture and breathing effort*	Re.axed appearance and posture, breathing effortless	Apprehension, restlessness, nasal flaring, intercostal retractions, accessory muscle use, "tripod position",
	Respirations-rate, pattern and chest expansion	Rate 12-20 breaths/min, smooth effort, even respiratory depth, rise and fall symmetrical	Respiratory rate less than 12 and greater than 20 bpm, retractions, frequent sighing
	Inspect nails, lips and skin color	Nail beds pink, skin tone consistent with ethnic background, lips pink	Cyanosis or pallor
	Inspect the posterior thorax for shape & symmetry	Ribs slope approx. 45dgrees, thorax symmetric AP:transverse diameter 1:2	Asymmetry Barrel chest
Palpation	*Palpate posterior thorax wall for masses, bulges or tenderness*	No masses, bulges or tenderness	Mass palpated, tender to palpation
	Palpate for thorax expansion	Expansion symmetrical bilaterally	Unequal chest expansion
	Palpate posterior thorax for tactile fremitus-"ninety-nine"	Vibrations felt equally bilaterally	Unequal vibrations felt on side to side comparison, Absent vibrations
Percussion	*Percuss (Greek key pattern) posterior and lateral thorax for tone*	Resonance heard throughout	Hyperresonance, flat or dull tones
	Percuss posterior thorax for diaphragmatic excursion	Excursion should be equal bilaterally	Decreased excursion
Auscultation	*Auscultation of posterior and lateral thorax*	Clear sounds bilaterally	Adventitious sounds-wheezes, crackles, rhonchi
	Auscultation of anterior thorax (will not be doing as part of the lab)	Clear sounds bilaterally	Adventitious sounds-wheezes, crackles, rhonchi
	Auscultation of voice sounds *Egophony-"eeee"* *Bronchophony-"Ninety-Nine" or "1-2-3"* *Whispered Pectoriloquy-"1-2-3"*	Egophony-eee tones muffled Bronchophony-sounds muffled Whispered Pectoriloquy-whispered sounds are muffled	Eee tone changes to an aaaa tone Clear sounds Loud and clear

HIERARCHY OF O2 DELIVERY SYSTEMS

METHOD

Nasal Cannula

1 lpm = 24% | 4 lpm = 36%
2 lpm = 28% | 5 lpm = 40%
3 lpm = 32% | 6 lpm = 44%

Simple Face Mask

5 lpm = 40% | 7 lpm = 50-55%
6 lpm = 45-50% | 8 lpm = 55-60%

Non-rebreather Mask

6 lpm = 60% | 9 lpm = 90%
7 lpm = 70% | 10 lpm = close to 100%
8 lpm = 80%

Venturi Mask

4 lpm = 24-28%
8 lpm = 35-40%
12 lpm = 50%

Trach Collar

21-70% at 10L

T-Piece

21-100% with flow rate at 2.5 times minute ventilation

CPAP

Positive airway pressure during spontaneous breaths

Bi-PAP

Positive pressure during spontaneous breaths and preset pressure to be maintained during expiration

SIMV

Preset Vt and f. Circuit remains open between mandatory breaths so pt can take additional breaths. Ventilator doesn't cycle during spontaneous breaths so Vt varies. Mandatory breaths synchronized so they do not occur during spontaneous breaths.

Assist Control

Preset Vt and f and inspiratory effort required to assist spontaneous breaths. Delivers control breaths. Cycles additionally if pt inspiratory effort is adequate. Same Vt delivered for spontaneous breaths.

Terms to Know:

Pressure support:
Preset inspiratory support level. When the pt initiates a breath, this positive pressure flows to assist the pts spontaneous breaths.

PEEP (positive end-expiatory pressure):
Maintenance of pressure above atmospheric at end expiration.

Auto-PEEP:
Trapping of gas in the lung caused by insufficient expiatory time (breath stacking). Increases risk of barotrauma.

PIP (peak inspiratory pressure):
Airway pressure at the peak of inspiration.

Minute ventilation (Ve):
Vt X f; volume of air expired per minute.

PaCO2 (35-45 mm Hg):
Amount of CO2 dissolved in arterial blood. Partial pressure of arterial CO2.

SaO2 (95-100%):
Percentage of oxygenated hemoglobin in arterial blood. Indirectly measured via SpO2 (pulse ox).

PaO2 (80-100 mm Hg):
Amount of oxygen dissolved in blood plasma.

EMPHYSEMA

"PINK PUFFER"

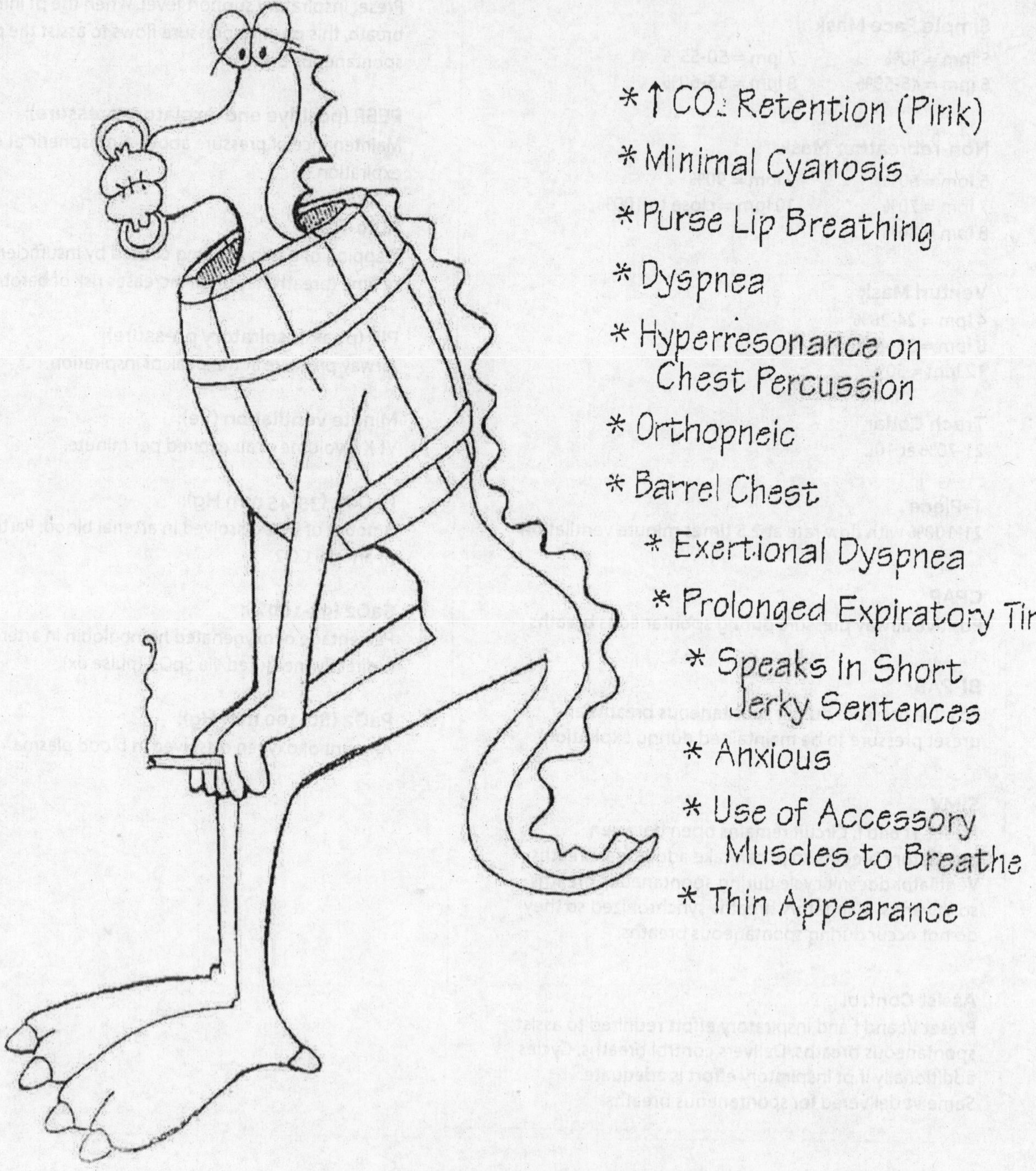
* ↑ CO_2 Retention (Pink)
* Minimal Cyanosis
* Purse Lip Breathing
* Dyspnea
* Hyperresonance on Chest Percussion
* Orthopneic
* Barrel Chest
* Exertional Dyspnea
* Prolonged Expiratory Ti
* Speaks in Short Jerky Sentences
* Anxious
* Use of Accessory Muscles to Breathe
* Thin Appearance

COPD

CHRONIC AIRFLOW LIMITATION

"EMPHYSEMA AND CHRONIC BRONCHITIS"

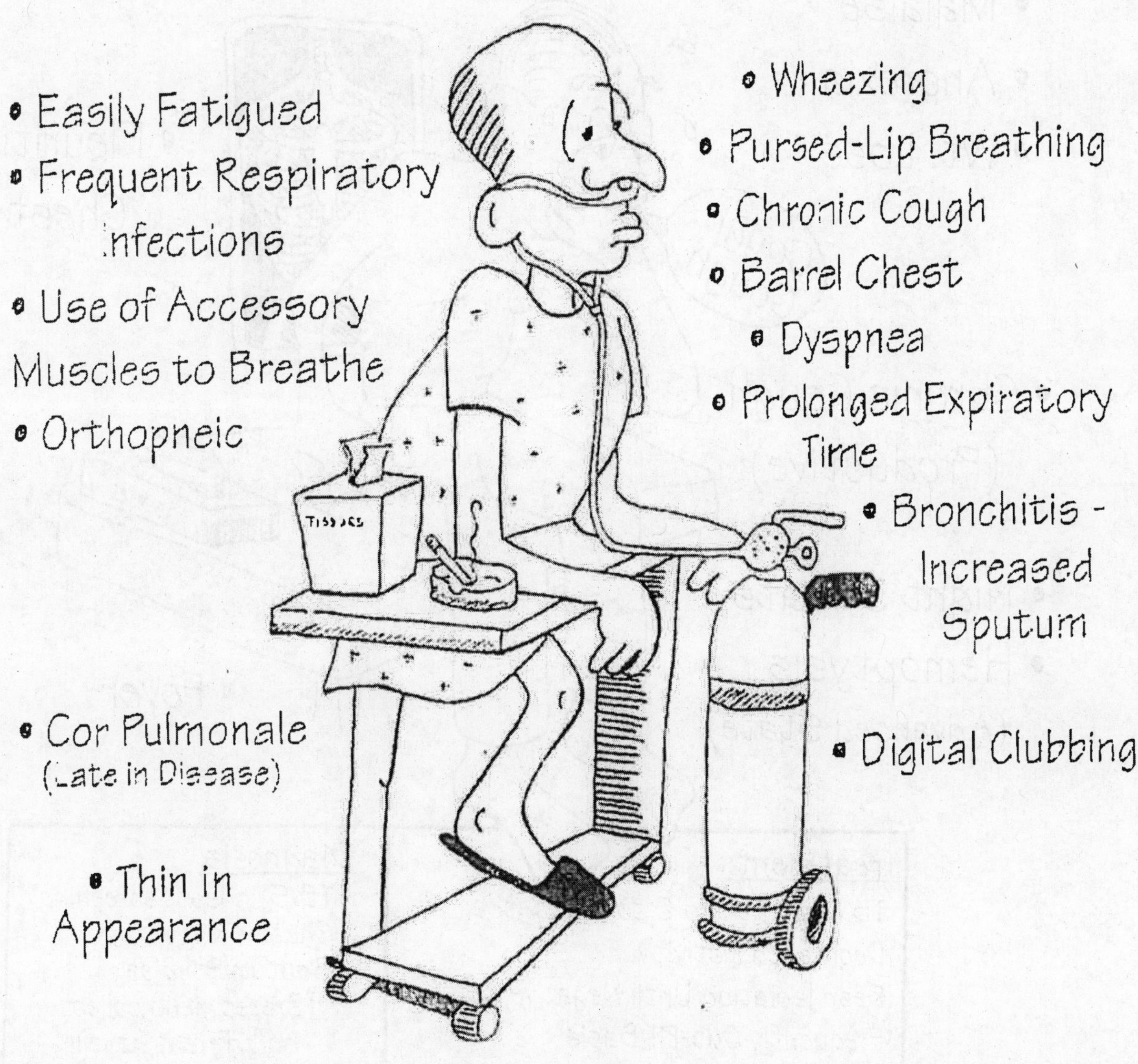

TUBERCULOSIS (TB)

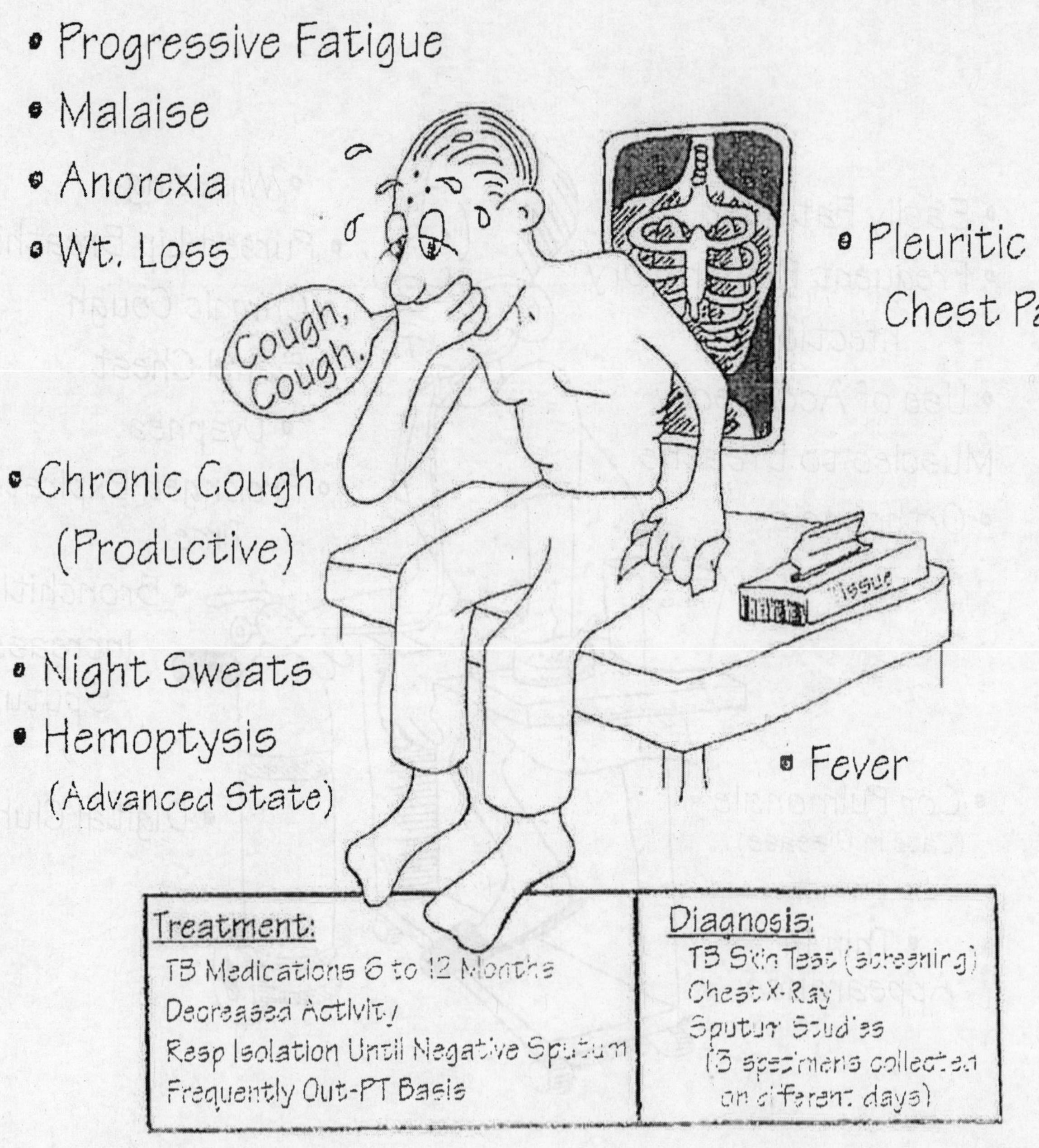
• Progressive Fatigue
• Malaise
• Anorexia
• Wt. Loss
Cough, Cough.
• Pleuritic Chest Pain
• Chronic Cough (Productive)
Tissue
• Night Sweats
• Hemoptysis (Advanced State)
• Fever
Treatment:
TB Medications 6 to 12 Months
Decreased Activity
Resp Isolation Until Negative Sputum
Frequently Out-PT Basis
Diagnosis:
TB Skin Test (screening)
Chest X-Ray
Sputum Studies
(3 specimens collected on different days)

ACUTE LARYNGOTRACHEOBRONCHITIS

LTB (Croup)

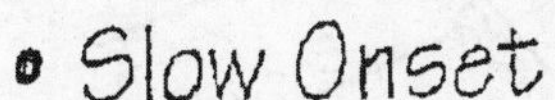

- Slow Onset
- Barking Cough
- "Crowing Sounds"

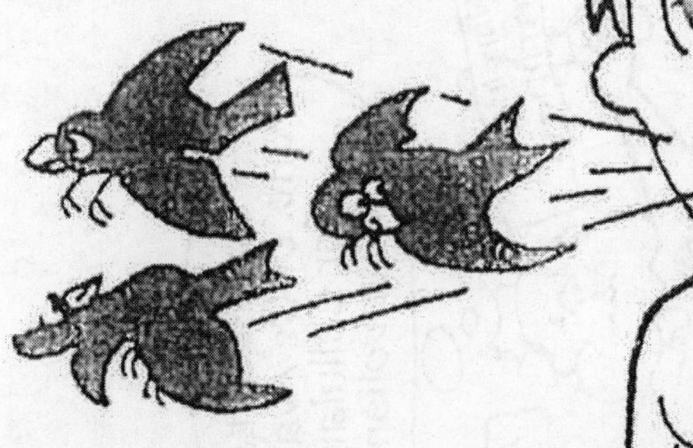

- Inspiratory Stridor
- Occurs at Night in Fall and Winter
- May Progress to Hypoxic State
- May Have Slight Temperature (<102°)

- Commonly Occurs Age 3 Months to 3 Years
- U.R.I.'s Frequently Precede LTB
- Restlessness
- Supra-sternal Retractions
- ↑Respiratory Rate

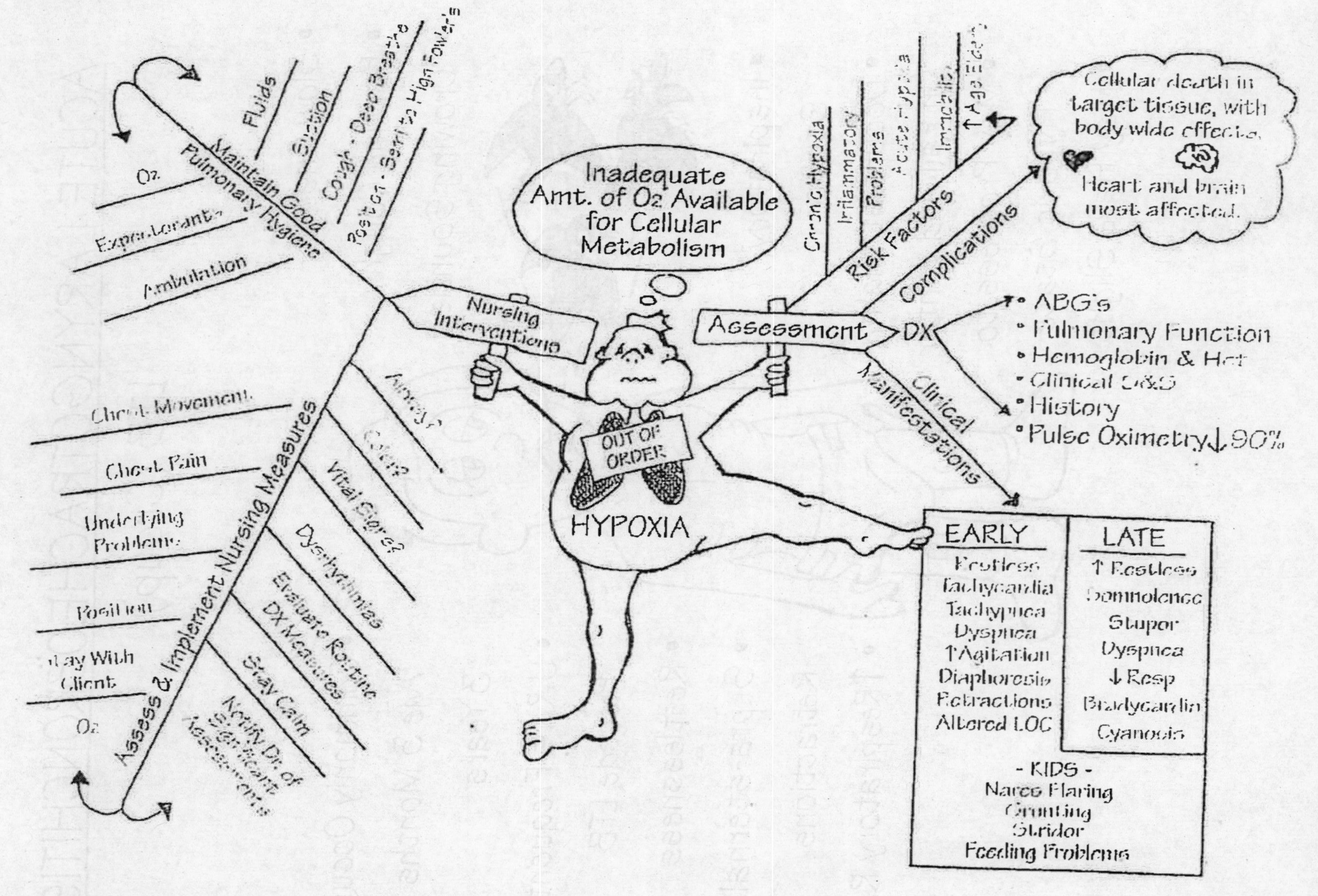

Inadequate Amt. of O_2 Available for Cellular Metabolism
HYPOXIA
OUT OF ORDER
Nursing Interventions
Maintain Good Pulmonary Hygiene
Fluids
Suction
Cough - Deep Breathe
Position - Semi to High Fowler's
O_2
Expectorants
Ambulation
Assess & Implement Nursing Measures
Chest Movement
Chest Pain
Underlying Problems
Position
Stay With Client
O_2
Colors
Vital Signs
Dysrhythmias
Evaluate Routine DX Measures
Stay Calm
Notify Dr. of Significant Assessments
Assessment
Risk Factors
Chronic Hypoxia
Inflammatory Problems
Acute Hypoxia
Immobility
↑ Age Elderly
Complications
Cellular death in target tissue, with body wide effects.
Heart and brain most affected.
DX
• ABG's
• Pulmonary Function
• Hemoglobin & Hct
• History
• Pulse Oximetry ↓ 90%
Clinical Manifestations
EARLY
Restless
Tachycardia
Tachypnea
Dyspnea
↑ Agitation
Diaphoresis
Retractions
Altered LOC
LATE
↑ Restless
Somnolence
Stupor
Dyspnea
↓ Resp
Bradycardia
Cyanosis
- KIDS -
Nares Flaring
Grunting
Stridor
Feeding Problems

CHRONIC BRONCHITIS

"BLUE BLOATER"

* Color Dusky to Cyanotic
* Recurrent Cough & $\uparrow$ Sputum Production
* Hypoxia
* Hypercapnia ($\uparrow pCO_2$)
* Respiratory Acidosis
* $\uparrow$ Hbg
* $\uparrow$ Resp Rate
* Exertional Dyspnea
* $\uparrow$ Incidence in Heavy Cigarette Smokers
* Digital Clubbing

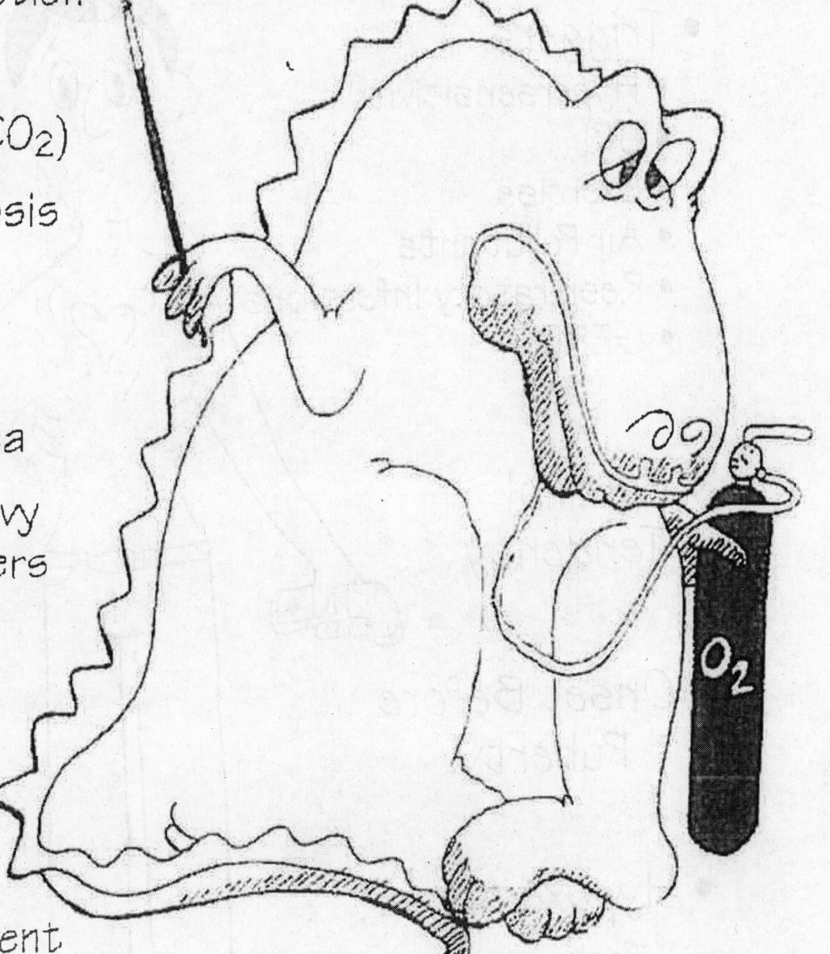

* Cardiac Enlargement
* Use of Accessory Muscles to Breathe
* Leads to Right-Sided Failure

ASTHMA

(Reactive Airway Disease)

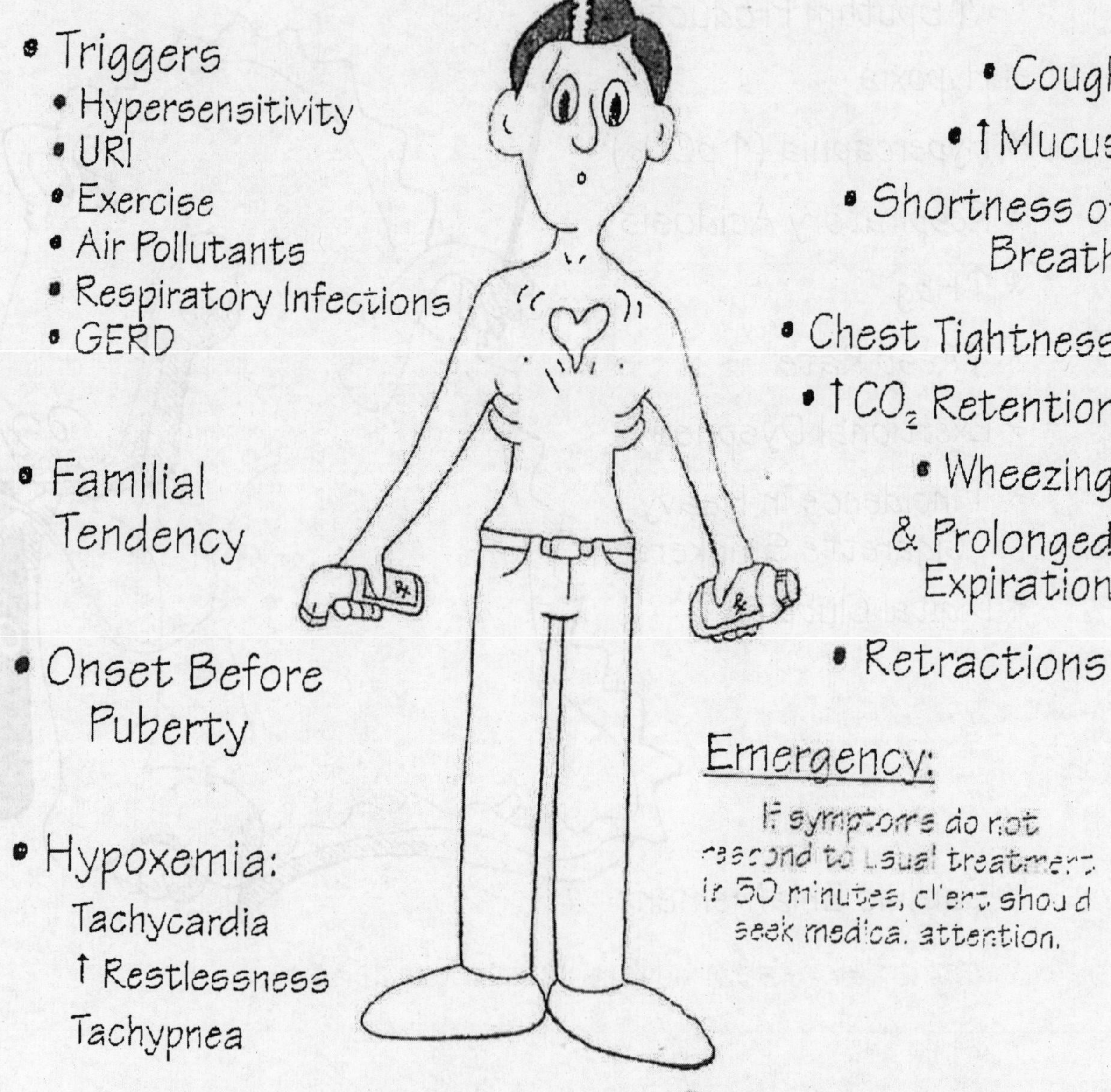

Status Asthmaticus

Can be life threatening!

ACUTE LARYNGOTRACHEOBRONCHITIS

LTB (Croup)

- Slow Onset
- Barking Cough
- "Crowing Sounds"

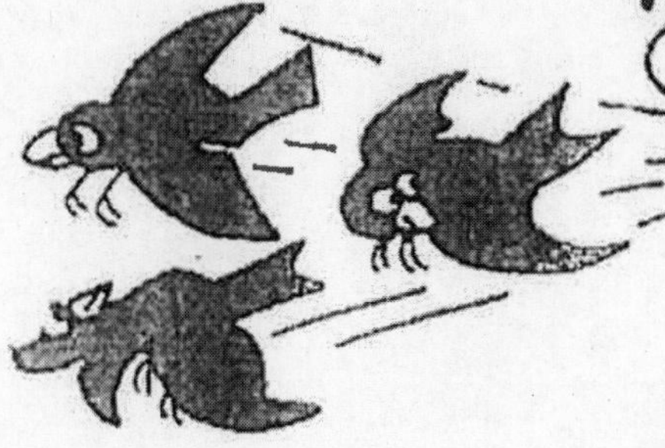

- Inspiratory Stridor
- Occurs at Night in Fall and Winter
- May Progress to Hypoxic State
- May Have Slight Temperature (<102°)

- Commonly Occurs Age 3 Months to 3 Years
- U.R.I.'s Frequently Precede LTB
- Restlessness
- Supra-sternal Retractions
- ↑Respiratory Rate

PULMONARY EDEMA

M Meds → Nipride, Morphine
A Airway
D Digitalis

D Diuretics (Lasix)
O Oxygen
G Blood Gases (ABG's)

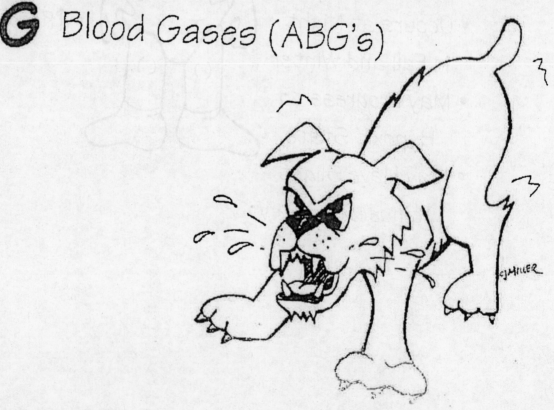

Sleep Apnea

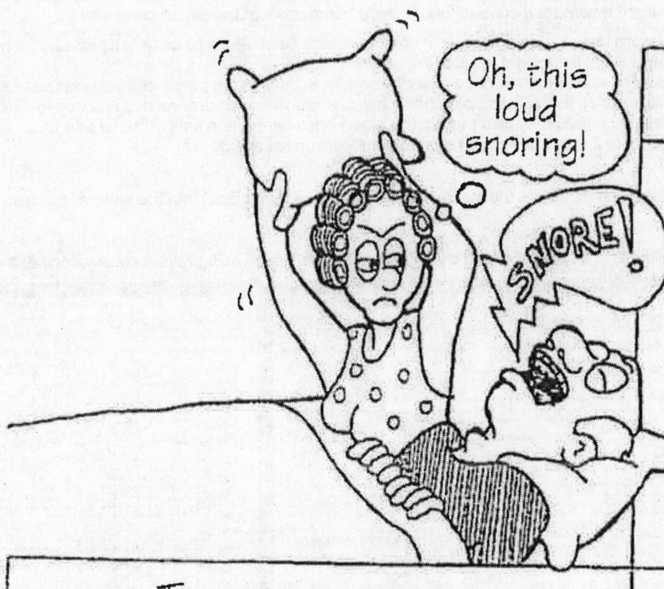

Symptoms

- Loud Snoring
- Excessive day time sleepiness
- Frequent episodes of obstructe breathing during sleep
- Morning headache
- Unrefreshing sleep
- Dry mouth upon awakening

Treatments

Non-Surgical
- Change sleep position
- Decrease weight
- CPAP (Constant Positive Airway Pressure)
- Drug Therapy

Surgical
- Adenoidectomy
- Uvulectomy
- Remodeling posterior oropharanx
- Tracheostomy

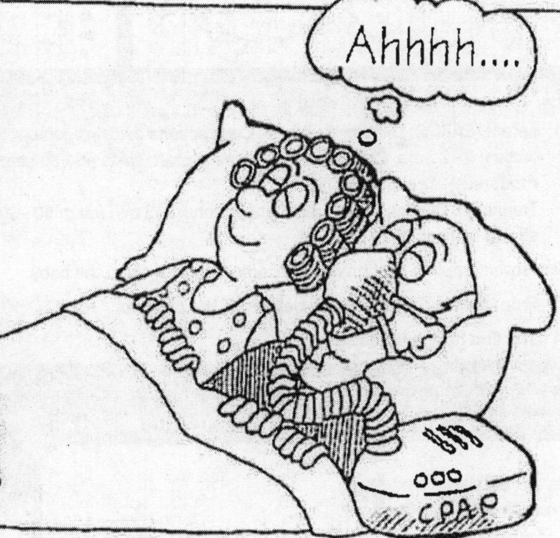

CJMILLER

OB & LABOR AND DELIVERY

Common Medications

Medication	Use	Mechanism of action	Rou
Pitocin	· Induction of term labor · Control of postpartum bleeding	Oxytocin is controlled by a positive feedback mechanism where release of the hormone causes an action which stimulates more of its own release.	· IV · IM
Misoprostol (Cytotec)	· Treat postpartum bleeding	Misoprostol, a prostaglandin analogue, binds to myometrial cells to cause strong myometrial contractions leading to expulsion of tissue. This agent also causes cervical ripening with softening and dilation of the cervix.	· Va · SL · PO
Cervadil (Dinoprostone)	· Cervical dilation	Dinoprostone cervical insert promotes cervical ripening by stimulating local receptors. The process of cervical ripening includes activation of the collagenase enzyme responsible for digestion of some of the structural collagen network of the cervix.	· Va
Methergine	· Treat bleeding during and after delivery · IV form is for emergency use only	Methergine is an ergot alkaloid uterine stimulant. It acts directly on the smooth muscle of the uterus and increases the tone, rate, and amplitude of rhythmic contractions. Thus, it induces a rapid and sustained titanic uterotonic effect which shortens the third stage of labor and reduces blood loss.	· IV · IM · PO
Hemabate	· Control bleeding post-partum	Stimulates in the gravid uterus myometrial contractions similar to labor contractions at the end of a full term pregnancy, they evacuate the products of conception from the uterus in most cases. Postpartum, the resultant myometrial contractions provide hemostasis at the site of placentation.	· IM
Magnesium Sulfate	· Delay Preterm birth by a few days. · Prevent seizures in preeclampsia	· Magnesium lowers calcium levels in uterine muscle cells. Since calcium is necessary for muscle cells to contract, this is thought to relax the uterine muscle. · Magnesium sulfate may act as a vasodilator, with actions in the peripheral vasculature or the cerebrovascular, to decrease peripheral vascular resistance and/or relieve vasoconstriction. · Magnesium sulfate may also protect the blood-brain barrier and limit cerebral edema formation, or it may act through a central anticonvulsant action.	· IV
Corticosteroid (betamethasone or dexamethasone)	· Reduces the risk of lung problems for babies between 29 and 34 weeks of pregnancy	Corticosteroids stimulate the synthesis and release of surfactants into the alveolar spaces.	· IM
Terbutaline	· Helps to delay preterm labor	Terbutaline is in a class of drugs called betamimetics, which help prevent contractions of the uterus.	· IM · IV

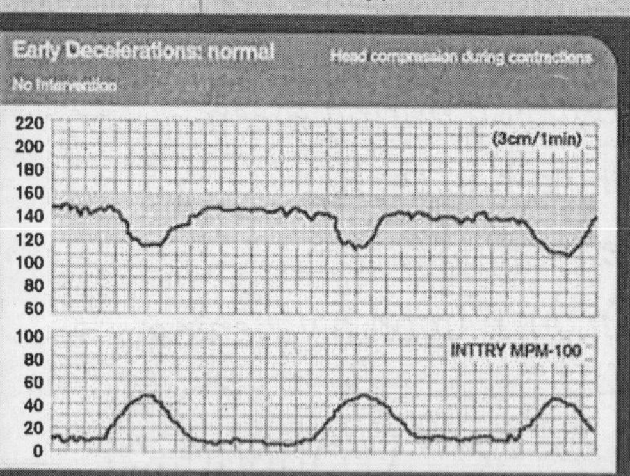

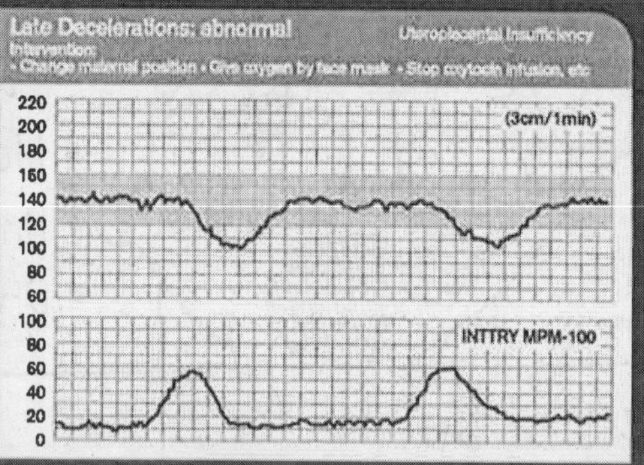

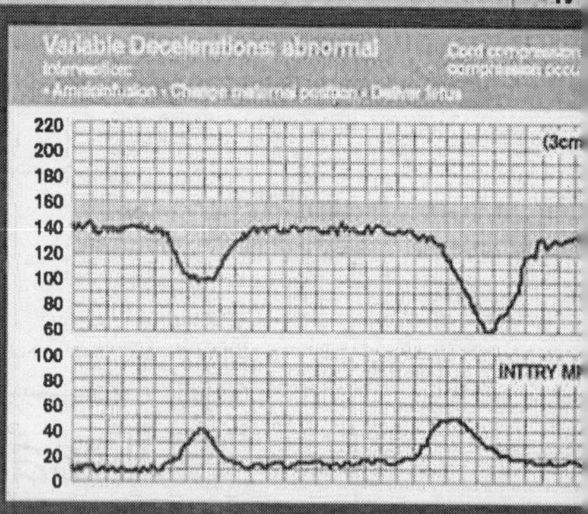

Variable Decelerations: abnormal
Intervention:
• Amnioinfusion • Change maternal position • Deliver fetus

Stages of Labor

Stage 1 · Latent (EARLY): Dilation 0 - 3 cms. Contractions mild/irregular.
· Active: 4 - 7 cms. Contractions 5 - 8 mins apart. Lasts 45 - 60 sec; moderate – strong intensity.
· Transition: Dilation 8 – 10 cms. Contractions 1 – 2 min apart; 60 – 90 sec; strong intensity.

Stage 2 · From complete dilation and effacement to delivery of the baby.

Stage 3 · From delivery of baby to the delivery of the placenta.

Stage 4 · The first hour after delivery.

GBS Positive - Antibiotic Guidelines

Recommended	Penicillin 5 units IV initial dose, then 2.5 - 3 million units IV every 4 hours until delivery
Alternative	Ampicillin, 2 g IV initial dose, 1 g IV every 4 hours until delivery
If penicillin allergic	-----
Patients not at high risk for anaphylaxis	Cefazolin, 2 g IV initial dose, then 1 g IV every 8 hours until delivery
Patients at high risk for anaphylaxis	-----
GBS susceptible to Clindamycin and Erythromycin	Clindamycin, 900 mg IV every 8 hours until delivery
GBS resistant to Clindamycin or erythromycin or susceptibility unknown	Vancomycin 1 g IV every 12 until delivery

Fetal Stations- FISHING

F	-3	Floating High
I	-2	In the Right Direction
S	-1	Settling In
H	0	Halfway There
I	+1	Inching Out
N	+2	Nearly There
G	+3	Get the Crown

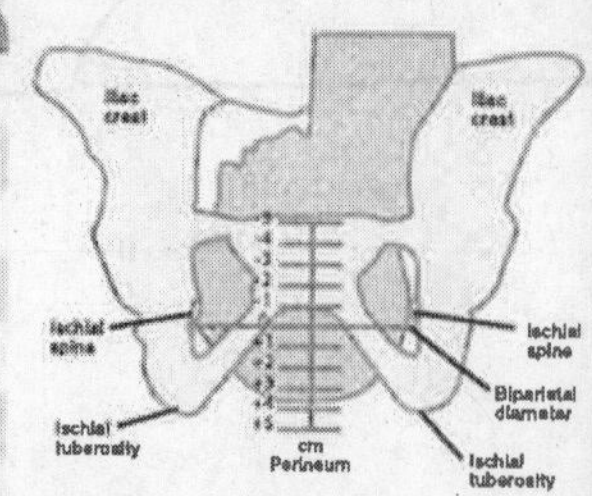

Antepartum Non Stress Test

Parameter	Normal NST (Previously "Reactive")	Atypical NST (Previously "Non-Reactive")	Abnormal NST (Previously "Non-Reactive")
Baseline	110 - 160 bpm	· 100 – 110 bpm · > 160 bpm < 30 min · Rising baseline	· Bradycardia <100 bpm · Tachycardia > 160 for > 30 min · Erratic baseline
Variability	· 6 – 25 bpm (moderate) · ≤ 5 (absent or minimal) for < 40 min	≤ 5 (absent or minimal) for 40 – 80 min	· ≤ 5 for ≥ 80 min · ≥ 25 bpm > 10 min · Sinusoidal
Decelerations	None or occasional variable < 30 sec	Variable decelerations 30 – 60 sec duration	· Variable decelerations > 60 sec duration · Late deceleration(s)
Accelerations Term Fetus	≥ 2 accelerations with acme of ≥15 bpm, lasting 15 sec < 40 min of testing	≤ 2 accelerations with acme of ≥ 15 bpm, lasting 15 sec in 40 – 80 min	≤ 2 accelerations with acme of ≥ 15 bpm, lasting 15 sec in > 80 min
Preterm Fetus (< 32 weeks)	≥ 2 accelerations with acme of ≥10 bpm, lasting 10 sec < 40 min of testing	≤ 2 accelerations of ≥ 10 bpm, lasting 10 sec in 40 – 80 min	≤ 2 accelerations of ≥ 10 bpm, lasting 10 sec in > 80 min

Intrapartum fetal heart rate monitoring - VEAL CHOP

Heart rate pattern	Cause
V - Variable decelerations	C - Cord compression/prolapse
E - Early decelerations	H - Head compression
A - Accelerations	O - Okay
L - Late decelerations	P - Placental insufficiency

Cervical Dilation (cm)

1 cm – cheerio, 3 cm – slice of banana, 5 cm – oreo, 7 cm – soda can, 10 cm – bagel

NEWBORN

agement of Glucose in At-Risk Infants:

rican Academy of Pediatric Guidelines – NML Infant Glucose 40-50 mg/dl

	When	What	Threshold	Intervention
tomatic*	<48 hrs	Any Screen	<40 mg/dl	IV Glucose/Dose: 200 mg/kg
ptomatic- SGA	0 - 4 hours (feed in 1st hr, screen glucose 30 min post feed)	Initial Screen	<25 mg/dl	Feed infant, recheck in 1 hr
		Subsequent Screenings	<25 mg/dl	IV Glucose/Dose: 200 mg/kg
			25 - 40 mg/dl	Refeed, IV glucose as needed
	4 - 24 hr (Continue feeds every 2-3 hr; screen before each feeding)	Initial Screen	<35 mg/dl	Feed infant, recheck in 1 hr
		Subsequent Screenings	<35 mg/dl	IV Glucose
			35 - 45 mg/dl	Refeed, IV glucose as needed
	24 - 48 hrs	Any Screen	<45 mg/dl	IV Glucose/Dose: 200 mg/kg
			≥ 45 mg/dl	Discharge when infant can maintain prior to feeding
fant treated V glucose	48 - 96 hrs	Any Screen	≥60 mg/dl	Discharge when infant can maintain prior to feeding

of Hypogycemia in infants: Apnea, Cardiac Arrest, Cyanosis, High-Pitched Cry, Hypothermia, Hypotonia, Irritability, iness, Lethargy, Poor Suck, Seizures, Tachypnea

Neonatal Infant Pain Scale

Variable	Finding	Points
Facial Expression	Relaxed	0
	Grimace	1
Cry	No cry	0
	Whimper	1
	Vigorous cry. If infant is intubated, score silent cry based on facial movement.	2
Breathing Pattern	Relaxed	0
	Change in breathing	1
Arms	Relaxed	0
	Flexed/Extended	1
Legs	Relaxed	0
	Flexed/Extended	1
State of Arousal	Sleeping/Awake	0
	Fussy	1
Heart Rate	Within 10% of baseline	0
	11 - 20% of baseline	1
	>20% of baseline	2
O_2 Saturation	No additional O_2 needed to maintain O_2 Saturation	0
	Additional O_2 needed to maintain O_2 Saturation	1

Limitations: The score can be false low if an infant is too ill to respond or receiving paralytic. (A score greater than 3 indicates pain)

VITAL SIGNS

= awake *s = sleeping

	Resp Rate	Heart Rate	Systolic BP	Diastolic BP
ate 3 days	30 - 50	a 100 - 205 s 90 - 160	60 - 80	35 - 55
t 2 mos	25 - 40	a 100 - 190 s 90 - 160	80 - 160	50 - 70

Normal Temperature Range by Method

Method	Normal Range (C°)	Normal Range (F°)
Rectal	36.6 - 38	97.9 - 100.4
Axillary	36.5 - 37.5	97.7 - 99.5

mon Newborn Meds and Labs

dard Newborn Meds/Labs	Recommendations
nin K	Prevent hemorrhage
biotic eye ointment	Prevent infection/blindness
Level	Within 24 hrs after 1st feeding
mbs Test	If mother is Rh-negative
unization	Hep-B

Gestational Age

Pre-Term	<37 wks
Term	37 - 41 wks
Post Term	> 42 wks

Weight Classifications

LGA	≥ 4000 g
AGA	2500 - 3999 g
SGA	< 2500 g

APGAR Scoring

ndicator	0 Points	1 Point	2 Points	Points totaled @ 1 min	5 mins
Activity (muscle tone)	Absent	Flexed arms and legs	Active		
Pulse	Absent	<100 bpm	>100 bpm		
Grimace (reflex irritability)	Floppy	Minimal response to stimulation	Prompt response to stimulation		
Appearance (skin color)	Blue: pale	Pink body, Blue extremities	Pink		
Respiration	Absent	Slow and irregular	Vigorous cry		

0-3 Severely depressed, 4-6 Moderately depressed, 7-10 Excellent condition

Total Score:

Appearance: pink, full ROM, strong cry

Fontanelles:
anterior (diamond shaped) – closes 7 - 19 mons
posterior (triangle shaped)– closes 2 - 3 mons

Mouth: Assess palate and lip for cleft and strong suck.

Bones: Assess clavicles.

Respirations: Assess rate, depth, effort, and auscultate.

Heart: Assess for murmur.

Umbilical Cord: 1 vein, 2 arteries, clamped.

Extremities: 10 fingers and toes of appropriate size/shape.

Genitals: Male: testes palpable. Female: mucous or bloody discharge WNL.

Skin: Document birthmarks.

Neonatal Resuscitation Algorithm from the American Academy of Pediatrics.

Birth

Term Gestation? Good Tone? Breathing or crying? — Yes → Infant stays with mother for routine care

No ↓

1 min

Warm and maintain normal temp, position airway, clear secretions, dry, and stimulate

Apnea or gasping? HR <100/min? — No → Labored breathing or persistent cyanosis?

- Yes → Position & Clear Airway; SpO2 Monitor; Supplementary O2 as needed; Consider CPAP

Yes ↓

PPV; SpO2 Monitor; Consider ECG Monitor

HR <100/min? — No → Postresuscitation care

Yes ↓

Check Chest Movement; Ventilation corrective steps if needed; ETT or laryngeal mask if needed

HR <60/min? — No → (back to HR <100/min?)

Yes ↓

Intubate if not already done; Chest Compressions; Coordinate with PPV, 100% O2; ECG Monitor; Consider Emergency UVC

HR <60/min?

Yes ↓

IV epinephrine; If HR Persistently below 60/min: Consider Hypovolemia; Consider PTX

Preductal SpO2 After Birth

1 min	60% - 65%
2 min	65% - 70%
3 min	70% - 75%
4 min	75% - 80%
5 min	80% - 85%
10 min	85% - 95%

Epinephrine
- Give Rapidly
- Concentration 1:10,000 (0.1mg/ml)
- ETT dose
  - 0.5 – 1 ml/kg
- UVC / IV dose
  - 0.1 – 0.3 ml/kg
    - Follow with a 0.5 – 1 ml flush NS
- Re-check heart rate after 1 min of compressions and ventilations
  - Maybe longer if given ETT
- Repeat dose every 3 – 5 mins
  - Epi can be given again immediately after UVC placement if given initially down ETT

NICU

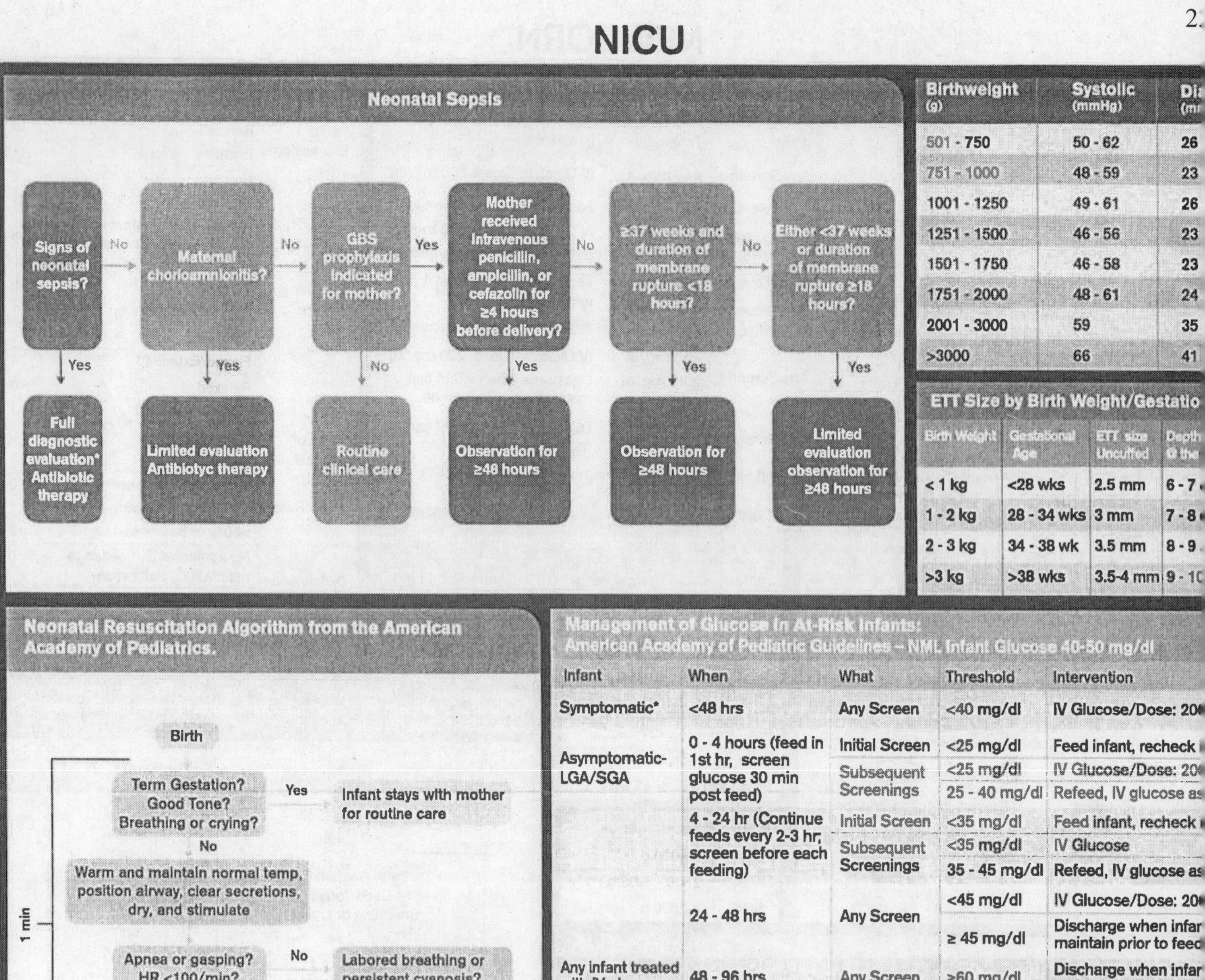

Birthweight (g)	Systolic (mmHg)	Di... (m...
501 - 750	50 - 62	26
751 - 1000	48 - 59	23
1001 - 1250	49 - 61	26
1251 - 1500	46 - 56	23
1501 - 1750	46 - 58	23
1751 - 2000	48 - 61	24
2001 - 3000	59	35
>3000	66	41

ETT Size by Birth Weight/Gestatio...

Birth Weight	Gestational Age	ETT size Uncuffed	Depth @ the...
< 1 kg	<28 wks	2.5 mm	6 - 7 ...
1 - 2 kg	28 - 34 wks	3 mm	7 - 8 ...
2 - 3 kg	34 - 38 wk	3.5 mm	8 - 9 ...
>3 kg	>38 wks	3.5-4 mm	9 - 10...

Neonatal Resuscitation Algorithm from the American Academy of Pediatrics.

Birth

1 min

Term Gestation? Good Tone? Breathing or crying? — Yes → Infant stays with mother for routine care

No

Warm and maintain normal temp, position airway, clear secretions, dry, and stimulate

Apnea or gasping? HR <100/min? — No → Labored breathing or persistent cyanosis?

Yes → PPV, SpO2 Monitor, Consider ECG Monitor

(Labored breathing) Yes → Position & Clear Airway, SpO2 Monitor, Supplementary O2 as needed, Consider CPAP

HR <100/min? — No → Postresusitation care

Yes

Check Chest Movement, Ventilation corrective steps if needed, ETT or laryngeal mask if needed

HR <60/min? — No (return to HR <100/min?)

Yes

Intubate if not already done, Chest Compressions, Coordinate with PPV, 100% O2, ECG Monitor, Consider Emergency UVC

HR <60/min?

Yes

IV epinephrine. If HR Persistently below 60/min: Consider Hypovolemia, Consider PTX

Preductal SpO2 After Birth	
1 min	60% - 65%
2 min	65% - 70%
3 min	70% - 75%
4 min	75% - 80%
5 min	80% - 85%
10 min	85% - 95%

Epinephrine
- Give Rapidly
- Concentration 1:10,000 (0.1mg/ml)
- ETT dose
  - 0.5 – 1 ml/kg
- UVC / IV dose
  - 0.1 – 0.3 ml/kg
  - Follow with a 0.5 – 1 ml flush NS
- Re-check heart rate after 1 min of compressions and ventilations
  - Maybe longer if given ETT
- Repeat dose every 3 – 5 mins
  - Epi can be given again immediately after UVC placement if given initially down ETT

Management of Glucose in At-Risk Infants: American Academy of Pediatric Guidelines – NML Infant Glucose 40-50 mg/dl

Infant	When	What	Threshold	Intervention
Symptomatic*	<48 hrs	Any Screen	<40 mg/dl	IV Glucose/Dose: 20...
Asymptomatic-LGA/SGA	0 - 4 hours (feed in 1st hr, screen glucose 30 min post feed)	Initial Screen	<25 mg/dl	Feed infant, recheck ...
		Subsequent Screenings	<25 mg/dl	IV Glucose/Dose: 20...
			25 - 40 mg/dl	Refeed, IV glucose as...
	4 - 24 hr (Continue feeds every 2-3 hr, screen before each feeding)	Initial Screen	<35 mg/dl	Feed infant, recheck ...
		Subsequent Screenings	<35 mg/dl	IV Glucose
			35 - 45 mg/dl	Refeed, IV glucose as...
	24 - 48 hrs	Any Screen	<45 mg/dl	IV Glucose/Dose: 20...
			≥ 45 mg/dl	Discharge when infar... maintain prior to feed...
Any infant treated with IV glucose	48 - 96 hrs	Any Screen	≥60 mg/dl	Discharge when infar... maintain prior to feed...

*S/S of Hypogycemia in Infants: Apnea, Cardiac Arrest, Cyanosis, High-Pitched Cry, Hypother... Hypotonia, Irritability, Jitteriness, Lethargy, Poor Suck, Seizures, Tachypnea

Skin Condition Score

Dryness	Erythema	Breakdown	N...
1 = Normal	1 = No evidence of erythema	1 = None evident	
2 = Dry skin, visible scaling	2 = Visible erythema, <50% body surface	2 = Small, localized areas	P... sc...
3 = Very dry skin, cracking/fissures	3 = Visible erythema, >50% body surface	3 = Extensive	W... sc...

Newborn Assessment

Appearance: pink, full ROM, strong cry

Fontanelles:
anterior (diamond shaped) – closes 7 - 19 mons
posterior (triangle shaped)– closes 2 - 3 mons

Mouth:
Assess palate and lip for cleft and strong suck.

Respirations:
Assess rate, depth, effort, and auscultate.

Extremities:
10 fingers and toes of appropriate size/shape.

Skin:
Document birthmarks.

B... A... clav...

Assess for mu...

Umbilical ... 1 vein, 2 ar... clar...

Ge... Male: testes pal... Female: m... or bloody discharge

PEDIATRICS

	*a = awake	VITAL SIGNS	*s = sleeping		
	Resp Rate (breaths/minute)	Heart Rate	Systolic BP	Diastolic BP	Systolic Hypotension
ate days	30 - 53	a 100-205 s 90-160	67 - 84	35 - 53	<60
t mons	25 - 40	a 100-190 s 90-160	72 - 104	37 - 56	<70
er rs	22 - 37	a 98-140 s 80-120	86 - 106	42 - 63	<70 + (age in years x 2)
hooler rs	20 - 28	a 80-120 s 65-100	89 - 112	46 - 72	<70 + (age in years x 2)
ol Age rs	18 - 25	a 75-118 s 58-90	97 - 115	57 - 76	<70 + (age in years x 2)
dolescent 2 yrs	18 - 25	a 75-118 s 58-90	102 - 120	61 - 80	<90
escent/Adult yrs	12 - 20	a 60-100 s 50-90	110 - 120	65 - 80	<90

Approximate Size and Depth for Placement of Endotracheal Tubes and Central Venous Lines

Ages 1-10 yrs
Uncuffed ETT size (mm) = (age in years/4) + 4
Cuffed ETT size (mm) = (age in years/4) + 3

Age	Uncuffed ETT mm	Cuffed ETT mm	Initial Depth cm	Central Line length/size
Newborn	3 - 3.5	3	9-10	5 - 8 cm/4 Fr
1-5 mons	3.5	3 - 3.5	10	5 - 8 cm/4 Fr
6-11 mons	3.5 - 4	3.5	11	8 - 12 cm/4 - 5 Fr
1 yr	4 - 4.5	4	12	8 - 12 cm/4 - 5 Fr
2-3 yrs	4.5 - 5	4 - 4.5	12-13	8 - 12 cm/4 - 5 Fr
4-5 yrs	5 - 5.5	4.5 - 5	13-15	8 - 12 cm/5.5 - 6 Fr
6-9 yrs	5.5 - 6	5 - 5.5	15	8 - 12 cm/5.5 - 6 Fr
10-12 yrs	6.5 - 7	6 - 6.5	17	12 - 15 cm/6 + Fr
13+ yrs	7 - 7.5	6.5 - 7	19	12 - 15 cm/6 + Fr

Immunization Schedule

ine	Birth	2 mons	4 mons	6 mons	12 mons	4-6 yrs	7-10 yrs	11-12 yrs	13-15 yrs	16-18 yrs
B										
(<7 yrs)					15 mons					
enza				Yearly	Yearly	Yearly	Yearly	Yearly	Yearly	Yearly
R										
cella										
A					1st dose >6 mons apart					
ingococcal								1st dose		Booster
≥7 yrs								(Tdap)		
								3-dose series		

Age	QRS interval (ms)	QTc (ms)**	PR (ms)
Birth - 2 yrs	30 - 80	<450	80 - 160*
3- 4 yrs	40 - 80	<450	80 - 160*
5 - 7 yrs	40 - 80	<450	80 - 160*
8 - 11 yrs	40 - 90	<450	80 - 160*
12 - 15 yrs	40 - 90	<450	<200
>15 yrs	50 - 100	refer to adult	<200

*Normal PR is 80-110ms in infants and smaller children but >=160 indicates block
**Please note QTc corrects for rate, but is less accurate as rate increases. Average is 410ms

Age	Hgb (g/dL)	Hct (%)
Term Newborn	13 - 20	40 - 58
1 mon	11 - 18	32 - 54
2 mons	10 - 15	28 - 44
1 - 2 yrs	10 - 13	32 - 40
> 2 yrs	11 - 14	33 - 42

iatric Fluid Management

ydration Type	Fluid Type
s	Normal Saline
tenance (<20 kg)	D5 ¼ Normal Saline
teniance (>20 kg)	D5 ½ Normal Saline

Pediatric Fluid Replacement

Weight	Hourly	Daily
<10 kg	4 mL/kg/hr	100 mL/kg/day
10-20 kg	40 mL + 2 mL/kg for every kg >10 kg	1000 mL + 50 mL/kg/day for every kg >10
>20 kg	60 mL + 1 mL/kg for every kg >20 kg	1500 mL + 20 mL/kg/day for every kg > 20

LAB	NORMAL
SERUM WBC ($x10^3/mm^3$)	Term Newborn: 8 – 30 >2 mons: 5 – 15
CSF WBC ($/mm^3$)	Term Newborn: 0-25 >2 wks: 0 - 5
Na (mmol/L)	Term: 132 – 142 >1 mon: 135 – 146
Cl (mmol/L)	95-108
BUN (mg/dL)	5-26
K (mmol/L)	Term: 3.8 – 6.1 >1 mon: 3.5 – 5.1
HCO_3 (mmol/L)	20-28
Cr (mg/dL)	0.2 – 1
Glucose (mg/dL)	Term: 32-100 >2 wks: 60 – 110

rmal Temperature Range by Method

hod	Normal Range (C°)	Normal Range (F°)
tal	36.6 - 38	97.9 - 100.4
panic	35.8 - 38	96.4 - 100.4
	35.5 - 37.5	95.9 - 99.5
ary	36.5 - 37.5	97.7 - 99.5

Donor's Blood Type

Patient's Blood Type	0-	0+	B-	B+	A-	A+	AB-	AB+
AB+	✓	✓	✓	✓	✓	✓	✓	✓
AB-	✓		✓		✓		✓	
A+	✓	✓			✓	✓		
A-	✓				✓			
B+	✓	✓	✓	✓				
B-	✓		✓					
0+	✓	✓						
0-	✓							

ic dosage calculation

esired dose) / mount on hand) x V (volume) = Dose

ips in mcg/minute

x $\frac{1,000 \text{ mcg}}{1 \text{ mL}}$ x $\frac{\text{mL}}{1 \text{ hour}}$ x $\frac{1 \text{ hour}}{60 \text{ minutes}}$ = mcg/minute

y kg to get mcg/kg/minute)

ips in units/hour

esired) / n hand) x V (volume) = units/hour (#mL x units/mL = dose)

PAIN ASSESSMENT TOOL

0 1 2 3 4 5 6 7 8 9 10

No Pain | Mild pain | Moderate Pain | Serious Pain | Severe Pain | Worst Pain Possible

Terminology for Physical Assessment of the Newborn

Acrocyanosis - A bluish discoloration of the hands and feet due to sluggish peripheral circulation.

Barlow's maneuver - A procedure to rule out congenital hip instability; flexion of the legs, abduction of the hips to approximately 90 degrees, then downward pressure is exerted while adducting the thighs. A positive sign is palpable dislocation during the maneuver.

Caput succedaneum - A collection of fluid in the soft tissues of the scalp that may override the suture lines. Caused by pressure on the presenting part of the head against the cervix during labor.

Cephalohematoma - A collection of blood between the periosteum and the cranial bone (usually the parietal bone) appearing as unilateral or bilateral and limited to the suture lines of the affected bone(s). A result of the extravasation of ruptured blood vessels from the pressure of birth.

Diastasis recti - Gap between abdominal recti muscles.

Epstein pearls - Small, white, round epithelial cysts on the hard palate and along the gum margins.

Erythema neonatorum toxicum - "Newborn rash" or flea bite rash. A generalized rash characterized by red, elevated papules appearing around 24-48 hours of age. Resolves without treatment.

Fontanelle - "Soft spot". An area of fibrous tissue over the juncture of the cranial bones.

Lanugo - Fine downy hair of varying distribution covering the body with exception of the palms of the hands and soles of the feet.

Milia - White, pinpoint papules on the chin and/or nose resulting from unopened sebaceous glands.

Molding - Shaping of the head caused by overriding of the cranial bones to facilitate movement through the birth canal.

Mongolian spots - "Oriental patches". An area of bluish-black pigmenta-tion over the buttocks and the lower back, commonly seen in non-Caucasian races.

Mottling - Discoloration of the skin in irregular areas resembling a lace-like pattern.

Occipital-frontal circumference (OFC) - The greatest circumference of the head, i.e., over the supraorbital ridges and the occipital prominence.

Ortolani's maneuver - A procedure to rule out congenital hip dislocation: flexion of the legs, abduction of the hips to approximately 90 degrees, then forward pressure from behind the greater trochanter while the thigh is abducted. A positive finding is a "click", which is palpable as the dislocation is reduced.

Pseudomenstruation - White or blood-tinged mucous discharge from the vaginal secondary to the withdrawal of maternal hormones.

Rugae - Folds of tissue over the scrotum that allow for expansion of the tissue.

Subconjunctival hemorrhage - An area of bleeding on the sclera due to changes in vascular tension during birth.

Telangiectatic nevi - "Stork bites" or capillary hemangiomas. A flat area of capillary dilatation appearing as small clusters of pink-red spots on the nose, nape of the neck, lower occipital bone, and eyelids, which blanc easily.

Vernix caseosa - A white cheese-like substance covering the body, particularly noticeable in the creases of the skin.

Reflexes in the Neonate

(See text for more reflexes)

REFLEX	STIMULUS	RESPONSE	SEEN	NOT SEEN
Moro	Infant lying on back, slightly raised head suddenly released; infant lowered abruptly	Arms extended, head thrown back, fingers fat out; arms brought back to center with hands clenched; legs extended	Birth	4 months
Rooting	Lightly stroke cheek with finger	Head turns toward stimulus	Birth	4 months
Sucking	Insert finger into infant's mouth	Rhythmic sucking	Birth	7 months
Startle	Loud noise	Similar to Moro response	Birth	4 months
Palmar (grasp)	Touch palm with finger or object	Grasp object, holds tightly	Birth	6 months
Tonic neck (fencing)	Head turned to one side while infant lies on back	Arm and leg extend on the side infant faces. Opposite arm and leg extend.	2 months	6 months
Blinking	Light flash	Eyelids close	Birth	-----
Stepping	Infant supported in an upright position with feet touching flat surface.	Rhythmic stepping movements	Birth	6 weeks
Babinski	Stroke the sole of foot from heel to toe laterally	Toes fan out	Birth	12 mo.

Component	Assessment Criteria	Normal Findings	Common Variations
Posture	Posture	Hands clenched, Flexion, adduction of extremities	Front breech may have extended legs and abducted thighs
Vital Signs: Temperature	Axillary: 36.5 - 37°C (97.7 - 98.6°F)		
Pulse	Rate	120-160 beats/minute	Varies with body temperature, period of reactivity, physical activity During sleep, as low as 100bpm; with crying, as high as 180bpm
	Quality	Strong	
	Rhythm	Regular	
	Heart Sounds	PMI: 4th-5th intercostal space left of midclavicular line	Often visible Apex of heart is at PMI in neonate
		Listen over entire precardium	Transient murmurs secondary to incomplete closure of ductus arteriosus or foramen ovale
Respirations	Rate	30-60 breaths/minute	Varies with body temperature, period of reactivity, physical activity
	Quality	Relaxed, synchronized movement of the chest and abdomen	
	Rhythm	Irregular—Assess for full minute	
	Breath Sounds	Bronchovesicular sounds with inspiration, expiration equal in duration	Sibilant and sonorous wheezes in immediate post delivery period
Blood Pressure		Systolic: 54-92 in males Diastolic: 38-72 in males Systolic: 46-84 in females Diastolic: 38-72 in females	
Bowel Sounds	Location	Present in all 4 quadrants	Bowel sounds may be absent during first period of reactivity.

Skin	Color	Caucasian: ruddy or pink-tinged Non-caucasian: consistent with racial background	Mottling Acrocyanosis Telangiectatic nevi Mongolian spots Jaundice may occur after 24 hours Ecchymosis or localized petechiae from birth trauma Harlequin coloring Plethora
	Texture	Soft, smooth, thin	Milia Mongolian spots Telangiectatic nevi Jaundice—significant if > 24hrs old Birthmarks: nevus flammeus—portwine stain strawberry hemangioma cavernous hemangioma café au lait spots
	Turgor	Elastic	
	Mucous membranes	Pink & moist	
Measurements	Head	33—33.5 cm (13-14- in.)	
	Chest	30.5 – 33 cm (12 – 13 in.)	
	Length	44 –53 cm (17.5 – 21 in)	

Worksheet for Complications of the Physical Assessment of the Newborn

Certain parameters are considered "abnormal" and need to be recognized early by the nurse. Use your texts to define and identify the significance of the following.

Head: Hydrocephaly

Microcephaly

Anencephaly

Forceps marks/abrasions/scalp electrode site

Eyes: Wide set eyes

Epicanthal folds

Conjunctivitis

Chemical conjunctivitis

Ears: Low set ears

Mouth: Extrusion of tongue

Chest: Abnormal respirations:

retractions
flaring nares
expiratory grunting

Abdomen: Umbilicus: if foul-smelling or discharge present

Back: Pilonidal sinus

Tuft of hair at base of spine

Male Genitalia:

Hydrocele
Congenital phimosis
Hypospadias/epispadias

Extremities:

Hands:

Simian crease
polydactyly
syndactyly

Feet:

positional deformity
club feet

Neurological:

Cry: Lusty
high-pitched
weak

Definition of Terms

Premature: Refers to an infant born after 20 weeks of gestation and before 38 weeks of gestation.

Postmature: Refers to an infant born after 42 weeks of gestation.

Small for Gestational Age: Refers to an infant whose length, head circumference, and weight fall at or below the tenth percentile for all babies at that gestational age.

Large for Gestational Age: Refers to an infant whose length, head circumference, and weight fall at or above the 90th percentile for all babies at that gestational age.

Appropriate for Gestational Age: A determination that the infant falls between the tenth and 90th percentile for all babies at that gestational age.

Predictable Problems Based on Gestational Age

Premature:

Respiratory Distress Syndrome
Hypothermia
Hypoglycemia
Infection
Apnea
Hypocalcemia
Hyperbilirubinemia
Intracranial hemorrhage

Postmature:

Birth asphyxia
Aspiration Syndrome
Hypoglycemia
Polycythemia
Small for Gestational Age

Small for Gestational Age:

Hypothermia
Hypoglycemia
Aspiration Syndrome
Birth asphyxia
Polycythemia
Intrauterine infection
Problems related to the etiology of the infant's poor growth

Large for Gestational Age:

Hypoglycemia
Birth trauma

Hypertensive Disorders

Hypertension in pregnancy predisposes the women to lethal complications (it is always serious!):
- Abruptio placenta*
- DIC
- Cerebral hemorrhage
- CVA
- Hepatic rupture*
- Acute renal failure
- Eclampsia*

* the leading causes of maternal death of HTN-complicated pregnancies

Hypertension in Pregnancy
- Defined as a Blood Pressure > than 140/90 or a mean arterial pressure > 105. Her baseline BP is not important...it's the amount of increase over the course of the pregnancy...an increase of 30/15 should be considered and watched carefully.
- Types of Hypertensive Disorders
  - Chronic Hypertension: BP >140/90
    - BEFORE twenty weeks of gestation
    - Occurs in 1-5% of pregnancies.
    - Not a good sign for things to come
  - Pregnancy induced hypertension (PIH) (aka Preeclampsia)
    - AFTER 20 weeks gestation.
    - Occurs in 5-8% of pregnancies.

Mom with PIH will have generalized edema. A lot of time you'll see it in the face and hands. You'll also hear wet lungs, may have multiples, will have protein in the urine, may have epigastric pain, may have headache, blurred vision. Will need to keep environment calm and soothing.

Chronic Hypertension
- Associated with ↑ incidence of abruption and preeclampsia.
- A woman with chronic hypertension is probably going to end up with PIH
- Many postpartum complications such as pulmonary edema, renal failure, hypertensive encephalopathy, heart failure
- Medical Management of Chronic Hypertension
  - Usually managed in consultation with primary care provider and perinatologist
  - Managed by
    - fetal and maternal assessment...may be every two weeks
    - lifestyle changes (exercise more)
    - nutrition (less salt)
    - Methyldopa (Aldomet)

Types of Pregnancy Induced Hypertension (PIH)
- Mild: BP> 140/90 and > 0.3 g protein in 24/h urine
- Severe BP>160/110 and > 2 g protein in 24 urine
- Eclampsia: either of the above with ***new onset seizures***
- HELLP: Hemolysis, elevated liver enzymes, low platelets (this is a SYNDROME!)
- Gestational: BP > 140/90 after 20 weeks gestation. No proteinurea in 24 hour urine.
  - Transient hypertension: Gestational hypertension - no signs of preeclampsia present at ??
  - May be 1st indicator of later hypertension
- Preeclampsia after 20 weeks

Preeclampsia
- Develops during pregnancy and disappears with expulsion of the placenta.
  - The treatment for this is essentially delivery of fetus and placenta.
- Cause remains unknown; there are no toxins in the body
- Many Risk factors:
  - primigravida, obesity, chronic HTN, renal disease, maternal age < 15 and > 40, diabetics, Rh incompatability,
- Progression of Disease

High Risk: Perinatal Infections

Most Common Perinatal Infections
- Toxoplasmosis
- Rubella
- Cytomegalovisrus (CMV)
- Herpes Simplex Virus (HSV)
- Group B Strep

Toxoplasmosis
- Can get this from cats...mom should not clean the litter box.
- Protozoan that is spread by exposure. It poses some pretty serious risks to mom and fetus.
- Symptoms
    - Either non existent or vague flu-like symptoms
    - Many women don't know they have it b/c symptoms are so vague
- Bad things that can happen
    - Retinochoroiditis ? (look this up)
    - Convulsions
    - Coma
    - Microcephaly
    - Hydrocephalus
- Prevention
    - Stay away from cat poop
    - Keep the cat off the bed
    - Wash hands
    - Don't garden without gloves
    - Don't run around barefoot

Rubella (measles)
- Prevention = immunization
- Check titer as part of first labs when mom comes in for prenatal visit to see if she has been immunized
- Spread by droplets
- Symptoms in mother
    - Most likely just have a very mild rash
    - Probably won't feel too bad, maybe a little headache and itchy
- Fetal Risks: Rubella
    - Congenital cataracts
    - Sensorineural deafness
    - Congenital Heart Defects

Chlamydia
- Very common STD
- Spread by intimate contact and thru birth
- Symptoms in the mother
    - Virtually no symptoms!
    - Mom doesn't even know most of the time
    - Often seen concurrently with gonorrhea which is very symptomatic
    - Over half the population of patients with STDs have it.
- Fetal Risks of chlamydia
    - Neuro complications
    - Anemia
    - Hyperbilirubinemia
    - Thrombocytopenia
    - Hepatosplenomegaly
    - SGA
    - At risk for PNA

High Risk: Perinatal Infections

- Breastfeeding safety is going to depend on mom being treated. I guess baby can't breastfeed safely unless mom gets treatment?
- Fetal demise is not uncommon :-(

Herpes
- Highly contagious and never goes away
- Spread by intimate contact and birth (via ascending infection as well...not sure what this means). If amniotic sac breaks, there is a < 4 hour window in which baby needs to be delivered. Women who have herpes are going to be tested throughout pregnancy and usually at 2 weeks to 1 month prior to delivery they'll get a thorough exam to check the status of lesions. May not be able to see all the lesions even with a vag exam. If woman has had active lesion in past month, they're going to go C/S route.
- Symptoms in the mother
  - Herpes lesions are very painful
  - The lesions can be in vaginal area or on mouth
  - First onset of herpes will usually have inguinal pain and enlarged lymph nodes
- Fetal Risks: Herpes
  - Preterm labor
  - Intrauterine growth restriction
  - Neonatal infection...these babies don't do very well.

Group B Strep
- This is an ascending infection
- When is the mother tested and how: tested during pregnancy
- Medications to treat the mother are given before she delivers
- Fetal Risks: GBS
  - Respiratory distress or pneumonia
  - Apnea
  - Shock
  - Meningitis
  - Long-term neuro complications
  - In nursery you may see: baby can't hold temp (early sign of a sick baby is an inability to hold temp), lungs sound a little gunky, color changes, irritable

Human Parvo-19 "slapped cheek disease", AKA "5th Disease"
- Causes a red rash
- Usually occurs in children, but can be transferred to adults where it is mild...not good news for fetus though
- How is it spread? It goes through the placenta in about 1/3 of the cases and has a fairly high fetal loss rate. May take 4-12 weeks post infection for the baby to die.
- When is it most detrimental to the developing fetus? She didn't say.
- Who is at risk? She didn't say. Maybe a pregnant woman who has school-age child? Don't know.
- Fetal Risks: Human B-19Parvo
  - Spontaneous abortion
  - Fetal hydrops
  - Stillbirth
- Diagnostic Testing
  - TORCH (an acronym for infections that are fetal toxic)
    - Toxoplasmosis, Other, Rubella, CMV, Hepatis/Herpes
  - Culture for chlamydia
  - Active lesions – could culture for HSV
  - Other lab tests (she didn't mention any specifically)

- Multisystem disease
- Diagnostic Signs
  - hypertension (in all cases)
  - proteinurea (in all cases)
  - edema (not in all cases)
  - May progress from mild→ severe → HELLP → convulsions → coma → death of mother and fetus
- Theories Regarding the Etiology of Preeclampsia
  - Vasoconstriction and vasospasm
  - Coagulation
  - Trophoblast invasion
  - Dietary deficiencies/excess: protein, Ca, N, Mag, Vit E, Vit A
  - Genetic predisposition (autosomal recessive)
  - Immune complex where maternal antibody system overwhelmed by fetal antigens in maternal blood. (an old idea...where the idea of "toxemia" came from)
  - Adverse immunologic response
    - Maternal antibody system being overwhelmed
    - Causes inappropriate endothelial cell activation (vasospasm)
    - Decreased production of Nitric Oxide (causes vasodilation)
  - Vasospasm
    - Caused by ↑ sensitivity to circulating vasopressors such as angiotension II and an imbalance between prostacyclin and thromboxane A2
    - Prostacyclin is produced by endothelial cells of blood vessels
    - Thromboxane is produced by platelets causes vasospasm
      - vasosopasm leads to ↑ BP
      - Endothelial cells dysfunction
      - Both of these contribute to capillary permeability
      - This leads to ↑ interstitial edema (3rd spacing) and ↓ decreased blood flow leading to poor perfusion in both mom and baby (placenta won't work well and won't transport nutrients the way it should be). This puts the fetus at jeopardy b/c the placenta is it's lifeline...if this isn't working well, baby can get into big trouble.
      - Baby is not well oxygenated, can get..
        - IUGR
        - If in labor, we start to see decelerations (late decelerations) "late decels" = utero placental insufficiency
      - Functions may becomes depressed....not just in placenta, but in liver, brain and kidneys as well. This depression can account for up to 40-60% of a decrease in function. The kidney dysfunction causes protein in the urine.
      - See flowchart to the right

Epidurals cause vasodilation; Induction drugs cause vasoconstriction.

The Endothelium (the capillary wall)

- The endothelium is usually impermeable to the plasma proteins and lipids. Under normal conditions, these stay within the plasma where they belong.
- Oncotic pressure changes
  - Most of the fluid within the capillaries is retained
  - Some filters through pores between the cells...pushed by a pressure gradient.
- Colloid Oncotic Pressure
  - Water and small solutes can pass freely through capillary pores into the interstitial fluid.
  - Protein does not leak into the interstitium...but protein pressure is going to draw water out of the interstitium and into the plasma. (look this fluid shift stuff up....she sped through this, not sure if I got it right)
  - Following injury, the capillaries can leak protein
  - Water follows protein into the interstitial space causing interstial edema (generalized edema)
  - Intravascular volume moves out results in hemoconcentration,and increased blood viscosity...this is a whole other category of problems d/t the thick blood.
  - Most of these woman have +4 pitting edema at the knee. Will also look at hands, arms, feet)

Vasospasm also leads to...
- Ruptured capillaries that leads to a release of clotting factors leading to risk fo blood clots, then to risk of DIC
- ↓ retinal perfusion which leads to visual disturbances (pt may say "I see bright lights" or "I see spots"...this is now SEVERE...we will expect her to have a seizure)
- ↓ organ perfusion and IUGR
- Cardiac failure is the worst outcome.

Potential Maternal/Fetal Complications
- Cardiovascular
- Renal
- Hematological
- Neurological
- Hepatic
- Uteroplacental

Cardiovascular effects...watch for this stuff!
- Severe hypertension
- Hypertensive crisis
- Pulmonary edema (will use Lasix on this mom)

Reduced Kidney Perfusion
- Decreased GFR...can even be oliguric.
- Protein is lost in the urine (albumin)
- BUN, serum creatinine, and serum uric acid increase
- Sodium and water are retained, leading to weight gain. Take daily weights...look for anything inconsistent with normal pregnancy weight gain.

When you have a PIH patie
think multisystem involveme
Watch for complaints of HA
epigastric pain, seeing spo
The next stop on this path i
convulsions!

Hematological Effects
- Hemolysis
- Decreased oxygen carrying capacity
- Thrombocytopenia
- DIC

Cerebral changes
- Increased CNS irritability. Signs&symptoms:
  - Cerebral edema/hemorrhage
  - Changes in mood, emotion, consciousness
  - Headache

Increased CNS irritability S&S, cont'd
  - Hyperreflexia/Clonus
  - Eclampsia-Seizures
  - CVA, amaurosis (blindness)

Decreased Liver Perfusion
  - Impaired function, hypoglycemia
  - Hepatic edema (liver will be tender if you can access it, but you'd actually use the lab values for this)
  - Subcapsular hemorrhage
  - ↑ liver enzymes AST,ALT
  - This is what is causing the epigastric pain.

Placental changes

- Decreased uteroplacental perfusion may lead to
  - IUGR
  - IUFD
  - Fetal intolerance to labor- fetal distress
  - Oligohydraminos
  - Abruptio placenta

Mild Preeclampsia Highlights/Review

- Criteria for diagnosis:
  - BP > 140/90 after 20 weeks
  - 1+or 2+ protein
  - Generalized edema of face, hands abdomen that does not disappear after 12 hours bed rest.

Severe Preecclampsia Highlights/Review

- BP>160/110
- Proteinuria >2+ or 3+ on random dip/ 2g/24 hours
- Signs & Symptoms:
  - Hyperreflexia,
  - Generalized edema
  - Oliguria
  - Cerebral/visual disturbances,
  - Liver involvement,
  - Thrombocytopenia

Eclampsia Highlights/Review

- Either mild or severe preeclampsia with a new onset of seizures
- Coma
- Fetal/Maternal death

HELLP

- H Hemolysis
- E elevated liver enzymes
- L (↑ AST/ALT)
- L low platelets
- Platelets (<100,000)
- May occur with mild or severe preeclampsia
- This person is now very very sick...will go to critical care unit.

Prenatal care

- Goal is to detect it early, so need ot know S/S of preeclampsia
- Other goals are to tabilize condition, deliver a healthy mom and baby
- Identify women at risk (if preeclampsia prior, then at least a 50% chance of having it again)
- Past obstetric / family history
- Accurate recording at each visit

Management of Mild Preeclampsia

- Frequent clinic F/U
- Assess wt, urine protein, BP, edema
- Monitor fetal movement NST
- Ultrasound
- Biophysical profile
- Home /bed rest (bedrest promotes diuresis)
- Diversional activities/ gentle exercise

- Nutrition

Biophysical Profile
- Fetal breathing movements
- Fetal body movements
- Fetal tone
- Fetal heart rate pattern by NST
- Amniotic fluid index (6-19 cm normal)
- Normal score is 8-10 (as long as AFI is adequate)

Health teaching
- Review signs/symptoms of preeclampsia
- Assess home environment to determine if home care viable option
- Teach women self assessment of clinical signs.
    - eg. BP, urine protein,daily weight, edema, I & O, assessment of fetal activity
- When to notify doctor
- Relaxation to ↓ BP and promote diuresis

Management of Severe Preeclampsia and HEELP
- Hospitalization with goal of stabilization and birth of baby.
- OB management in consult with Perinatologist and Neonatologist
- Specialized Nursing care
    - Bed rest, decreased stimulation, low lights, limit visitors
    - Critical care: VS, I+O, cardiac monitoring, IVs, weight, reflexes, looking for clonus (?)
    - Continuous fetal and uterine monitoring maybe, but once stabilized will let mom have an hour or so off the monitor.
    - Medication to stabilize condition and improve outcomes
- Laboratory Monitoring
    - Blood: CBC, 'lytes, uric acid
    - Coagulation Profile: PT, PTT, fibrinogen
    - Urine: test for protein, look at Cr clearance
- Drug Treatment
    - Goals of therapy:
        - Decrease chance of seizures
        - Decrease BP to diastolic of 100-90
        - Promote fetal lung maturity
        - Stabilize patient to prolong pregnancy as long as possible
        - Delivery if unable to stabilize mom
- **Eclampsia (the seizure sequence)**
    - Onset of seizures
    - Eyes are fixed
    - Twitching of facial muscles
    - All body muscles are in tonic contraction
    - Muscles relax, respirations are long, deep, noisy inhalation
    - Followed by coma

- **Management of Eclampsia (woman has had a seizure and can't take care of herself, so you do this...)**
    - Airway management: suction and O2
    - Protect from injury during seizure
    - Record time, duration, type of seizure
    - R/O abruption (ultrasound eval) uterine tone
    - Chest X-ray, blood gases, labs
    - Pulmonary, renal function
    - Hygiene:Urine/ fecal incontinence, oral care

- Stabilize with Magnesium Sulfate
- Control BP
- Assess fetal status
- If birth can be delayed administer Betamethasone
- If situation critical prepare for emergency Cesarean section

HELLP SYNDROME

- Severe form of preeclampsia occurs in 1/1000 pregnancies
- May occur in 2nd or 3rd trimester
- Maternal symptoms: malaise, epigastric pain, N+V, Flu-like sx (docs with think this is the flu)
- Labs: hemolysis, ↑LFTs, ↓platelets
- HELLP is associated with increased risk for
    - Abruption
    - DIC
    - Renal failure
    - Hepatic rupture
    - Recurrent preeclampsia
    - Fetal and maternal mortality

Common lab changes in Preeclampsia

- See attachment!

Medications used in treatment

- Anticonvulsants, Blood Pressure Meds, Betamethasone

Magnesium Sulfate (MgSO4)

- Drug of choice to prevent seizure activity
- Decreases neuromuscular irritability
- Depresses CNS irritability
- Usually also ↓ diastolic BP slightly
- Another name for it is "Epsom Salts"
- Mom will feel like her body is a brick...very heavy! Need to remind her to turn b/c she is not going to feel like moving at all. She'll feel like a slug! If she's getting both Mag Sulfate and Terbutaline, she'll feel like she's stuck in cement with a racing heart...not fun!
- **Action:** CNS/Neuromuscular depressant
- **Indication:** Prevention of seizures, ↓contx
- **Dose:** 40 g MgSo4 in 1000 ml LR
    - Loading dose: 4-6 g over 15-30 min
    - Maintenance dose- infuse at 2-4 g/ hour
- **Adverse reactions:** ↓ muscle tone, uterine atony, ↓respirations, HA, Flushing, N+V, ↓maternal temp, cardiac arrest...this is a serious medication!

- Nursing Care of MgSo4 Patient
    - Establish primary IV
    - Magnesium is *always* piggybacked to primary using Infusion pump
    - Keep antidote (calcium gluconate) at bedside- 1g of 10% solution at bedside
    - Assess VS (especially RR), Urine output, deep tendon reflexes
    - Continuous fetal monitoring (Maternal VS and FHR checked Q 15 min during bolus)
    - Nurse remains at bedside during bolus infusion
- Nursing care during continuous infusion
    - DTRs/Clonus Q 1-2 hours
    - BP, RR: Q 30-60 min -O2 sat monitoring
    - Breath sounds Q 4 hours- eval for pulmonary edema
    - Monitor I+O hourly
    - Assess for signs of toxicity(↓ RR/apnea, ↓ LOC)

- Asses for worsening of Preeclampsia
- Mag levels as ordered
- May need Pitocin for augmentation/ atony
- Magnesium Toxicity Signs
  - Loss of DTRs
  - Respiratory depression <12/min,
  - Oliguria < 30 cc/hr
  - SOB/chest pain
  - Cardiac arrest
- Nursing priorities when Mag toxicity occurs
  - STOP MAG SULFATE IMMEDIATELY
  - Notify MD
  - Give calcium gluconate 1g (10ml of 10% solution) slooooowly until calcium begins to antagonize effects of magnesium
  - Have bag and mask ready for assisted respirations if RR < 10
  - May need to intubate

Blood Pressure Medications
- Used if BP > 160/110
- These are used to prevent cerebral vascular events in mother and to decrease chance of Abruptio placentae
- Goal is BP diastolic of 90-100mm Hg
- BP < 90 diastolic may lead to uteroplacental insufficiency
- Hydralazine Hydrochloride is the treatment of choice by ACOG
  - Action: arteriolar vasodilator
  - Indication: BP >160/110
  - Dose: depends on response
  - Adverse reaction: flushing, HA, Maternal/fetal tachycardia, Palpitations,uteroplacental insufficiency, Late decels,distress
- Labetalol
  - Action: decreases BP by vasodilatation, decreases heart rate
  - Indication: BP> 160/110
  - Dose: depends on response- usually 5-10 mg over 2-3 minutes
  - Repeat doses at 10 min intervals prn
  - Adverse reactions: hypotension, fetal/ maternal bradycardia, hypoglycemia, bronchospasm
  - Pt needs continuous cardiac monitoring. Contraindicated in patients with asthma or heart block > 1st degree
- Nursing actions
  - Monitor fetal and maternal response
  - Continuous monitoring
  - Frequent BP+ HR monitoring. Q 5 minutes during bolus, then Q 15 minutes until stable
  - Assess urine output
  - Side lying bed rest/Side rails up
- Betamethasone
  - Action: used to stimulate fetal lung maturity and production or release of fetal surfactant
  - Indication: to reduce or prevent the severity of respiratory distress syndrome in the preterm infant(24-36 weeks gestation)
  - Dose: Betamethasone 12mg IM x 2 doses 24° apart if possible.
  - Adverse reactions: maternal infection, pulmonary edema, worsening DM or BP
  - Give deep IM in gluteal muscle
  - Assess for pulmonary edema, worsening blood sugar,worsening hypertension
  - Do not give if the women has infection
  - Usually given if women is in preterm labor 24-36 weeks gestation
  - It takes at least 24° to develop lung maturity. Administer early!

Neonatal Infections

Neonatal Sepsis
Infection spreads rapidly through blood, and one of the most common we see in the nursery is staph or strep. If it's strep it's usually because somebody has a cold such as staff, nurse or even mom. Staph comes from the skin and is a result of poor hygiene, so practice good handwashing! There are about 1-5 incidences per 1000 births and the risks go up with the little babies in NICU. Sadly, infections in the neonate have a high mortality rate.

Sepsis: Risk Factors
- Maternal low SES
- Prolonged labor
- Premature labor
- Maternal UTI
- PROM
- Twin gestation
- there are others, but these are the main ones.

Sepsis: Signs & Symptoms
- Apnea, bradycardia
- Tachypnea, grunting, nasal flaring, retractions, low O2 saturations...basically signs of respiratory distress.
- Sepsis, which shows as acidosis, decreased cardiac output, hypotension, fever, elevated white count, decreased perfusion, decreased urine output, coagulopathies, etc.. For more information about sepsis, see the Sepsis Latte at www.straightanursingstudent.com

Diagnostic Tests for Neonatal Sepsis
- CBC with diff
- Chest X-ray
- Gram stains
- Pan cultures...blood (2), urine, sputum, spinal fluid, skin...basically anything and everything.

Therapy for Neonatal Sepsis
- Instituted before results of workup are obtained
- Two antibiotics, usually ampicillin and gentamicin given for about 7 to 14 days with the goal of maintaining respirations, optimizing hemodynamics, supporting nutritionally and achieving metabolic homeostasis.

TORCH Infections
- Toxoplasmosis S&S: convulsions, coma, hydrocephalus, microcephaly Survivors are often blind, severely retarded or deaf. Cats are carriers (pregnant women should not clean the litter box!)
- Rubella: can cause congenital cataracts and heart defects, deafness. Babies are infectious at birth and must be put into isolation. The treatment for this is to basically prevent it...mom must get the vaccine right before she leaves the hospital and she absolutely cannot get pregnant for three months!
- Cytomegalovirus infects a small number of newborns (0.5-2.5%), but is has a significant mortality rate of up to 30%. It causes a lot of problems including mental deficits, microcephaly, hydrocephaly, cerebral palsy, hearing deficits.
- Herpes Simplex is passed to the baby during the birthing process as baby passes through the vaginal canal. If mom has a present lesion she has to have a C/S because the risk of transmission is so high (50%). Babies get symptoms soon after birth, about 2-12 days and will have temperature regulation problems (too high or too low), jaundice, won't eat well, will have lesions and possibly even seizures. You'll treat with medication!

Other Infections
- Gonorrhea: babies will have neonatal conjunctivitis (aka ophthalmia neonatorum), corneal ulcerations and discharge and may even get septic. You'll treat prophylactically with erythromycin ointment.
- Syphilis: Baby will have a red or copper-colored rash, fissures at his mouth, be cranky, look edematous, have rhinitis and possibly othes. You need to isolate these babes and give them penicillin.

- Hepatitis B is passed from mom to babe during childbirth, and can be prevented with a routine vaccine. If a baby is born to an infected mom, he will get immunoprophylaxis.
- HIV is an opportunistic disease with a vertical transmission of 13-40%. If you suspect HIV in your babe, you'll test them before they are 48-hrs old and can get results via PCR in 24-hours. You'll test again at 1-2 months and once more at 4-6 months. The signs of HIV are numerous and can include recurrent respiratory infections, rhinorrhea, enlarged glands/spleen/liver, and pneumonia (there are lots more). You will treat this baby by providing optimal nutrition to facilitate growth, protect him from infections, promote attachment with mom, provide good skin care and comfort the poor little guy.

Bacterial Infections

- Group B Strep signs/symptoms are respiratory distress and pneumonia, apnea (not breathing), shock states, meningitis (late-onset). Long-term youll see neurologic complications. Risk factors for this infection are being premature, a maternal fever at time of birth, ROM >24 hrs, an infant that was previously infected and GBS bacteriuria in current pregnancy. Babies are screened and treated with prophylactic abx.
- Chlamydia Trachomatis will show as newborn conjunctivitis and pneumonia. You'll give these babes the erythromycin ointment (I think all babies get this actually).
- Other Bacterial Infections include TB (if active don't let baby have direct contact with mom), e. Coli, fungal infections, listeriosis and candidiasis (thrush, diaper rash...give Nystatin)

Low Risk Pregnancy

Uterine Changes

Think of pregnancy as 1,2, 3 trimester.

- Enlargement of uterus due to cell hypertrophy. When you think of a cell as a round cell with nucleus in center...the way the uterus is able to enlarge, the cells elongate (they don't increase in number). There is no other organ in the body that can change shape and grow like the uterus can.
- Thickening of the walls
- Increase in vascular and lymphatic system. Think of the uterus as a "mother organ", in that all the nutrients that enable egg to implant are inside on the endometrial lining. So, we need to have an awesome vascular and lymphatic system in order for the pregnancy to be healthy.
- Height of fundus changes as pregnancy goes along...the change tells us how far along they are. By the time you can feel the fundus at the umbilicus, you are about halfway (20 weeks). Baby "drops" at 40 weeks into the pelvis (will be about two finger-breadths below xiphoid)
- Formula for calculating due date:
- If you calculate she's at 20 weeks, but only measures 16..the first thing you should think is that the dates are off. Keep it simple!
  - Look at mom's nutrition and lifestyle habits if you suspect that the baby is small for gestational age.

Cervical Changes

- Development of mucous plug. Serves as a barrier to keep pathogens from migrating up into fundus and affecting fetus. Communication between vagina and uterus is the cervix (only about an inch). If something lives in vagina, it's going to seek out a better environment in the uterus. The plug helps keep this from happening. It is released toward the end of pregnancy (around a week to a day prior to delivery). Losing the plug is a sign that the cervix is softening up.
- Goodell's sign - softening. We examine the cervix to see if she is pregnant...it will feel soft. In a non-pregnant woman it feels like a button.
- Chadwick's sign - bluish-purple discoloration d/t hypervascularization r/t pregnancy.

Vaginal Changes

- Hypertrophy, increased vascularization, hyperplasia due to estrogen. Looks really bright pink d/t blood supply. The hyperplasia due to estrogen causes an overgrowth of cell and enables elasticity of the vagina.
- Increase in secretions, loosening of connective tissue. All of this is d/t hormonal response regulated by anterior and posterior pituitary. Anytime there is an increase in estrogen you have an increase in secretions.

Breast Changes

- Glandular hyperplasia and hypertrophy. Breasts start to enlarge...gain 1-2 pounds of breast tissue on average (1-2 cup sizes).
- Darkened areolae, superficial veins prominent.
- Striae may develop d/t breast tissue stretching.
- Colostrum is secreted usually around 30 weeks.

Respiratory Changes

- Tidal volume increases to meet oxygen demands of the fetus. Body becomes more efficient oxygen machine!
- Oxygen consumption increases
- Breathing changes from abdominal to thoracic. As diaphragm is pushed by an enlarging fetus, there is less lung expansion into abdominal space.
- Vascular congestion of nasal mucosa. When you get hypervascularization in the nose, you get stuffy noses and nose bleeds. Who knew?

Cardiac Changes

The gigantic uterus is sitting on the pelvic vasculature...why doesn't it collapse? In order to accommodate, we have to increase the blood volume and circulating volume.

- Blood volume increases 40 to 45% (with twins it can go up to 60%). This does not increase blood pressure...in fact, many women experience a drop in blood pressure when pregnant. This also increases oxygen carrying capacity of the blood. When mom delivers the baby, she now has a "cushion" so she doesn't bleed to death.
- Decrease in systemic and pulmonary vascular resistance so blood can get where it needs to go.
- Increase in cardiac output, basically the heart becomes a more efficient pump.

GI Changes
- Nausea and vomiting happens in early pregnancy. Shouldn't be vomiting after about 14 weeks.
- Hyperemia, softening and bleeding of gums (d/t vascularization)
- Constipation. As uterus enlarges we have a mechanical compression of the colon AND we have a bolus of progesterone (the hormone of relaxation...it's a smooth muscle relaxant) which causes smooth muscle to relax including GI tract. The woman needs to eat lots and lots of fiber.
  - FYI! The progesterone is systemic...the smooth muscle relaxant is another reason the BP stays low, vericose veins, peripheral edema.
- Heartburn d/t relaxation of sphincter and growth of the fundus.
- Hemorrhoids b/c woman isn't taking in enough fiber, vasodilation of vascular system, straining.

FYI:
If a non-pregnant person lose 500 ml of blood, it drops Hgb down by 1 and Hct down by 3

Urinary Changes
- Pressure on bladder causes frequency
- Dilatation of kidneys and ureteres
- Increased GFR and renal plasma flow. We pay attention to this to determine if mom is spilling sugar or protein into urine. Increased BP + protein in urine are precursers for pre-eclampsia. Sugar in urine = gestational diabetes.

Skin Changes
- Hyperpigmentation...can't do anything about it and is d/t genetics. *Linea negra* is the line that goes up the belly from umbilicus to pubis.
- Striae
- Chloasma is the "raccoon mask" on the face. This can also happen with BC pills.
- Vascular spider nevi...little vessels on legs.
- Decreased hair growth or increased...depends on hair cycle.
- Hyperactive sweat and sebaceous glands.

Musculoskeletal Changes
Progesterone also works on ligaments and tendons
- Pelvic joints relax, gets loose. Feels like "hinged together with rubber bands."
- Center of gravity changes (safety issue). If a woman wears high heels this will make backache worse. Backache is due to attachments of uterus...two of them tie directly into the back.
- Separation of rectus abdominus. These muscles hold you upright and are very important! Babies need to spend all their time on their tummy unless sleeping. This is the only way the baby develops back, neck and abdominal muscles. The rectus abdominus supports the back. In pregnancy, the muscle has to stretch and thin and for some women it separates...that's called the rectus diastesis. Palpate at umbilcus...walk fingers across abdomen and if they "fall into the ditch" then they have a separation here. Exercise: walk a lot...do side-lying leg raises.

Eye, Cognitive, and Metabolic Changes
- Decreased intraocular pressure d/t vasodilation
- Thickening of cornea
- Reports of decreased attention, concentration, and memory
- Extra water, fat, and protein are stored
- Fats more completely absorbed

Endocrine Changes

- T4 and BMR increase, TSH decreases.
  - If we have a woman with thyroid problems, we have to stay on top of this! If you are hypothyroid, you can produce microcephaly in the fetus leading to permanent brain damage. No bueno. This baby will get on thyroid hormone as soon as born, and mom will be on it also during pregnancy.
- Concentration of parathyroid hormone increases
- Thyrotropin and adrenotropin alter maternal metabolism. Mom uses fat more efficiently and may be hungry a lot.
- Prolactin is responsible for lactation. It is released AFTER delivery of placenta.
- Oxytocin (secreted from pituitary and it causes uterine contractions) and vasopressin are secreted. At some point a bolus of oxytocin is released and this starts labor.
- Increased aldosterone

Physical Symptoms of Pregnancy

- Braxton Hicks contractions...the uterus stretching. Usually go away if get up and walk.
- Increased vaginal discharge and risk of infection. d/t hypervascularity of vagina...the secretsions can act as a wick for pathogens.
- Leaking of colostrum, especially if already had a baby.
- Hyperventilation d/t shallow breathing r/t huge fundus.
- Nasal stuffiness and nosebleeds
- Lower extremity edema
- Postural hypotension
- Supine hypotensive syndrome...mom lies on back and presses on vena cava → loss of consciousness/faint. Have mom lie on her left side or sit her up.
- Nausea and vomiting
- Bleeding of gums
- Constipation and hemorrhoids
- Pruritus
- Figure 14–1 Vena caval syndrome. The gravid uterus compresses the vena cava when the woman is supine. This reduces the blood flow returning to the heart and may cause maternal hypotension.
- Physical Symptoms of Pregnancy (cont'd)
- Urinary frequency
- Hyperpigmentation (linea nigra)
- Striae
- Vascular spider nevi
- Decreased rate of hair growth
- Heavy perspiration, night sweats, acne
- Waddling gait
- Backache
- Difficulty wearing contact lenses d/t changes in intraocular pressure.

Presumptive Signs of Pregnancy

- Amenorrhea
- Nausea and vomiting
- Excessive fatigue
- Urinary frequency
- Breast changes
- Quickening (may feel fetal movement)

Probable Signs of Pregnancy

- Changes in the pelvic organs
- Enlargement of the abdomen
- Braxton Hicks contractions can be felt
- Abdominal striae

- Uterine souffle (listen with Doppler, can hear sound of uterus). This is the mother's pulse in the vasculature of the placenta. This is NOT the fetal heart rate!
- Changes in skin pigmentation
- Hegar's sign, a softening of the isthmus of the uterus, can be determined by the examiner during a vaginal examination. (picture to right)
- Early uterine changes of pregnancy. **A**, Ladin's sign, a soft spot anteriorly in the middle of the uterus near the junction of the body of the uterus and the cervix. *(see picture on bottom)* **B**, Braun von Fernwald's sign, irregular softening and enlargement at the site of implantation. **C**, Piskacek's sign, a tumorlike, asymmetric enlargement (B and C not pictured)
- Ballottement. Can push up on cervix and feel something bob up and down...that is the fetal head.
- Positive pregnancy tests

Positive Signs of Pregnancy
- Auscultation of fetal heartbeat
- Fetal movement (woman can feel it and gets more intense as pregnancy goes on...others can begin to feel it from outside...it eventually becomes uncomfortable for mom.)
- Visualization of the fetus via ultrasound.

Pregnancy Tests (look up each of these in book)
- Hemagglutination-inhibition (HI) test
- Latex agglutination test
- β-subunit radioimmunoassay (RIA)
- Immunoradiometric assay (IRMA)
- Enzyme-linked immunosorbent assay (ELISA)
- Fluoroimmunoassay (FIA)
- Home Pregnancy Tests
    - Enzyme immunoassay tests:
    - False-positive results low
    - False-negative results higher

Mother's Response to Pregnancy
- Ambivalence is very common
- Acceptance
- Introversion
- Mood swings
- Changes in body image can be good or bad. It depends. This is not a reversible change...cervix is changed forever, uterus shrinks but can expand more easily, striae remain, vericose veins may get worse.

Rubin's (1984) Tasks of Pregnancy
- Ensuring safe passage through pregnancy, labor, and birth
- Seeking of acceptance of this child by others
- Seeking of commitment and acceptance of self as mother to the infant (binding-in). Women have to go through the process of seeing themselves as a mother and this needs to happen during pregnancy. If it doesn't, there are probs...will see with substance abusing moms fo sho.
- Learning to give of oneself on behalf of one's child

Father's Response to Pregnancy
- Confused by partner's mood changes
- Feels left out of pregnancy...need to help dad see he is a partner. Moms need to communicate with dads.
- Resents attention given to the woman
- Resents changes in their relationship
- Needs to resolve conflicts about fathering...need to take on mantle of fatherhood.
- Couvade...man experiences things wife is experiencing...abdominal discomfort, constipation, back hurts.

High Risk L&D

Taking care of patients who have non-reasurring pattern

- A non-reassuring pattern is:
  - no variability
  - less than 2 accelerations
  - decelerations
- In antepartum setting, you are looking at variable and accelerations
- Parameters for 28-32 weeks is different than 32 weeks or greater
- What about in labor?
  - looking for late decels (these are bad)
  - variability is THE most important thing!
    - moderate variability shows the CNS is intact
    - absent variability is no bueno...this would be a big issue if it was moderate before and now has become absent. If pt had medication, then this may not be so much of a concern b/c the meds affects the baby.
    - minimal may be bad (probably is)
    - marked is also not good
- Category 1: has variablity, maybe a random decel (but most likely none), has accelerations
- Category 2: starting to get into a little gray area; physician can proceed forward with usual plan of care; moderate or minimal variability; may have recurring decels (of any type);
- Category3 : absent or minimal variability with repetitive late decels; baby is not coping
- What's the first thing you would do if pt had repetitive variable decels?
  - reposition, increase IV, put Oxygen on mom, call doc (You will reposition b/c the variable decels are d/t cord compression).
  - You would give O2 if she had decreased variability (according to Dr. Ferguson)
  - Baby can get late decels from mom lying on her back (so position change), or from having low BP (so give IV bolus).

Things you need for precipitous birth

- IV
- Oxygen
- BOA kit (Birth on Arrival kit)

What kind of risks are involved with precipitous birth?

- Tearing at perineum
- Hemorrhage d/t lacerations and such
- Pneumothorax (not in boook!). This can happen to baby when he takes his first breath.
- Low APGAR scores
- Meconium aspiration
- Brachial palsy

What is considered a post-date birth? 42 weeks...

- These women will get misoprostal or pitocin induction (make sure contractions aren't too close together, monitor for fetal distress; mom will need an epidural b/c pitocin hurts; potential post-delivery problems for baby r/t epidural; hemorrhage can happen PP b/c sites are saturated with pitocin already and mom isn't going to contract very well; non-reassuring patterns b/c BOW broken causes temps to go up, resting tone too high and contractions too close together can cause fetal distress;
  - High-Dose and Low-Dose Pitocin
  - Start out at around 4, and go up in "jumps" to get woman in labor...or can go up gradually I guess? See book. Basically RNs utilize a protocol for this, but the idea is to start low and titrate accordingly.
  - Baby is most likely going to be large with post-date moms
    - Shoulder dystocia, brachial palsy (whatever it's called)
- May have amniotomy (infection)
- C/S...and all the complications
- Maternal anxiety

Twin presentation
- One can be vertex and the other can be breech
- What they can do for the breech twin is do an internal rotation of the baby. This is usually the 2nd baby.

Macrosomia (> 4500 grams)
- Shoulder dystocia
- hemorrhage
- Don't know if pelvis is adequate, mom may need C/S
- McRobert's maneuver if head comes out and shoulder doesn't.
    - Pull mom's legs back to open pelvis more, this can help get baby out; also put pressure above pubic bone to dislodge the shoulder (but can break the clavicle)
- U/S is not reliable in establishing fetal weight

Amniotic Fluid Embolus
- pretty rare, but mortality rate is very high (61-81%)
- mom gets amniotic fluid from baby that has crossed over into maternal circulation
- Causes circulatory collapse and system-wide problems that go into DIC
- Occurrence = 1:20,000 to 1:30,000 live births
- Moms usually end up going to ICU, will probably be on vent
- Teach mom to tell you if she has any difficulty breathing...this is serious!

Hydramnios (fluid > 2000 ml)
- May be related to congenital abnormalities
- Diabetes mom if BS is out of control; baby pees a lot b/c there is too much glucose
- Twins can have this also
- Can be chronic or acute (20-24 weeks)
- Mom may have difficulty breathing d/t big uterus; may remove some of the fluid
- Big issue in labor is that baby is floating around a lot and don't engage real well. If baby doesn't engage, then can have cord prolapse when BOW ruptures.

Olligohydramnios (fluid < 500 ml)
- Cause unknown
- Seen in post-maturity and IUGR (IUGR is usually r/t malformation in placenta, can be r/t PIH and placenta not getting good blood flow, so smoking can cause this also; two types of IUGR...assymetrical and symmetrical. Symmetrical means baby is small but proportionate (< 10% in growth); with assymetrical, the head is bigger than the abdomen and femur length...baby looks really skinny like a little old man; with IUGR the blood is spared for the most important organs (brain, heart, adrenal glands)...so abdomen is not going to get bigger but head is! Kidneys aren't getting enough blood so the kidneys aren't making enough urine which leads to oligohydramnios.
- If mom is post-date: will be induced
    - Mom will have variables (decelerations) b/c she doesn't have a lot of extra fluids so the vein is compressed.
    - May get amnioinfusion to get some of the pressure off the cord
- If mom is 28 weeks, she will be monitored via antepartum testing (fluid tested weekly or biweekly), NST, maybe biophysical profile.

Analgesic Agents
- Administration- based on
    - woman's request
    - established labor pattern
    - baseline assessment of mom & baby
    - progress of labor
- Types
    - Sedatives: barbituates (Seconal, Ambien); benzos (valium, versed) flumazenil is benzo reversal agent; H-1 Receptor antagonists (Phenergan, Vistaril, Benadryl); Narcotics (Stadol, Nubain, Demerol); Narcan is reversal for opioids

- Narcotic (Stadol, Nubain, Demoral...IV administration preferred, may precipitate drug withdrawal)
- H1-Receptor agonists: Phenergen, Vistaril, Benadryl
- Nursing Management
  - Determine Stage of Labor
  - Evaluate contraction frequency, duration, & intensity,
  - Established fetal well being
  - Desired effect & side effects
  - Safe form of transportation
  - Red Flags – Multipara greater than 8 cm, Advanced dilation primipara

Regional Anesthesia
- Temporary and reversible loss of sensation
- Types
  - Lumbar epidural – Uterus, Cervix, Vagina, & Perineum
  - Pudendal – Perineum & lower Vagina- Given in Second Stage, just before birth
  - Local infiltration –Perineum Given just before birth
  - Spinal – Uterus, Cervix, Vagina, & Perineum
- Risk- less than general anesthesia – produced by injecting anesthetic into specific area-agent direct contact with nervous tissue

Lumbar Epidural
- Administration
  - Injection of local anesthetic agent into epidural space
- Continuous block
  - Block continuous – usually administered during active labor, 85% achieve complete relief, 15% partial, & 3% no relief
- Advantages & Disadvantages
  - Advantages: Adequate pain relief, Woman fully awake during labor and birth process, Allows for internal rotation, Adjusted to allow for laboring down
  - Disadvantages: Hypotension, Severe Complications -Postdural puncture, seizure, meningitis, cardio-respiratory arrest, vertigo
  - Problems- Major problem Hypotension, Inadequate block-One sided block, Pruritus, Break through pain, Maternal temperature
  - Headaches, migraine headaches, neckaches, & tingling of the hands and fingers (Cunningham et al., 2005), Systemic toxic reaction
  - Redflags- drop in maternal blood pressure, fetal deceleration, respiratory depression, post delivery headache-worse with ambulation
- Contraindications
  - Local or systemic infection
  - Coagulation disorder or low PLT count
  - Anticipated maternal hemorrhage
  - Abuptio placentae, Placenta previa
  - Allergy to a specific class of local anesthetics
  - Women with heart failure or aortic stenosis

Spinal Block
- Local anesthetic into spinal fluid (subarachnoid space)
  - Injected directly into the spinal fluid
  - Failure rate is low
  - Allows the drug to immediately mix with cerebrospinal fluid
  - Eliminates window (whatever that means). Usually used for operative delivery (C/S)
- Advantages & Disadvantages
  - Advantages: immediate onset, smaller drug volume, relative ease of administration
  - Disadvantages: intense blockade of sympathetic fibers, greater potential for fetal hypoxia, uterine tone is maintained, short acting so difficult to maintain

- Complications
  - Hypotension (prehydrate 500-2000 ml)
  - Ephedrine drug reaction- total spinal neurological sequelae (not sure what this means)
  - Anesthesia occurs at C3-C5 level
  - Respiratory function impaired
  - Spinal headache in 1-3%
  - Lasts up to 7 days
  - Blood patch performed, helps spinal headache

Pudendal Block
- Perineal anesthesia for second stage labor, birth & episiotomy repair; injected below pudendal plexus
- Advantages & Disadvantages
  - Adv: ease of administration, absence of hypoT, allows use of vacuum or low forceps delivery
  - Dis: urge to bear down may be decreased; burning sensation when block administered

Local Infiltration
- Intracutaneous, subcutaneous, & intramuscular
  - Injected into the perineum
- Advantages & Disadvantages
  - Adv: least amount of anesthetic agent used; done just prior to birth
  - Dis: large amounts of solution used; burning sensation at time of injection

General Anesthesia
- Methods Used
  - IV Injection
    - Pentothal –short acting Narcosis 30 seconds after IV administration
    - Ketamine – intermediate acting, contraindicated with preeclampsia or chronic hypertension
  - Inhalation of anesthetic agent
    - Nitrous oxide -Fetal uptake in 20 minutes; Isofluorane, halothane, sevoflurane, desflurane, enflurane – (may be in combination with Nitrous), May be used in combination with spinal or epidural anesthesia
  - Combination of both of the above
- Administration considerations
  - Preterm: susceptible to depressant drugs; poorly developed BBB; medication will attain higher concentration in CNS; decreased ability to metabolize and excrete drug after birth; use smallest dose possible
  - Preeclampsia: regional anesthesia preferred
  - Diabetes: reduction in placental blood flow, hypoT likely, CV depression during block, higher sympathetic blockade
  - Cardiac disease
    - Mild Stenosis: preferred method is continuous epidural and low forceps delivery, no valsava maneuvers;
    - Hypotension, controlled IV fluids, epidural or general anesthesia for C/S; avoid ketamine b/c it causes tachycardia
  - Bleeding:
    - If there is no active bleeding, FHR is good, and mom;s CV status is stable, then epidural is OK
    - if there is active bleeding, then treat hypovolemia; regional block is contraindicated in active bleeding, general anesthesia-Pentothal (a cardiac depressant and vasodilator) and Ketamine are recommended.
- Complications
  - General anesthesia has risk of aggravating maternal HTN
  - Intubation may be difficult, may cause mucosal edema in oral cavity and glottis
  - Fetal depression...anesthetic agent reaches fetus in about 2 minutes
  - Uterine relaxation, uterine atony
  - Decreased gastric motility (undigested food makes for production of more gastric juices which can be aspirated (Mendelson's syndrome/chemical pneumonitis). This is a leading cause of maternal death and it is due to the failure to establish a patent airway
  - Red flags for intubation is obesity!

Dysfunctional Labor Patterns (slide 12)
- Abnormal labor pattern
- MOST COMMON INDICATION FOR C/S
- It is termed 'dystocia"...an abnormal labor pattern resulting in prolonged labor
- The abnormality occurs with one of these three Ps (or maybe all): Power (contractions), Passenger (fetus) or Passageway (soft tissue or pelvis)
- **Hypertonic Labor Patterns**
  - Ineffective uterine contractions in the latent phase, resting tone is increased
  - Contractions are painful but ineffective. There is no cervical dilation or effacement
  - Contractions more frequent
  - Clinical Therapy = bedrest, sedation, oxytocin or amniotomy, rule out CPD or malpresentation.
- **Hyptonic Labor Patterns**
  - Cause -Unknown
    - Genetic factors which control normal physiologic process of labor
    - C-section and operative deliveries run in families
    - Advanced maternal age
  - Definition = uterine contractions irregular, low amplitude, less than 1 cm dilation per hour (protracted labor) OR no change of cervical dilation for 2 hours (arrest of progress)
  - Clinical Management
    - Oxytocin or AROM
  - Nursing Care
    - Assess VS, contractions, FHR
    - Vag exam to determine dilation, descent, check for caput (it increases as hypotonic labor goes on)
    - Assess mom for stress and anxiety
  - Red flags
    - PROM
    - Maternal temp
    - Increased incidence of chorioamninotis

Precipitous Labor and Birth
- Rapid birth process: occurs within 3 hours
- Cause: low resistance in maternal soft tissues, rapid dilation, rapid descent, strong contractions
- Maternal Risks: Abruptio placenta, extensive laceration of cervix, vag and perineum
- Fetal Risks: Meconium, low apgar, brachial palsy, intracranial trauma

Postterm Pregnancy
- Definition = pregnancy that extends more than 294 days or 42 full weeks (from last menstrual period)
- Incidence = 7% of all pregnancies
- Cause = unknown; possibly error in dating; associated with previous postterm pregnancy, primiparity, placenta sulfatase deficienty, fetal ancephaly, male fetus, genetic predisposition
- Maternal Risks = labor induction, macrosomic or LGA baby, increased use of vacuum or forceps, maternal hemorrhage, increased risk of C/S; mom has anxiety, fatigue, irritability
- Fetal Risk = Decreased uterine-placental circulation; decreased blood supply, oxygen and nutrition; mortality rate goes up; potential for dysmaturity syndrome is 20%; increased risk of oligohydramnios and umbilical cord compression
- Clinical Management = Nonstress test biweekly; amniotic fluid index weekly; possible biophysical profile

Fetal Malposition
- Persistent Posterior Occiput
  - Most common fetal malposition
  - 15% in early labor...as labor progresses, it may cease or the fetus is born in the OP position 5% of the time
- Maternal symptmos: intense back pain in the small of the back throughout labor
- Maternal/Fetal Risks

- third or fourth degree laceration
- higher incidence of operative delivery
- if failure to rotate, then fetal mortality

- Clinical Management
  - close monitoring of fetus
  - safest method of delivery is spontaneous birth with manual rotation
  - forceps assisted delivery with rotation is "Scanzoni maneuver"

Fetal Malpresentations

- Brow (the least common)
  - Cause: high parity, placenta previa, uterine anomaly, hydramnios, fetal anomaly, low birthweight, large fetus
  - Mechanics: forehead of fetus is the presenting part; the head is slightly extended and the fetal head enters the birth canal with its widest diameter...OUCH!
  - Maternal Risk: prolonged labor or arrested labor; C/S
  - Fetal Risk: birth injury, cerebral and neck compression, damage to trachea and larynx.
- Face
  - Occurrence: multiparous women, women with a pendulous abdomen (Yellow Dot!)
  - Contributing factors: contracted pelvis 10-40% (I have no idea what the percentages mean); ancephaly 30%, fetal malformations 60%
  - Mechanics: face of fetus is presenting part and head is hyperextended
  - Success rate for vaginal delivery
    - 60-70%
    - no attempt to manually rotate
    - mentum posterior can become wedged on anterior surface of sacrum
    - can place FSE on mentum (fetal scalp electrode can go on the chin)
- Breech
  - Incidence: 4% overall; for gestational age of 25-26 weeks it's 25%; for gestational age of 32 weeks it's 7%
  - Associated with...
    - Placenta previa
    - implantation of placenta in cornual area
    - hydramnios
    - high parity
    - oligohydramnios
    - hydrocephaly
    - anencephaly
    - previous breech presentation
    - uterine anomalies
    - pelvic tumors
    - multiple gestations
    - fetal anomalies

  - Types of Breech Presentation
    - Frank Breech (50-70%) most common; flexed and extended hips
    - Footling Breech (10-30%) one or both hips extended, foot is presenting part, occurs more frequently with preterm labor
    - Complete Breech (5-10%) sacrum is presenting part
  - Complications: cord prolapse, head entrapment (oh boy!)
  - Medical Management:
    - External version: attempted at 37-38 weeks
    - Planned C/S
    - Alternative therapies = mugwort (Chinese)
- Shoulder
  - Definition: Infant's long axis lies across abdomen
  - Associated with...

- grandmultiparity
- lax uterine muscles
- obstructions of bony pelvis
- placenta previa
- neoplasms
- fetal anomalies
- hydramnios
- preterm fetus
- Incidence: 1 in 300; not uncommon in multiple gestations
- Clinical Management: external version if baby is 28 weeks or greater
- Complications: cord prolapse, uterine rupture

Fetal Macrosomia
- Definition: fetal weight greater than 4500 grams
- Incidence: women who are obese are more likely to have macrosomic baby
- Complication: shoulder dystocia, adequate pelvis for normal birth but not for biiig baby, possible brachial plexus injury
- Clinical Management:
  - McRobert's maneuver (lie on back with knees at chest)
  - Ultrasound for fetal weight, early induction

Multiple Gestations
- Incidence
  - Twins account for 3.2% of all pregnancies
  - Triplets account for 1.8% of all pregnancies
- Terminology
  - Dizygotic -Two separate ova (Faternal twins) 67%, Monozygotic Single ovum (Identical twin) 33%
  - Dichorionic-diamniotic twin (Single ovum) – division occurs within 72 hours after fertilization 30% of monozygotic twins
  - Monochoronic-diamniotic – division occurs at blastocyst stage 4 to 8 days after fertilization 68% of monozygotic twins
  - Monochorionic-monoamniotic – division occurs in primitive germ disk 9 to 13 days past fertilization 2% of monozygotic twins
- Maternal Complications
  - spontaneous abortion, gestational diabetes, HTN, pulmonary edema, maternal anemia, hydramnios, PROM, incompetent cervix, IUGR, preterm birth
  - uterine dysfunction, uterine atony or hemorrhage
- Clinical Management
  - Decision is made based on presence of complications and presentation of fetus
  - If no complications and both are vertex, then vag birth
  - Placenta is examined after and sent to pathology to determine if mono or dizygotic twins

Placenta Problems
- Types
  - Developmental: placenta lesions, succenturiate placenta, circumvaliate placenta, battledore placenta
  - Degenerative: infarct and placental calcifications
- Placental Problems (Developmental)
  - Succenturiate Placenta
    - One or more accessory lobes is attached to the main placenta by fetal vessels
    - Complications: PP hemorrhage; no complications for baby
  - Circumvallate Placenta
    - Fetal surface of placenta exposed through an opening around the umbilical cord; vessel descends from cord and ends at margin (I have absolutely NO IDEA what this means)
    - Maternal Complications are linked to threatened abortion: PTL, painless bleeding after 20 weeks, placental insufficiency, intrapartum hemorrhage

- Fetal Complications: IUGR, prematurity, death
- Developmental Problems of the Placenta
  - Definition: insertion of the cord within 1.5 cm of the margin
  - Incidence: 5-7% of all pregnancies
  - Maternal Complications: PTL, bleeding in labor, vessel rupture
  - Fetal Complications: prematurity and fetal distress
- Degenerative Changes of Placenta
  - Definition: excessive calcifications or infarcts
  - Affects uterine/placental fetal exchange
  - Causes: HTN (PIH or chronic), smoking
  - Grade 0: lasts 1st trimester through early 2nd trimester only; uniform moderate ethnogenicity; smooth chorionic plate without indentations
  - Grade 1: mid 2nd trimester through early 3rd trimester (18-29 weeks), subtle indentations of chorionic plate, small and diffuse calcifications (hyperechoic) that are randomly dispersed in the placenta
  - Grade 2: late 3rd trimester (around 30 weeks through delivery); larger indentations along the chorionic plate; larger calcifications in a dot-dash configuration along the basilar plate
  - Grade 3: 39 weeks to post dates; complete indentations of chorionic plate through to the basilar plate creating "cotyledons"...these are portions of the placenta separated by the indentations; there are more irregular calcifications with significant shadowing; may signify placental dysmaturity which can cause IUGR; associated with smoking, chronic HTN, SLE and diabetes

Umbilical Cord Abnormalities
- Types
  - Umbilical vein: true knot, hypercoiled cord, short cord, long cord
  - Insertion variations: velamentous insertion, vasa previa
- Valementous Insertion
  - Incidence: 1-2% of all placentas
  - Definition: cord insertion into membranes; vessels run between amnion and chorion
  - Maternal complication: hemorrhage if one of the vessels is torn
  - Fetal complications: fetal stress, hemorrhage

Amniotic Fluid Embolism
- Definition: bolus of amniotic fluid enters maternal circulation and lungs causing a massive immune response to occur
- Cause: unknown
- Mortality rate: 61-86% of women die; 50-61% of fetuses die; it is the SECOND LEADING CAUSE of maternal death
- Signs of symptoms: respiratory distress, restlessness, dyspnea, cyanosis, pulmonary edema, respiratory arrest
- Signs of circulatory collapse: tachyC, hypoT, shock, cardiac arrest
- Nursing response: optimize perfusion and oxygenation, maximize cardiac output and BP, deliver a live fetus!

Hydraminos
- Definition: greater than 2000 ml of fluid (aka "polyhydramnios")
- Cause: unknown; occurs in major congenital anomalies, gestational diabetes, anencephaly, twins
- Types
  - Chronic: fluid builds gradually
  - Acute: fluid builds suddenly between 20-24 weeks
- Clinical Management: needle amniotomy to decrease symptoms of maternal dyspnea and pain
- Red flag: watch for prolapsed cord in labor!

Oligohydramnios
- Definition: less than 500 ml amniotic fluid
- Cause: unknown, found in postmaturity and IUGR
- Clinical Management: biophysical profile, NST, serial ultrasounds

- Considerations in labor: amnioinfusion

Cephalopelvic Disproportion (CPD)
- Definition: a contracture in any of the following:
  - maternal bony pelvis (beginning at inlet where the ischial tuberous has a diameter of < 8cm, and ending at outlet)
  - maternal soft tissues
- Medical Management:
  - trial of labor...mom labors down and the forces of labor push the biparietal diameter of the fetal head beyond the interspinous obstruction
  - If mom has an infection, then labor is prolonged....or she meant that prolonged labor leads to infection.
- Treatment: C/S for no progress
- Red Flags
  - unengaged head in early labor with primigravidas
  - hypotonic uterine contractions
  - deflexion of fetal head
  - uncontrolled pushing before compete dilation
  - failure to descend
  - edema of anterior portion of cervix

Birth Related Procedures
- Version
  - Definition – turning the fetus to change the presentation by abdominal or intrauterine manipulation, in which the fetus is changed from a breech, transverse, or oblique lie to a cephalic presentation by external manipulation
  - Success rate – 60%
  - Types
    - external cephalic version – may be attempted after 36 to 37 weeks applying pressure to the fetal head and buttocks so that the fetus completes a backward flip or forward roll
    - Podalic version – used in second twin deliveries during a vaginal birth; obstetrician places hands inside of uterus, grabs the fetus feet and then turns the fetus from transverse or non cephalic presentation to a breech presentation
  - Criteria – single fetus, fetal breech not engaged, adequate amniotic fluid, reactive nonstress test, fetus must be at 36 to 37 weeks,
  - Contraindications
    - suspected IUGR, fetal anomalies, presence of abnormal FHR, rupture membranes, cesarean birth indicated anyway, maternal problems –gestational diabetes (requiring insulin), uncontrolled hypertension, preeclampsia, maternal cardiac disease
    - Amniotic fluid abnormalities – oligo or poly, previous lower uterine segment c-section, nuchal cord, multiple gestation, third trimester bleeding, uterine malformation

Induction of Labor
- Types
  - Stripping Membranes –sweeping motion separate amniotic membranes from lower uterine segment and internal os – thought to release prostaglandins
  - Oxytocin Infusion – High dose vs low dose
  - Cervical Ripening Agents – cytotec, cervidil, prepdil
  - Mechanical – Balloon catheter, laminaria
  - Complementary – intercouse, nipple stimulation, Herbs, castor oil, accupressure
- Indication for Induction -Diabetes Mellitus, renal disease, preeclampsia, hypertensive disorders, PROM, Chorioamnionitis, fetal demise, postterm gestation, IUGR, Isoimmunization, history of rapid delivery, mild abruption placenta, nonreassuring antepartal testing, severe oligohydramnios
- Contraindications -Abnormal fetal heart rate pattern, breech presentation, unknown fetal presentation, multiple gestation, polyhydramnios, presenting part above maternal pelvic inlet, severe hypertension, maternal heart

disease, complete placenta previa, vasa previa, abruptio placentae, prolapsed cord, previous myomectomy, vaginal bleeding unknown cause, transverse lie, more than 1 previous c-section, cpd, active genital herpes

- Prelabor Status Evaluation- Bishop score
  - 5 criteria; cervial dilation, cervical effacement, fetal station, cervical consistency, cervical position

Amniotomy

- Definition: artificial rupture of membranes (AROM); uses a hook inserted through the cervix to break the bag of water
- Advantages:
  - contractions elicited are similar to spontaneous labor
  - usually there is no risk of hypertonus or ruptured uterus
  - does not require intensive monitoring
  - EFM facilitated due to ability to place the fetal scalp electrode
  - color and composition of amniotic fluid can be evaluated
- Disadvantages
  - Increased incidence of infection, cord prolapse compression and molding of fetal head
  - variable decels
  - fetal injury
  - bleeding if undiagnosed vasa previa is present
- Red flags: amniotomy with undescended fetal head can lead to cord prolapse

Amnioinfusion

- Introduction of warmed normal saline into amniotic cavity through an IUPC
- Indications
  - oligohydramnios
  - fetal cord compression
  - severe variable decels or prolonged decels
  - meconium stained fluid
- Contraindications
  - Amnionitis
  - hydramnios
  - uterine hypertonus
  - multiple gestation
  - known fetal anomaly
  - uterine anomaly
  - nonreassuring fetal status requiring birth
  - nonvertex presentation
- Procedure: inflation of fluid bolus from 250-500 ml over 20-30 mins followed by a continuous infusion; monitor I&O
- Red flags: increasing uterine size without output or bleeding

Episiotomy

- Definition- surgical incision of the perineal body
- Types
  - Midline – performed along the median raphe of the perineum – extends down from the vaginal orifice to the fibers of the rectal sphincter
    - Disadvantage- tear will extend through anal sphincter and rectum
  - Mediolateral – begins in the midline of the posterior couchette and extends at a 45-degree angle downward to the right or left
    - Disadvantage- greater blood loss, longer healing period, postpartal discomfort, repair more difficult
  - Predisposition – large or macrosomic fetus, occiput-posterior, use of forceps or vacuum extractor, shoulder dystocia, and white race- other factors use of lithotomy position (excessive perineal stretching, encouraging or requiring sustained breath holding during second-stage pushing, time limits

- Considerations -No maternal advantage, does not protect perineum, perineal lacerations heal quicker, greater likely hood of extension
- Questions as to whether should be performed in LGA births
- Complications -Blood loss, infection, perineal discomfort, dyspareunia, flatal incontinence

Forcep-Assisted Delivery

- Definition: instrument delivery with two curved spoon-like blades; these assist in delivery of the fetal head using traction applied with contractions
- Indications:
    - Fetal distress during labor
    - Abnormal presentation
    - Breech delivery – instrument delivery of head
    - Arrest of rotation
    - Any condition that threatens the mother or fetus that can be relieved by birth
- Prerequisites -Empty bladder, fully dilated, fetal head engaged, adequate anesthesia

Vacuum Extraction

- INVOLVES THE USE OF A CUPLIKE SUCTION DEVICE THAT IS ATTACHED TO THE FETAL HEAD. TRACTION IS APPLIED DURING CONTRACTIONS TO ASSIST IN THE DESCENT AND BIRTH OF THE HEAD, AFTER WHICH, THE VACUUM CUP IS RELEASED AND REMOVED PRECEDING DELIVERY OF THE FETAL BODY.
- Accounts for 68% of all operative births
- Pump creates negative pressure -50 to 60 mmHg depends on hospital protocol
- Indications
    - Maternal exhaustion
    - fetal distress during second stage labor
    - prolonged second state or nonreassuring heart rate pattern
- Conditions
    - Presenting part must be vertex at 0 station
    - only performed by experienced practitioner
    - terminated if device pops off after three attempts and delivery does not occur
- Risks: Cephalohematoma, scalp lacerations, subdural hematoma, maternal lacerations to cervix, vagina, or perineum

Cesarean Birth

- Indications: Complete placenta previa, CPD, placental abruption, active genital herpes, umbilical cord prolapse, failure to progress, nonreassurring fetal status, breech, anomalies, previous C/S, maternal preference.
- Incisions:
    - Skin=Transverse – suboptimal visualization, does not allow for extension, Vertical - quicker
    - Uterine =Depends on need for cesarean, Lower uterine segment, Upper segment of uterine corpus
- Preoperatively
    - Consents, shave, indwelling catheter, prepare site, provide emotional support
- Intraoperatively
    - Assist in positioning of patient, fetal heart rate, instrument counts
- Postoperatively
    - Monitoring vital signs, provide pain relief, dressing and perineal pad checks, assist mother and baby with bonding

Vaginal Birth After Cesarean (VBAC)

- Success rate:
    - highest for C/S performed for breech (91%)
    - nonreassuring FHR pattern (84% success rate)
    - previous dystocia before 5 cm (67%)
    - previous dystocia 6-9 cm (73%)

- second stage dystocia (75%)
- Guidelines by ACOG: one previous C/S birth with low transverse incision, adequate pelvis, no other uterine scar or previous rupture
- Complications:
  - uterine rupture and dehiscence
    - 0.1% to 0.7% risk of rupture
  - hysterectomy
  - uterine infection
  - maternal and neonatal death
    - higher rates of stillbirth and hypoxia infants
    - transfusion

High-Risk Pregnancy

Contrast the etiology, medical therapy, and nursing interventions for the various bleeding problems associated with the first trimester of pregnancy.

- Spontaneous Abortion (Miscarriage)...first trimester
  - Etiology: 60% of first trimester SAs are due to chromosomal abnormalities: other causes are inherited thrombophelias, teratogenic drugs, faulty implantation, weakened cervix, placental abormalities, chronic disease, endocrine imbalance, polycistic ovarian syndrome, dysfunctional folate metabolism and maternal infections. Lots on pg 482.
  - Signs and Symptoms:
    - Reliable indicator = pelvic cramping and backache
    - 25% of first trimester SAs have bleeding
  - Evaluation:
    - Pelvic exam to determine the presence of cervical polyps or cervical erosion
    - Ultrasound to check for fetal heart activity and presence of gestational sac or crown-rump length that is SGA. If there is a FHR this is a good sign the pregnancy will continue (86% chance!)
    - hCG cannot confirm a live fetus b/c the levels fall slowly after fetal death
    - H & H to determine blood loss; type and cross
  - Therapy
    - Bed rest, no sex, maybe sedation.
    - Woman may be hospitalized if bleeding persists or if abortion is imminent or incomplete.
    - IV therapy and blood transfusions to replace fluid
    - D&C or suction evacuation if need to get the products out (can be outpatient if no complications)
    - Rh is woman is Rh-neg...given within 72 hours
    - If beyond 12 weeks gestation, and products of conception are not expelled then woman is induced by IV oxytocin and prostaglandins or misoprostol.
  - Nursing Interventions
    - Assess amount and apperance of vaginal bleeding
    - Monitor VS and pain
    - Ensure woman's blood type and Rh factor are identified
    - Assess FHR if > 10-12 weeks (Doppler)
    - Assess the woman's response to the crisis; evaluate coping mechanisms
    - Dx= fear, acute pain, anticipatory grieving
  - Community-Based Care
    - If woman is in first trimester and begins cramping or spotting, she may be evaluated as an outpatient
    - Guilt is a common emotion
    - Grieving period is 6-24 months
    - Referall to support group helps
- Ectopic Pregnancy (first trimester)
  - What is it?
    - Implantation of ovum in a site other than the endometrial lining of the uterus.
    - Most common location is the ampulla of the tube
  - What are the risk factors?
    - Tubal damage caused by PID; previous pelvic or tubal surgery; emdometriosis; previous ectopic pregnancy; presence of an IUD; high levels of progesterone (alters motility of egg); congenital anomalies of the tube; use of ovulation-inducing drugs; primary infertility; smoking; advanced maternal age
  - Signs & Symptoms
    - Normal S&S of pregnancy initially (including Chadwick's and Hegar's); hCG is present
    - Slow vaginal bleeding d/t fluctuating hormone levels...can lead to hypovolemic shock if really bad
    - If bleeding has occured into the pelvic cavity then a vag exam is extremely painful; may be able to palpate a mass of blood in the cul-de-sac of Douglas
    - Possibly one-sided lower abdominal pain and fainting or dizziness (50% have referred right shoulder pain)
    - 1/4 involve uterine enlargement
    - Adnexal tenderness on physical exam; 50% have palpable adnexal mass
    - Low H&H, rising leukocyte levels
    - hCG rising more slowly than usual

- Evaluation
  - Differentiate between ectopic pregnancy and other disorders (SA, ruptured corpus luteum cyst, appendicitis, salpingitis, torsion of the ovary, ovarian cysts, UTI)
  - Menstrual history
  - Pelvic exam (check for masses and tenderness)
  - Lab tests
  - Ultrasound to check for gestational sac...if you see one then it's not an ectopic pregnancy
  - Laparascopy if you can't figure it out otherwise
- Therapy
  - Methotrexate if woman wants future pregnancy and the ectopic pregnancy is not ruptured and smaller than 3.5 cm (and stable condition). There must be no fetal cardiac activity and no evidence of maternal thrombocytopenia, leukopenia, kidney disease or liver disease. The med is given IM and may be repeated in 7 days (though the one-dose regime is more common)
  - If surgery is indicated and woman wants future pregnancy, then a laparascopic linear salpingostomy is done to evacuate the ectopic pregnancy gently and preserve the tube.
  - If tube is ruptured or no future pregnancies are wanted, then a laparoscopic salpingectomy is done.
  - il woman is in shock, then an abd incision is made
- Nursing Interventions
  - First, you assess the apperance and amount of vaginal bleeding
  - Monitor VS (esp BP and pulse), and watch for signs of shock
  - Assess emotional status, etc...
  - Nursing Dx= anticipatory grieving, pain, health-seeking behavior
  - If given Methotrexate, woman is monitored as an outpatient:
    - Monitor woman for increasing abdominal pain (generally lasts 24-48 hours and is mild). More severe pain could mean the treatment failed and follow-up is needed.
      Teach mom want to report: heavy bleeding, dizziness, tachycardia
    - Monitor hCG levels...will go up for 1-4 days then decrease
  - In the hospital:
    - Start an IV and begin preop teaching
    - Watch for signs of developing shock
    - Give pain meds if needed
- Gestational Trophoblast Disease (first trimester)
  - What is it: a pathologic proliferation of trophoblastic cells
    - Hydatidiform mole (can be complete or partial)
    - Invasive mole
    - Choriocarcinoma
  - Signs and Symptoms of hydratidiform mole:
    - Vaginal bleeding as early as 4th week or as late as 2nd trimester; brownish (prune juice color), but could be bright red
    - Anemia s/t blood loss
    - Hydropic vessicles may be passed (with partial mole they are small and may not be noticed)
    - Uterine enlargement greater than expected for gestational age (in 50% of cases)
    - Absence of fetal heart sounds in the presence of other signs of pregnancy
    - Markedly elevated hCG (usually it increases from time of conception and peaks in 60-70 days then reaches a low point at 100-130 days)
    - Very low levels of MSAFP
    - Hyperemesis gravidarum (probably due to high levels of hCG)
    - Preeclampsia (esp if it continues into 2nd trimester)
    - Hyperthyroidism can occur, but is rare.
  - Evaluation
    - Ultrasound after 6-8 weeks to identify vesicular enlargement
  - Clinical Therapy
    - Suction evacuation of the mole and curettage of the uterus to remove placental fragments
    - Hysterectomy if no more kids or woman is bleeding excessively

- Treatment for choriocarcinoma:
    - These develop in 20% of women after the mole is removed
    - Women need follow up care in order to watch for this...baseline CXR to detect metastasis + a repeat CXR if chemo is needed. Also CT scan, and brain CT to rule out metastatic spread.
    - Continued high hCG is a sign of this, so the hCG is monitored every 1-2 weeks until two negatives in a row, then q 1-2 months for a year.
    - Pelvic exams q 4 weeks until remission (if getting chemo) and then q 3 months for 1 year
    - Woman needs to be on birth control during this time that hCG levels are out of whack or getting chemo
- Nursing Interventions
    - If hospitalized...monitor VS, bleeding and signs of hemorrhage.
    - Type and cross match
    - Administer oxytocin to prevent hemorrhage
    - Rh if woman is Rh negative and not sensitized.
    - Nursing Dx = fear, health-seeking behavior, anticipatory grieving

Identify the medical therapy and nursing interventions indicated in caring for a woman with an incompetent cervix.

- What is it: Painless dilation of the cervix without contractions d/t a structural or functional defect
- Contributing factors
    - Congenital factors; may be found in women exposed to DES or those with bicornuate uterus
    - Acquired factors r/t inflammation, infection, subclinical uterine activity, cervical trauma, cone biopsy or late abortions, or increased uterine volume (multiples).
    - Biochemical (hormonal) factors = increased relaxin levels
- Risk factors
    - Multiple gestations, multiple 2nd term losses, previous preterm birth, short labors...others pg 489.
- Signs and Symptoms
    - Woman is usually unaware of any contractions and presents with advanced effacement and dilatation, maybe bulging membranes
- Treatment
    - Medical Management
        - Close monitoring of cervical length via transvaginal US at 16-24 weeks
        - Bed rest
        - Progesterone supplements
        - Anti-inflammatory drugs and abx
    - Surgical Management
        - Cerclage procedures (a heavy suture to reinforce the cervix at the internal os)
            - McDonald cerclage uses a purse-string technique high up on the cervix
            - Shirodkar method uses a submucosal band placed at level of internal os
            - Abdominal cerclage may be needed for women with short or amputated cervix (others pg 490)
        - Tocolytics, Abx and anti-inflammatory drugs are given peri-operatively and for ongoing tx
        - Emergency cerclage requires 5-7 days in hospital, others are done outpatient
        - The suture can be cut after 37 weeks for vaginal birth; or left in place and C/S
- Nursing intervention
    - Treat mom signs of impending birth: lower back pain, pelvic pressure, changes in discharge

Discuss the medical therapy and nursing care of a woman with hyperemesis gravidarum.

- What is it:
    - N/V so severe it affects hydration and nutrition status
    - Occurs in 0.5 to 2% of pregnancies
    - Occurs more frequently in nulliparous women, adolescents, women with multiples, obese women, certain ethnic groups, pregnancies complicated by GTD or fetal abnormalities, and women with a family history of it.

- What causes it?
  - Still not sure, but possible culprits are hCG, estradiol, displacement of GI tract, hypofunction of pituitary and adrenal cortex, abnormalities of corpus luteum, h. pylori infection and pyshologic factors
- Diagnostic criteria
  - Hx of intractable vomiting in first half of pregnancy
  - Dehydration
  - Ketonuria
  - Loss of 5% of body weight
- Evaluation
  - Ultrasound to exclude possibility of molar pregnancy
- Clinical Therapy
  - First line: frequent small meals of simple CHOs and occasional use of antiemetics
  - If that doesn't work she may require IV fluids as an outpatient
  - If that doesn't help, she may need to be hospitalized
  - Initially, women is NPO, then given IV fluids to correct dehydration, then K to prevent hypokalemia. Woman will also get thiamine…(don't give dextrose before thiamine...this can cause Wernicke encephalopathy)
  - Desired urine output is 1000 ml/24 hours
  - Ginger can help as can acupuncture and acupressure
  - If woman does not respond to this treatment, then she gets TPN until she can take oral feedings.
    - Six small dry feedings followed by clear liquids; or…
    - 1 oz water each hour, followed as tolerated by clear liquids then nourishing liquids, advance as tolerated
- Nursing Interventions
  - Assess amount and character of emesis
  - I & O
  - FHR
  - Maternal VS
  - Weight
  - Signs of jaundice and bleeding
  - Teach about home care: small CHO meals with high protein and no fatty foods; rest with feet elevated; slowly sip carbonated beverages when nauseated. Herbal tea may help;
  - Teach woman to avoid odors, exposure to fresh air, very hot or cold liquids, ice and straws
  - In the hospital: same stuff you do for chemo patient

Discuss the nursing care for a woman experiencing premature rupture of the membranes.

- Consider PROM if a woman complains of a watery vaginal discharge or sudden gush of fluid
- Ask her about time of initial fluid loss, if the leak is continuous, the color/odor/amount/consistency of the fluid.
- Check any leaking fluid with nitrazine paper (amniotic fluid is more alkaline than normal vag secretions). The paper will change to blue-green or blue if ROM (but some things can cause a false negative, see pg 493). Can also do a fern test
- Sterile speculum exam if more evaluation is needed...looking for gross pooling in the vagina when she bears down.
- US can look for reduced amniotic fluid
- Amniocentis if you can't figure it out...they put a blue dye in there and then put in a tampon to see if it turns blue. Urine will be green!
- Assess FHR via heart rate tracing or biophysical profile
- Calculate gestational age of fetus to determine plan
  - > 36 weeks, labor will start in 50% of women within 12 hours
- Management of PROM in absence of infection and < 37 weeks is conservative
  - Amniocentesis maybe
  - Fetal lung maturity test if nearing 34 weeks gestation
  - BR and hospitalized
  - Complete CBC and UA on admission
  - Regular non-stress tests or biphysical profiles to monitor fetal well being
  - Maternal BP, pulse and temp q 4 hours
  - Labs to detect maternal infection

- After initial treatment and observation some women can go home if the leak stops or if the fetus has not reached age of viability. Woman is advised to continue BR with bathroom privileges; monitor temp QID, keep a fetal movement record and go on pelvic rests. She may get twice weekly non-stress tests and CBS, and weekly US and cervical visualization.
- Prophylatic abx with any woman with unknown strep status or history of a positive culture during pregnancy
- IMMEDIATE BIRTH IS INDICATED IF AMNIOTIC FLUID SHOWS:
    - low glucose level
    - high WBC
    - positive gram stain
    - organisms in the fluid
- Betamethasone decreases likelihood of neonatal respiratory distress syndrome, necrotizing enterocolitis, intraventricular hemorrhage and perinatal death
    - 12 mg IM followed by second doze in 24 hours
    - ...or dexamethasone 6 mg IM q 12 hours for 4 doses
- Tocolytics usually not indicated...but may be used short-term to allow the short course of steroids to be administered.
- Encourage woman to rest on right or left side

Contrast the etiology, medical therapy, and nursing interventions for preterm labor.

- Signs and Symptoms
    - abdominal pain
    - back pain
    - pelvic pain
    - menstrual-like cramps
    - vaginal bleeding
    - increased vag discharge (may be pinkish or mucus-like)
    - pelvic pressure
    - urinary frequency
    - diarrhea
- Evaluation
    - Assess for fFN...the presence of fFN after 20 weeks gestation and before term is abnormal
    - Assess contraction frequency, but this alone is not enough info
    - Digital cervical exam once ROM has been ruled out
        - 3cm or more dilated or 80% or more effaced with regular contractions = PTL
    - Assess cervical length by endovaginal US
        - length of less than 20 mm with regular contractions = PTL
    - Primary Intervention to reduce preterm birth = dx and treat infections, perform cervical cerclage and give progesterone
    - Secondary Intervention = abx and tocolytics
        - Tocolytics
            - May delay birth for 2-7 days so that you can give betamethasone for fetal surfactant induction or get mom to another facility
            - Effect of tocolytics is reduced if cervix is more than 4-5 cm dilated or if there is subclinical amnionitis
            - The only tocolytic approved by FDA is Yutopar, but there are others that are currently used...
            - B-adrenergic agonists (aka B-mimetics): often choses as first-line Thx, but can affect maternal CV and metabolic physiology (hypoT, arrhythmias, tachyC, palpitations, myocardial ischemia, pulmonary edema and maternal hyperG)
            - Mag sulfate: has fewer side effects than those above;
                - Loading dose is 4-6 g IV in 100 ml over 20 minutes
                - Maintenance dose is 1-4 g/hour titrated to deep tendon reflexes and serum Mag levels
                - Therapy lasts 12 hours
                - Maternal serum level is usually 5.5 - 7.5 mg/dL
                - Loading dose SE: flushing, feeling warm, HA, nystagmus, nausea, dry mouth, dizziness

- Other SE: sluggishness, risk of pulmonary edema (if infection or multiple gestation, too much IV fluid or concurrent B-mimetic Thx)
- Fetal SE: hypotonia and lethargy for 1-2 days, hypoG, hypocalcemia
- CCB (Nifedipine)
  - Inhibits contractile activity
  - Common SE: hypoT, tachyC, facial flushing, HA
  - Coadministration with terbutaline or ritodrine (B-adrenergics) is effective
  - Coadministration with Mag sulfate is bad...can cause seriously low Ca levels and maternal CV collapse
- Prostaglandin synthetase inhibitors (celecoxib, sulindac, indomethacin, ketorolac)
  - Few maternal SE: dyspepsia, N/V, depression, dizziness (psychosis and renal failure are RARE)
  - Best to give with an antacid or taken with meals
  - Do not use in women with drug-induced asthma, coagulation probs, hepatic or renal insufficiency or PUD.
  - Indomethacin crosses placenta...can lead to oligohydramnios and premature closure of fetal ductus arteriosus. Associated with some other probs...not widely used.
- Corticosteroids (betamethasine or dexamethasone) should be administered antenatally if woman is at risk for PTL.

- NO ATTEMPT TO STOP LABOR IF...
  - fetal demise
  - lethal fetal anomaly
  - severe preeclampsia/eclampsia
  - hemorrhage/abruptio placentae
  - chorioamnionitis
  - severe fetal growth restriction
  - fetal maturity
  - acute nonreassuring fetal status
- Nursing Care for PTL
  - Nsng Dx = Health-seeking behavior, fear, ineffective coping
  - Once uterine activity stops, woman is sometimes placed on oral tocolysis and discharged
  - Teaching for self care:
    - Teach S&S of PTL:
      - Contractions that occur a 10 mins or less (may not be painful)
      - Miild menstrual-like cramps low in abd
      - Pelvic pressure
      - ROM
      - Low, dull backache
      - Change in vag discharge
      - Abd cramping with or without diarrhea
    - Evaluate contraction activity 1-2 x a day by lying down tilted to one side. Place fingertips on fundus and chack for contractions for 1 hour.
    - If she has PTL symptoms for > 15 mins she needs to:
      - Empty bladder and lie down (tilt to the side)
      - Drink 3-4 cups of fluid
      - Palpate for uterine contractions for 1 hour (if they are 10 mins apart, she needs to call doc)
      - Soak in a warm tub bath with uterus completely submerged
      - Rest for 30 mins after symptoms subside; gradually resume activity
      - Call doc if symptoms persist, even if no contractions.
  - Hospital based care
    - Promote bed rest, monitor VS, measure I &O, continuously monitor FHR and contractions
    - Place woman on left side to promote maternal-fetal circulation
    - Minimal vag exams
    - Monitor for adverse affects of tocolytics (if used)

	Abruptio Placentae	Placenta Previa
What is it?	Premature separation of a normally implanted placenta from the uterine wall. Classification is based on the extent of the abruption (Class 0-3)	Placenta is improperly implanted on lower uterine segment. Classified in 4 degrees (total, partial, marginal, low-lying)
Etiology	More frequent in pregnancies complicated by smoking, PROM, HTN; risk of recurrence is 10x higher if a previous abruption has occurred; cause is unknown, can occur in trauma.	Cause is unknown; occurs in 1 in 200 pregnancies; factors = multiparity, increasing age, placenta accreta, defective development of blood vessels in decidua, prior C/S, smoking, recent SA or TA, large placenta.
Signs & Symptoms	-Sudden onset -Bleeding can be internal or concealed -Dark venous blood -Anemia is greater than apparent blood loss -Shock is greater than apparent blood loss -Toxemia may be present -Severe and steady pain -Uterus is tender -Uterus is firm to stony hard -Uterus may enlarge and change shape -Fetal heart tones are present or absent -Engagement may be present -No relationship to fetal presentation	-Quiet and sneaky onset -Bleeding is external -Blood is bright red -Anemia = blood loss -Shock = blood loss -Toxemia is absent -Pain is present only if in labor -Uterus is not tender -Uterus is soft and relaxed -Uterine contour is normal -Fetal heart tones are usually present -Engagement is absent -Fetal presentation may be abnormal
Treatment	-Coagulation tests -Maintain CV status of mom -Develop plan for birth -If separation is mild and near term, induce for vag birth; C/S if no labor in short time -If moderate to severe, C/S after hypofibrinogenemia has been treated by cryopreciptate of FFP -Whole blood if hypovolemic to a Hct of 30% -Lactated Ringers	-Determine if PP or advanced labor with copious bloody show -Localize placenta via tests that do not require vag exam (transabdominal US) -If < 37 weeks: try to delay birth (try to stop bleeding. If bleeding recurs or complete previa or labor is present or signs of distress, then C/S -If > 37 weeks, C/S if bleeding continues or complete previa; otherwise induce. -BR with bathroom privileges only if not bleeding -No vag exams -Betamethasone if premature -Lactated Ringers -Possible blood transfusion
Nursing Interventions	Type and cross Establish large bore IV Continuous external fetal monitoring CVP monitoring Monitor urine output Monitor contractions and resting tone Abd girth measurements hourly Place mark at top of fundus and check q hr Reinforce positive aspects of condition Monitor VS Complete BR Keep mom NPO Betamethasone if baby premature Assess amount of blood loss	Maintain mom on BR Monitor blood loss, pain, uterine contractility Evaluate FHR monitoring (external) Monitor mom's VS Evaluate H&H, Rh, UA I&O Check newborn's Hbg, cell volume, erythrocytes
Complications	DIC Couvelaire uterus	Hemorrhage Shock

Rh/ABO Incompatibility

The RH factor
- RH Incompatibility Disorder
- Etiology: RH negative mother becomes sensitized to RH positive blood during pregnancy with a RH positive fetus. This is a big issue for mom and fetus, though we tend to treat it well these days.
- Incidence: 15% of all women are RH negative.
- Diagnosis
  - Lab test: Indirect Coombs: Test of maternal blood for RH antibody titre against RH positive blood cells.
  - Lab Test: Direct Coombs: Test of newborn blood for RH antibodies coating newborn's RBCs.
- Management
  - Goal: Prevent mother from coming in contact with fetal RH positive RBCs in pregnancy/post delivery.
  - Monitor maternal blood during pregnancy/post delivery
  - Goal is to have no fetal harm come due to this dissonance between blood types...want to keep mom from coming into contact with the fetal RBCs
- Repeat Indirect Coombs blood test at 28 wks.
- Give Rhogam at 28 wks prophylatically.
- Give Rhogam within 72 hrs after birth.

Some Rhogam Scenarios
If a woman is having her first baby and she's Rn-, and baby is Rh+...she is not going to get Rhogam in pregnancy. No reason to. What if she had a ThAb? Absolutely, she would get Rhogam...it is the second pregnancy where this comes into play. Most of the time a woman was Rh- and has a TAB or SAB, she'll get Rhogam prophylactically.

A mother is Rh-, she is having her second baby. Her first one was Rh- also. Is there any threat to the first pregnancy? NONE! Second baby is Rh +...is she going to get Rhogam? Decision made at 28 weeks....but theoretically she should be OK b/c sensitization has not been triggered.

We have a mom, she is having second baby. baby is RH+, mom is Rh-...she says this is her last baby. Does she need Rhogam? What if she gets tubes tied? She'll still get Rhogam becuase can't predict what will happen in the future. What if she goes to donate blood and she's Rh-? Let's say that unit of Rh- blood is transfused into a woman who has not yet had a baby...now that primagravida has a Rh problem b/c that blood is sensitized. EVERYBODY gets Rhogam after an Rh+ baby if they are Rh-.

Mom is Rh- at first pregnancy, she has twins and they are both Rh+, but she loses one of them early in the pregnancy...does she become sensitized and is there a risk to the surviving twin? Dr. HS says she'd probably get Rhogam.

RH disease (erythroblastosis)
- Most people have RH + blood, meaning they have an inherited protein found on their RBCs.
- About 15% of White population and 7% of the African American population lack this factor, and are considered RH-
- If a RH – Mother and a RH + father conceive a child, the fetus may inherit the RH+ blood type of the father...usually the baby's blood turns out to be like mom's...but the RH part is the wild card.
- During pregnancy, labor, or expulsion of the placenta, fetal RBCs enter the maternal circulation.
- These RBCs are recognized as foreign, and the mother tries to fight off these by developing antibodies.
- If mom has had Rhogam, then body doesn't make the antibodies, because it thinks it already has them.
- In each subsequent pregnancy the antibodies cross the placenta and attack the fetal RBCs.

Rhogam
- Rhogam is synthesized...the body reads it as "I've already done the work to make the antibodies, so I don't have to do it."
- RH Immune Globulin from sensitized person.
- Action: suppresses antibody formation in RH- mother with RH+ infant.
- Dosage: 1 vial (300ug) IM or microdose of 50ug IM.
- Precautions: must be given within 72 hours after delivery to prevent antibody formation by immune system.

- Other indications: miscarriage, abortion, abdominal trauma during pregnancy, chorionic villi sampling, ectopic pregnancy, amniocentesis.

Mom makes antibodies
- Mother develops antibodies against the RH + fetal RBCs
- Mother now has RH + antibody titer
- The RH+ antibodies cross the placenta
- In subsequent pregnancies these antibodies will lyse any Fetal RH + RBCs. If next baby is Rh- there is no issue here. The issue is if the baby is Rh+.

What if it goes untreatead?
- Untreated leads to fetal anemia, ↑immature fetal RBCs, fetal jaundice, hepatospleenomegaly, cardiac decompensation, death if severe

Management goals
- Prevent mother from producing RH+ antibodies
- Maintain RH+ fetal well being throughout pregnancy
- Evaluated by blood type, RH factor and Coombs testing
- Conduct Coombs Testing
  - Lab tests that reveal antigen-antibody reaction. Detects antibodies in blood
  - Direct coombs:detects the presence of cell bound antibodies that may damage RBCs. Venous blood or blood from umbilicus
  - Indirect Coombs reveals the presence of RH antibodies in maternal blood

If RH negative Mother is Sensitized:
- Pathologic jaundice occurs in fetus
- Management includes:
  - Amniocentesis tests during pregnancy to determine amt. of fetal bilirubin in fluid (delta OD level).
  - Give fetal blood transfusions (PUB) with O negative blood prn during pregnancy.
  - At birth, send vial of fetal cord blood to lab
  - Direct Coombs is a test to determine level of RH antibodies in fetal blood...it looks for the presence of cell-bound antibodies that cause damage to the RBCs. We use venous or umbilicus blood in the fetus. (Indirect: looks at mom's blood)
  - Ratio 1:64, blood transfusions are done.
  - Phototherapy treatments
- Treatment
  - Rhogam given routinely at 28 weeks GA and within 72 hours of delivery
  - Rhogam given other times if possible exposure to fetal blood: trauma,miscarriage, amniocentesis,abortion,
  - Goal is to prevent mother from developing antibodies

If RH negative Mother is Sensitized
- Management includes: Amniocentesis tests during pregnancy to determine amt. of fetal bilirubin in fluid (delta OD level).
- Give fetal blood transfusions (PUB) with O negative blood prn during pregnancy. Use US to get to the fetal abdomen and give the blood cells through there...the blood gets in to the right place! Think of peritoneal dialysis.
- At birth, we send vial of fetal cord blood to lab
- Direct Coombs test to determine level of RH antibodies in fetal blood Ratio 1:64, blood transfusions are done. Phototherapy treatments
- Once a mom is sensitized, every Rh+ pregnancy is vulnerable. They will give the Rhogam to try to minimize the effects.

Untreated RH Sensitization in Pregnancy
- Pathologic jaundice in fetus
  - RH positive fetus develops:
    - Anemia

- Produces immature RBCs (liver)
  - Develops hepatosplenomegaly
  - Cardiac decompensations and cardiomegaly
  - Ascites
  - Death
- Erhthroblastyosis fetalis hydrops fetalis

What is Rhogam?
- Immune Globulin or antibodies to RH+ blood
- Given to prevent development of maternal antibodies
- A 1:1000 dilution of Immune globulin is cross matched to mother's blood to insure compatibility
- Blood product precautions
- Indications for dosing of Rhogam
- 50 ug: after CVS, ectopic pregnancy, miscarriage or abortion < 13 weeks
- 300 ug: miscarriage/abortion>13 weeks, amniocentesis, abruption,trauma, bleeding, at 28 wks, within 72 hr of deliv
- >300 ug after large placenta hemorrhage or mismatched blood transfusion

ABO Incompatibility
- Etiology: Mother is O blood type, infant is A or B blood type.
  - May occur with first or any infant as mother with O blood type naturally has anti-A and anti-B antibodies naturally in the blood.
  - Antibodies are larger, more difficult to cross the placental membrane.
- Management:
  - Direct Coombs test on fetal cord blood
  - Phototherapy if > 4 mg bilirubin in infant blood at birth. Most babies under the lights are there b/c of the ABO compatability issues.
- ABO incompatibilities are more common than RH incompatibilities
- If a baby is born and within 24 hours is jaundiced...this is called pathological jaundice. This is d/t ABO compatability. Physiologic jaundice is "normal" and this happens around day 2-3 b/c liver isn't working at full steam yet (peak bili around Day 4...the bad number for bili is > 18.....this is when the nurses start to freak out. So if you have a baby at 16 on Day 4, you need mom to feed that bay to flush it out...you can also place baby in sunny window...if getting high then it needs to be under the lights. Home phototherapy is preferred...it's a little glow-y blue pad. Remember to keep baby under lights to the point that bili is lower than you want...b/c when you take them out it rebounds a bit. Other nursing interventions with light...cover the eyes, monitor temperature, can take baby out for half an hour to let mom breastfeed. Most babies are under lights for 3 days or so.
- KEY MESSAGE = IF JAUNDICED IN FIRST 24 HOURS THIS IS PATHOLOGICAL!
- Third type of jaundice is breastmilk jaundice...around day 10
  - If really bad, pull them off breast every other day
  - For the most part, it just goes away on its own

ABO incompatabilities
- More common than Rh incompatibilities
- 4 major blood groups are A,B,AB, and O
- Type A has A antigens and has antibodies to Type B
- Type B has B antigens and has antibodies to Type A
- Type AB has A+B antigens and has NO antibodies
- Type O has no antigens and has antibodies to both A and B
- If mother has different blood type antibodies can cross the placental barrier into fetal circulation

Results of ABO incompatibilities
- Usually milder fetal effect
- Weakly positive Direct Coombs (not as definitive a dx as with Rh issues)
- Common cause of jaundice in neonate
- Treatment is usually phototherapy

High Risk Pregnancy: Anemia HIV, Heart Disease

Iron Deficiency Anemia: Maternal problems associated with deficiency
- Infections
- Fatigue
- Preeclampsia
- Postpartum hemorrhage
- Decreased blood loss tolerance
- Iron deficiency anemia is totally fixable for the most part...nutrition! Iron supplements are usually given to women in the prenatal period

Iron Deficiency Anemia: Fetus
- Low birth weight babies b/c they have not gotten perfused as much with oxygen-rich blood
- Prematurity
- Stillbirth
- Neonatal death
- The placenta is "stringy" or skinny

Iron Deficiency
- Prevention: 27 mg of iron daily
- Treatment: 60-120 mg of iron daily; prenatal vitamins have iron in them

Folate Deficiency (Vit B9?)
- Maternal: Nausea, vomiting, anorexia
- Fetal: Neural tube defects such as spina bifida, opened-up spine...all kinds of things.

Folate Deficiency
- Prevention: 0.4mg folic acid daily
- Treatment: 1mg folic acid daily plus iron supplements

Sickle Cell : Maternal
- Vaso-occlusive crisis...put baby on monitor 24/7 until crisis passes.
- Infections (can trigger an event)
- Congestive Heart Failure
- Renal Failure
- The sickled cells don't carry oxygen as well...
- Ensure hydration status is good...give oxygen also to increase flow to fetus. Probably put her on ABX and analgesics
- Mom is probably going to be induced and have oxygen on the whole time. Don't want to do a C-Section unless you absolutely have to.

Sickle Cell : Fetus
- Death (high incidence of SAB)
- Prematurity
- IUGR (intrauterine growth restriction)
- Treatment
    - Folic Acid for mom
    - Prompt infection control
    - Prompt response to vaso-occlusive crisis

Thalassemia
- This is an autosomal recessive disorder
- It's not very common
- The cells are teeny tiny (microcytic red cells). The anemia can cause really low Hgb levels (around 5)...really need to transfuse them at this point...that is LOW!
- The cells don't live very long. Prone to having hepatosplenalmegoly!

- Treatment
  - Folic Acid
  - Transfusion
  - Chelation therapy
- Nursing care is all about trying to prevent infections, work on the anemia, keep the fetus healthy, monitor fetus frequently with ultrasound.

HIV in Pregnancy: Maternal
- Asymptomatic women – pregnancy has not effected this.
- Women with low CD 4 will experience acceleration of the disease.
- Zidovudine (ZDV) therapy diminishes risk of transmission to fetus (BIG ISSUE)
- Breastmilk transmission...HIV goes right straight through the breastmilk. Transmission via breastmilk usually doesn't happen until after 3 months.
- Half of all infection is during L/D

HIV Effects on Fetus
- Infants often have positive antibody titer
- Infected infants are usually asymptomatic, but are often:
  - Premature
  - Low Birth Weight
  - Small for Gestational Age (SGA)

Treatment : Pregnancy
- Counseling...tell moms they should not be eating garlic b/c it interferes with the medication.
- Antiretroviral therapy
- Fetal testing can be done
- C-Section for delivery

Cardiac Disorders in Pregnancy
- Congenital Heart Disease
- Marfan Syndrome (autosomal dominant)
  - Disorder of CT of heart
  - Will have to watch this mom very carefully
- Peripartum Cardiomyopathy
  - Dysfunction of left ventricle...tends to occur toward end of pregnancy (last 4-6 weeks) and even postpartum.
  - Usually presents with anemia and infection.
  - This defect has remained unknown until pregnancy when increased demand make the impairment evident.
  - 1:3000 live births
  - Mortality up to 50%
  - S&S are related to congestive heart failure
- Eisenmenger Syndrome
  - Left to right shunting occurs in people who are born with septal defects
  - Cannot be corrected
  - Shunting results in pulmonary HTN
  - Mortality rates up to 50%
- Mitral Valve Prolapse
  - Usually asymptomatic; < 20% of people have it
  - Once the valve starts to prolapse into left atrium...then woman starts to get a lot of irregular heart rhythms and some mitral regurgitation.
  - Women will tolerate pregnancy pretty well...but be very careful that they do not get infections
  - Prognosis is "fine"
  - Will probably be most bothered by symptoms of heart palpitations, may have pain and SOB caused by cardiac arrhythmias.
  - Helps mom to limit caffeine intake to help with palpitations

- Probably put them on Enderol
- Do NOT give prophylactic abx...that's old school. Now we treat episodically.

Clinical Therapies: Criteria Committee of the New York Heart Association
- Class 1: person has no limitations; probably asymptomatic; no fatigue or palpitations with activity; things that would make it bothersome would be extra exertion in pregnancy (beyond the norm)
- Class 2: slight limitations; ordinary physical activity doesn't cause undue fatigue or pain, but do have cardiac insufficiency; when start adding more stress/work they will have more symptoms.
- Class 3: marked limitation; would discourage this person from even getting pregnant 25 years ago; comfortable at rest, but anything other than ordinary physical activity is going to cause fatigue, angina, dyspnea, palpitations. They can go grocery shopping, but probably can't carry the groceries; won't be climbing stairs
- Class 4: inability to carry on any physical activity w/o discomfort; even at rest will have pain, palpitations, discomfort, dyspnea. Just walking around the house is too much.

- **Labor and Childbirth**
  Class 1 & Class 2: spontaneous labor and adequate pain relief is recommended...pretty normal pregnancies
- Class 3 & 4: may need to be hospitalized before onset of labor for cardio stabilization.
  - Will be reducing anemia to relieve strain on the heart
  - Will take care of all infections ASAP
  - Will screen every month for asymptomatic bacteriuria (sp?)
  - High incidence of developing pyelonephritis (which puts a direct load on the heart)
  - Will be on cardiac drugs: heparin does not cross placenta, probably on a diuretic to decrease CHF symptoms (recall that pregnancy increases fluid volume by 50%)

Nursing Assessment
- Functional capacity
- Pulse, respirations, B/P compared to normal
- Monitor activity level including rest
- Look for signs of strain on heart
- Watchful for CHF...listen to lungs, check for edema (not ankle edema...look at hands and face!), monitor I&Os, daily weights etc...

Nursing Plan: Antenatal
- Meet physio and psych needs
- Teach recognition of signs of complications
- Dietary needs and changes
  - Essential nutritional counseling is vital!
- Bi weekly visits

Nursing Plan: Labor/ Delivery
- Close monitoring of vital signs
- Auscultation of lungs...they can get noisy fast.
- Ensure cardiac emptying
- Oxygenation – semi Fowlers position
- Support
- EFM (fetal monitoring)

Nursing Plan: Postpartum
- Very close monitoring...not out of the woods yet!
- Attend to psychosocial needs: "Is the baby ok?"
- Diet and stool softeners...do not want them to strain
- Breastfeeding is good for them...will need help with this. Get her comfy in a semi-Fowler's...she will be tired but can't lie down!
- Manage fatigue...get others on board to help with baby care.

LABOR AND DELIVERY

Ampicillin Sodium

Dosage/Range: IM, IV 500 mg to 3 g q 6 hrs, PO 250-500mg q 6 hrs
Onset /Peak/ Duration: rapid/ 1-2 hr/ 4-6 hr /
Indication: Anti- infective Binds to bacterial cell wall, resulting in cell death.
Contraindications: Hypersensitivity to penicillins, Use cautiously in lactation: distributed into breast milk. Can cause rash, diarrhea, and sensitization in the infant.
Nursing Considerations: Assess for infection- vitals wound appearance, sputum, urine, stool, and WBC. Obtain history to determine previous use and reaction to penicillin.
AE: seizures, diarrhea, rashes, allergic rxn

Betamethasone

Dosage/Range: IM: 12mg daily for 2-3 days
Onset/Peak/Duration: 1-3hr/unk/1 week
Indication: used to prevent respiratory distress in preterm newborn (helps lungs produce surfactant)
Contraindication: active untreated infections; traumatic brain injury; hypersensitivity to bisulfates
Nursing Considerations: Give in the morning to coincide with body's natural release of cortisol; shake IM suspension well before drawing up
AE: depression, euphoria, HTN, peptic ulceration, anoreixa, nausea, adrenal suppression

Bupivacaine Hydrochloride 125% (Marcaine, Sensorcaine)

Dosage/Range: Epidural10-20mL administer in increments of 3 -5ml allowing sufficient time to detect toxic signs
Onset /Peak/ Duration: 10-30 min/ unk/ 2-8 hr
Indication: Local anesthetics
Contraindications: Hypersensitivity, Contains bisulfites &should be avoided in patients with known intolerance. Obstetrical paracervical block anesthesia. Use cautiously in concurrent use of anticoagulants
Nursing Considerations: Assess for systemic toxicity (tingling &numbness, ringing in ears, metallic taste, dizziness, slow speech. Monitor BP, HR, and RR .Monitor for return of sensation after procedure
AE: seizures, cardiovascular collapse

Dinoprostone (Prepidil, Cervidil)

Dosage/Range: 0.3 mg/hour over a 12 hour period
Onset /Peak/ Duration: rapid/ 30-45 min/ unknown
Indication: Inducing labor (ripening of cervix)
Contraindications/Nursing Considerations: Hypersensitivity to prostaglandins. Evidence of fetal distress where delivery is not imminent; remove insert at onset of active labor, before amniotomy or after 12 hours
AE: abnormal uterine contractions

Clindamycin phosphate (Cleocin Phosphate)

Dosage/Range: PO 150-450 mg q 6hrs IM, IV 300-600 mg q 6-8 hrs
Onset /Peak/ Duration: PO Rapid/ 60 min/ 6-8 hrs IM Rapid/1-3hr min/6-8 hrs IV Rapid, end of infusion, 6-8 hrs
Indication: Tx of infection
Contraindications: Hypersensitivity, present in breastmilk.
Nursing Considerations: Assess for diarrhea, cramping, fever or bloody stools.
AE: diarrhea, vertigo, rashes, phlebitis

Fentanyl citrate(Sublimaze)

Dosage/Range: IM, IV: 50-100mcg
Onset /Peak/ Duration: :7-15 min/ 20-30min/1-2 hrs
Indication: Regional anesthesia during labor
Contraindications/ Nursing Considerations: Can interact w/MAO-I's, grapefruit juice, other CNS depressants; O2, Narcan & resusc equip need to be avail. IV:admin over 1-3 min
AE: apnea, laryngospasm, itching, respiratory depression.

Gentamicin sulfate (Cidomycin, Garamycin)
Dosage/Range: IM, IV: <1200g: 2.5mg/kg/dose q24h.Premature: <1000g: 3.5mg/kg/dose q24h.
Onset /Peak/ Duration: IM: rapid/ 30-90 min / 8-24hr IV: rapid/ 15-30 min/ 8-24hrs
Indication: Tx of susceptible bacterial infections.
Contraindications/Nursing Considerations: Use caution:enters breast milk in small amounts. DON'Tuse in pts with hypersensitivity to gentamicin or other aminoglycosides. Risk of nephrotoxicity and ototoxicity. Use in caution w/ neonates d/t renal immaturity,& pts w/preexisting renal impairment,auditory or vestibular impairment, hypocalcemia, & myasthenia gravis.
AE: ataxia, vertigo, ototoxicity, nephrotoxicity

(Hemabate) Carboprost tromethramine
Dosage/Range: IM: 250 mcg, prn q 15-90min, not to exceed 2mg (8 doses). IM: 250mcg, prn q1.5-3.5h, not to exceed 12mg.
Onset /Peak/Duration: unk/ 16 hr/ unk
Indication: Tx of postpartum hemorrhage d/t uterine atony. Aborting pregnancy between 13th & 20th weeks of gestation.
Contraindications/Nursing Considerations: Use w/caution in pts with a hx of asthma, hypo- or HTN, cardiovascular, renal, or hepatic disease, anemia, jaundice, diabetes, epilepsy, or pts with compromised (scarred) uterus. Monitor BP, pulse, watch for hemorrhage. Examine for cervical trauma. Possible teratogenic effects on fetus; 20% of abortions may be incomplete. Do not use in pts with acute PID, active cardiac, pulmonary, renal or hepatic disease. May result in excessive uterine tone, causing decreased uterine blood flow and fetal distress.
AE: diarrhea, N/V, uterine rupture, fever

Ibuprofen (Motrin)
Dosage/Range: IV: 500-1500g, 10mg/kg. PO Analgesic: 4-10mg/kg/dose q6-8h, max 40mg/kg/day
Onset /Peak/ Duration PO (antipyretic) 0.5-2.5hr/2-4hr/ 6-8 hrPO: (analgesic):30min/ 1-2 hr/ 4-6 hrPO (anti-infl): 7days/1-2 wk/unk
Indication: Tx of inflammatory diseases and rheumatoid d/o's, mild to moderate pain, fever, dysmenorrheal, gout.
Contraindications/Nursing Considerations: Use caution: enters breast milk in small amounts. Do not use in pts with hypersensitivity to ibuprofen, aspirin, or other NSAIDs. May increase risk of GI bleeding, irritation, ulceration, and perforation. Not recommended for pregnant patients; has been associated with persistent pulmonary HTN in infants.
AE: GI bleed, hepatitis, headache, allergic reactions, N/V

Indocin (Indomethacin)
Dosage/Range: PO: 25-50 mg 2-4 x a day or 75 mg extended tablet 1-2x day;
Onset/Peak/Duration: 30 mins/0.5-2hr/4-6 hr
Indication: a tocolytic used to stop preterm labor
Contraindications: known alcohol intolerance, active GI bleeding, ulcer disease, recent history of rectal bleeding, intraventriucular hemorrhage, thrombocytopenia
Nursing Considerations: Give PO after meals or with food; monitor BUN and Cr; monitor LFTs; pt should stay upright for 30 mins after taking PO; this one crosses the placenta and can close PDA prematurely, can also lead to oligohydramnios; not widely used.
AE: dizziness, pyschic disturbances, drug-induced hepatitis, GI bleeds, constipation, dyspepsia, N/V

Lactated Ringers
Dosage/Range: IV: 20-30ml/kg body weight/hour
Onset /Peak/ Duration: Enters blood immediately.
Indication: Isotonic solution for fluid and electrolyte replenishment, usually after blood loss. Contains Na, Cl, K, Ca, lactate.
Contraindications/Considerations: Not used for maintenance fluids, b/c sodium content is too high.Monitor electrolytes (esp K) & hydration status.Contraindicated in tx of lactic acidosis d/t lactate content.Never give LR in same IV as blood

Lidocaine hydrochloride (Xylocaine)
Dosage/Range: IV: 50-100 mg (1mg/kg) infusion up to 4.5 mg/kg or 300 mg in 1h. Topical: apply as needed (not to exceed 35g/day as cream).
Onset /Peak/ Duration: IV: immed./ 10-20min-several hrs IM: 5-15min, 2-3 hr Local: Rapid, 1-3 hrs.
Indication: IV: ventricular arrhythmias.IM: infiltration/mucosal/topical anesthetic
Contraindications/Nursing Considerations: Do not use in pts with hypersensitivity, advanced AV block. Use cautiously in pts with liver disease, CHF, resp. depression, shock, pregnancy/lactation (safety not established).
AE: seizures, confusion, cardiac arrest, stinging at IV site

Magnesium Sulfate
Dosage/Range: Loading Dose = 4-6 g IV in 100 ml over 2 mins; Maintenance Dose = 1-4 g/hour titrated to DTR and serum Mag levels
Indication: Used to stop pre-term labor (tocolytic)
Contraindications/Nursing Considerations: Effect of tocolytics is reduced if cervix is more than 4-5 cm dilated; Mag has fewer side effects than other tocolytics
AE: initially a feeling of warmth, HA, nystagmus, nausea, dry mouth, dizziness; risk of pulmonary edema, sluggishness; in fetus = hypotonia and lethargy for 1-2 days, hypoG, hypoC

(Methergine) Methylergonovine Maleate
Dosage/Range: PO: 200-400 mcg (0.4-0.6 mg) q 6-12hr for 2-7 days IM/IV: 200 mcg (0.2mg) q 2-4 hr for up to 5 doses
Onset /Peak/ Duration: PO: 5-15 min/ unk/3 hr IM:2-5 min/unk/3 hr IV: immed/unk/45min-3 hr
Indication: To produce uterine contractions and prevent postpartum hemorrhage due to uterine atony. Also used in management of subinvolution
Contraindications: known hypersensitivity to drug, hypersensitivity to phenol, HTN, sever hepatic or renal disease, sepsis
Nursing Considerations: excessive vasoconstriction may result when used with heavy cig smoking or other vasopressors (ie. dopamine) Admin at a rate of 0.2mg over at least 1 min
AE: HTN, N/V, cramps

Misoprostol (Cytotec)
Dosage/Range: 25-50 mcg for induction of labor term
Onset /Peak/ Duration: 30 min/ unk/3-6 hr
Indication: Induce labor (Cervical ripening)
Contraindications: Preterm Pregnancy, component allergy
Nursing Considerations: Take the full course. May have diarrhea. Notify doctor if it last longer than I week.
AE: abd pain, diarrhea, miscarriage

Mineral Oil
Dosage/Range: 5-45mL PO
Onset /Peak/ Duration: PO 6-8hr/ unk/ unk Rectal: 2-15hr/ Unk/unk
Indication: Used to soften feces, management of constipation
Contraindications: Hypersensitivity
Nursing Considerations: May cause diarrhea, assess color, consistency, and amount of stool produced
AE: no major AEs, may cause diarrhea

Morphine (Duramorph)
Dosage/Range: IV,IM,SC: 4-10 mg q 3-4 hour
Onset/Peak/Duration: IV: rapid/20 mins/4-5 hr; IM: 10-30m/300-60m/4-5hr; SC: 20 m/50-90m/4-5hr
Indication: severe pain
Contraindications: hypersensitivity
Nursing Considerations: ATC may be more effective than prn; do not administer discolored solution; assess LOC, BP, HR and RR before and during; assess bowel function routinely; narcan is reversal
AE: sedation, respiratory depression, hypotension, constipation, bradycardia

(Mylanta) Aluminum Hydroxide
Dosage/Range: 10-30 mL or 300-1200 mg PO q4-6 hr.
Onset /Peak/ Duration: Immed/ unk/ 3 hr
Indication: Relief of heartburn, upset or sour stomach, or acid indigestion
Contraindications/ Nursing Considerations: Separate other drug administration by 2 hours, increase effictiveness of liquid form; OK in renal failure
AE: constipation

Narcan (Nalaxone)
Dosage/Range: 0.4 mg IV, IM, SC (or 10 mcg/kg), may repeat a 2-3 mins.
Onset/Peak/Duration: IV: 1-2 mins/unk/45 mins
Indication: opioid overdose
Contraindications: Hypersensitivity
Nursing Considerations: monitor RR, rhythm and depth, HR, ECG, BP and LOC for 3-4 after dose given; pt may be extremely sensitive to narcan
AE: HTN, hypoT, v-fib, v-tach, N/V

Nubain (Nalbuphine)
Dosage/Range: 10 mg q 3-6 hours IM, SC, IV (NTE 160 mg)
Onset/Peak/Duration: IV: 2-3 mins/30 mins/3-6 hr; SC: <15 min/unk/3-6hr; IM < 15 min/60 mins/3-6hr
Indication: moderate to severe pain; analgesia during labor
Contraindications: Physically dependent patients
Nursing Considerations: Give IM deep into well-developed muscle; assess BP, P and RR before and during administration; Narcan is the reversal
AE: sedation, respiratory depression, dry mouth, N/V, urinary urgency, blurred vision

Oxytocin (Pitocin)
Dosage/Range: Induction of Labor IV: 0.5-2 milliunits/min Postpartum Hemorrhage: 10 units
Onset /Peak/ Duration: IV: Immediate/ N/A/ 1hr IM: few mins/ N/A/ 20 min
Indication: Induction of labor, postpartum control of bleeding after expulsion of the placenta
Contraindications: Hypersensitivity, anticipated non-vaginal delivery
Nursing Considerations: Can cause painful contractions. Assess fetal maturity & presentation prior to admin.Assess character, frequency of contractions; if <2min apart, last 60-90 sec or longer, or change in fetal HR develops, stop admin & place pt on left side Frequency of fundal checks is determined by physician/ CNM order's, the woman's condition, and the status of the fundus q 15 min for the first hour; q 30 for the second postpartum hour; q 4-8 hours until discharge. When oxytocic drugs are used to prevent or reverse uterine atony, a physician/CNM should be immediately available to manage complications. When the drug is administered, the uterus should remain in strong, continuous contraction. The woman may complain of uterine pain or cramping. Be prepared to administer analgesics for pain relief if cramping is intense. When the uterus remains atonic (not contracted), the dose of the drug or rate of the IV infusion may be insufficient to effectively control uterine bleeding. Notify physician/ CNM immediately. Be prepared to administer additional doses to increase I Assess for diarrhea, cramping, fever or bloody stools. infusion rate.
AE: coma, seizures, intracranial hemorrhage, asphyxia, increased uterine motility, painful contractions

(Reglan) Metoclopramide Hydrochloride
Dosage/Range: Post-op n/v:IM, IV: 10-20mg, prn q6-8 hr
Onset /Peak/ Duration: PO: 30-60 min/1-2 hrs. IM: 10-15 min/1-2 hrs. IV: 1-3 min/ 1-2 hrs.
Indication: Prevention of chemotherapy induced emesis. Post surgical and diabetic gastric stasis. Post-op n/v.
Contraindications/Nursing Considerations: Do not use in pts with hypersensitivity, possible GI obstruction, hemorrhage, or Parkinson's disease. Use cautiously in pts with a h/o depression, diabetic, pregnancy/lactation.
AE: neuroleptic malignant syndrome, drowsiness, EPS, restlessness

Terbutaline

Dosage/Range: SC: 250 mcg q 1 hour; IV: 10 mcg/min infusion, increase by 5 mcg/min q 10 mins until contractions stop

Onset/Peak/Duration: SC: <15 min/0.5-1hr/1.5-4hr

Indication: Management of preterm labor

Contraindications: Hypersensitivity to adrenergic amines

Nursing Considerations: Give SC in lateral deltoid area; may dilute continuous infusion in D5W, NS or 1/2 NS; monitor mom's BP, contractions and fetal heart rate; monitor mom and neonate for signs of hypoglycemia; signs of toxicity include persistent agitation, chest pain or discomfort, decreased BP, dizziness, hyperG, hypoK, seizures, tachyarhythmias, persistent trembling and vomiting.

AE: nervousness, angina, HTN, tachyC, N/V, hyperglycemia

(Zofran) Ondansetron hydrochloride

Dosage/Range: PO: 8mg IM: 4mg IV: 4mg

Onset /Peak/ Duration: PO: rapid/ 15-30 min/4-8 hrs IM: rapid/ 40 min/ unk
IV: rapid/ 15-30 min/4-8 hrs

Indication: Prevention and tx of N/V

Contraindications: Hypersensitivity, orally disintegrating tablets should not be used in pts with phenylketonuria.

Nursing Considerations: SE include headache, constipation, and diarrhea. Assess pt for extra pyramidal SE following administration

AE: HA, constipation, diarrhea, EPS

POSTPARTUM

Acetaminophen (Tylenol)
Dosage/Range: 650 mg PO or PR q 4-6 hr or 1000 mg PO q 6 hr; 4g/24h
Onset /Peak/ Duration: 0.5-1 hr/ 1-3 hr/ 3-8 hr
Indication: Mild- moderate pain, HA, fever
Contraindications/Nursing Considerations: Delayed absorption if given with food. Don't use with alcohol, teach S/ S of hepatotoxicity, consult healthcare provider if temp is greater than 103 for more than 3 days
AE: hepatic and renal failure, rash, uticaria

(Benadryl)Diphenhydramine hydrochloride
Dosage/Range: 25-50 mg PO,IM pr IV bid-tid
Onset /Peak/ Duration: PO: 15-60 min/2-4 hr/4 -8 hr IM: 20-30 min/2-4 hr/4-8 hr IV: Rapid / unknown/ 4-8 hr
Indication: Prevent allergic reactions, motion sickness, potentiate narcotics, sedation, cough suppression
Contraindications: acute asthma
Nursing Considerations: Increase risk of photosensitivity- use sunscreen; may cause drowsiness.
AE: drowsiness, anorexia, dry mouth

Benzocaine Menthol
Dosage/Range: bid
Onset /Peak/ Duration: ~1min/ unk/ 15-20 min
Indication: hemorrhoids
Contraindications/Nursing Considerations: use cautiously in large or severely abraded areas of skin or mucous membrane
AE: stinging, allergic rxn, uticaria

Colace -Dioctyl sodium sulfosuccinate (Docusate Sodium)
Dosage/Range: 50-500 mg PO divided qid
Onset/Peak/Duration: PO: 24-48 hrs/ unk/ unk
Indication: Constipation; adjunct to painful anorectal conditions (hemorrhoids)
Contraindications: Don't use with mineral oil; intestinal obstruction, acute abdominal pain, N/V
Nursing Considerations: Take with full glass of water; no laxative action; do not use > 1 week
AE: throat irritation, mild craps, rash

Hydrocortisone 1%
Dosage/Range: Rectal: Aerosol foam – 90 mg 1-2X/day for 2-3 wk; then adjusted
Onset /Peak/ Duration: mins-hrs/ hrs-days/ hrs-days
Indication: Mgmt of inflammation
Contraindications/Nursing Considerations: shake well and spray on affected area; hold container 3-6" away. Spray for about 2sec to cover an area the size of a hand. Do not inhale
AE: burning, dryness, irritation

Lanolin Ointment (Lansinoh)
Indication: Sore, cracked nipples
Contraindications/Nursing Considerations: Area may burn, sting or become red

(Milk of Magnesia) Magnesium hydroxide
Dosage/Range: PO: 30-60 ml single or divided dose or 10-20ml as concentrate
Onset /Peak/ Duration: 3-6 hr/ unk/unk
Indication: Laxative / antacid
Contraindications: hyperMg, hypoC, Anuria, heart block. Use cautiously in any degree of renal insuff.
Nursing Considerations: Shake solution well before admin; admin on empty stomach. Do not admin at bedtime or late in day. Follow PO doses with glass of water
AE: diarrhea, flushing, sweating

(Methergine) Methylergonovine maleate

Dosage/Range: PO: 200-400 mcg (0.4-0.6 mg) q 6-12hr for 2-7 days IM/IV: 200 mcg (0.2mg) q 2-4 hr for up to 5 doses **Onset /Peak/ Duration:** PO: 5-15 min/ unk/3 hr IM:2-5 min/unk/3 hr IV: immed/unk/45min-3 hr
Indication: To produce uterine contractions and prevent postpartum hemorrhage due to uterine atony. Also used in management of subinvolution
Contraindications: known hypersensitivity to drug, hypersensitivity to phenol, HTN, severe hepatic or renal disease, sepsis
Nursing Considerations: excessive vasoconstriction may result when used with heavy cig smoking or other vasopressors (ie. dopamine) Admin at a rate of 0.2mg over at least 1 min
AE: HTN, N/V, cramps

(Maalox) Calcium Carbonate

Dosage/Range: 0.5-1.5g PRN
Onset /Peak/ Duration: PO: unk IV: immed/ immed/ 0.5-2 hr
Indication: Relief of acid indigestion or heartburn
Contraindications: hyperC, renal calculi, V.fib Use cautiously in : pts rec' dig, renal disease, cardiac disease
Nursing Considerations: May interact with cereals, spinach or rhubarb may <absorption. Admin 1-1.5 hr after meals. Follow oral doses with a glass of water
AE: constipation, diarrhea

Oxytocin (Pitocin)

Dosage/Range: Induction of Labor IV: 0.5-2 milliunits/min Postpartum Hemorrhage: 10 units
Onset /Peak/ Duration: IV: Immediate/ N/A/ 1hr IM: few mins/ N/A/ 20 min
Indication: Induction of labor, postpartum control of bleeding after expulsion of the placenta
Contraindications: Hypersensitivity, anticipated non-vaginal delivery
Nursing Considerations: Can cause painful contractions. Assess fetal maturity & presentation prior to admin. Assess character, frequency of contractions; if <2min apart, last 60-90 sec or longer, or change in fetal HR develops, stop admin & place pt on left side Frequency of fundal checks is determined by physician/ CNM order's, the woman's condition, and the status of the fundus q 15 min for the first hour; q 30 for the second postpartum hour; q 4-8 hours until discharge. When oxytocic drugs are used to prevent or reverse uterine atony, a physician/CNM should be immediately available to manage complications. When the drug is administered, the uterus should remain in strong, continuous contraction. The woman may complain of uterine pain or cramping. Be prepared to administer analgesics for pain relief if cramping is intense. When the uterus remains atonic (not contracted), the dose of the drug or rate of the IV infusion may be insufficient to effectively control uterine bleeding. Notify physician/ CNM immediately. Be prepared to administer additional doses to increase I Assess for diarrhea, cramping, fever or bloody stools. infusion rate.
AE: coma, seizures, intracranial hemorrhage, asphyxia, increased uterine motility, painful contractions

Rhogam Rh (D) Immune Globulin

Dosage/Range: Rh Immune Globulin for IM only: 1 vial standard dose (300 mcg) w/in 72 hrs of delivery Rh Immune Globulin IV (for IM or IV use)WinRho – 600 IU (120mcg) OR Rhophylac – 1500 IU (300 mcg) w/in 72 hr of delivery
Onset /Peak/ Duration IM: rapid/ 5-10 days/ unk; IV: unk/2 hr /unk
Indication: Admin to Rh- pts who have been exposed to Rh+ blood
Contraindications: prior allergic rxn to human immunoglobulin
Nursing Considerations: Do not confuse IM and IV formulations. Rh Immune Globulin (microdose and standard dose) is for IM use only and cannot be given IV. Rh Immune Globulin IV may be given IM. Admin at room temp IM into deltoid – should be given within 3 hrs but may be given up to 72 hr after delivery IV admin over 3-5 min
AE: anemia, diarrhea, rash, vomiting, pain at site, fever

Rubella virus vaccine

Dosage/Range: 0.5 mL Subcutaneous Onset /Peak/ Duration: 2-4 weeks/ unk/unk
Indication: Prevents infection by the Rubella virus by stimulating the body to produce antibodies
Contraindications: Do not become pregnant for three months following immunization
Nursing Considerations: Assess pts for signs of allergic reaction following administration

Simethicone chew tablets (Mylicon)
Dosage/Range: PO40-125mg QID
Onset /Peak/ Duration: immediate/ N/A/ 3 hrs
Indication: Relief of pain caused by gas in the GI tract
Contraindications: None
Nursing Considerations: Assess abd pain, bowel sounds, and distention during therapy. Assess frequent belching and passage of flatus
AE: no significant side effects

Sodium chloride .9%
Dosage/Range: 1-2L 100mL/hr IV
Onset /Peak/ Duration: rapid/ end of infusion/ unk
Indication: Hydration and maintenance of fluid and electrolyte status
Contraindications: Pts with elevated or decreased serum sodium
Nursing Considerations: Assess for fluid overload during infusion. Assess pt for signs of hyponatremia during infusion

Tucks Pads (Witch Hazel-Glycerin)
Dosage/Range: Apply pads to perineum after cleansing after each void or BM.
Onset /Peak/ Duration: Unk
Indication: Promotes healing of hemorrhoids and perineal pain. Relieves inflammation.
Contraindications: unknown
Nursing Considerations: Assess for perineal and hemorrhoidal pain and itching. Assess for skin integrity.

(Vicodin 5-500mg) Acetaminophen & Hydrocodone bitrate
Dosage/Range: 2.5 to 10 mg q 3 to 6 hours prn pain. Not to exceed 4 g acetaminophen per day.
Onset /Peak/ Duration: Onset: 10 to 30 minutes. Duration: 4 to 6 hours.
Indication: Management of moderate to severe pain.
Contraindications: Hypersensitivity to drug, bleeding disorders, severe hepatic or renal disease.
Nursing Considerations: Assess VS. Assess for sedation, constipation, and pain relief.
AE: sedation, hypoT, constipation, nausea, dyspepsia, respiratory depression

NEWBORN

Erythromycin Ointment (Ilotycin)
Dosage/Range: 0.5 to 1 cm strip along lower conjunctival surface of each eye, inner canthus to outer canthus.
Onset /Peak/ Duration: Onset/Duration: unlisted for topical medications. It is safe to wipe away excess medication after 1 hour.
Indication: Prevention of infection with neonatal conjunctivitis and ophthalmic neonatorum, which may be passed to infant from mother during birth.
Contraindications/Nursing Considerations: Wash hands before applying. Observe for hypersensitivity. Possible side effects include sensitivity reaction, inability to focus (temporarily), edema, inflammation. Apply before 1 hour after birth.
AE: rash, allergic rxn

Hepatitis B vaccine Recombinate
Dosage/Range: Children and Adolescents 0 to 19 yr of age. IM 5 mcg at 0, 1, and 6 mo.
Onset /Peak/ Duration: Duration: prolonged immunity (years).
Indication: Results in endogenous production of antibodies to protect against HBV for those who are now or may be at risk of contracting HBV in the future.
Contraindications: hypersensitivity to previous hepatitis vaccine, to preservatives, or other additives (may contain thimerisol, neomycin, and/or egg protein).
Nursing Considerations: Assess for fever >39.5, dyspnea, hives, urticaria, severe lethargy or weakness, convulsions, or swelling of eyes, face, or inside of nose.
AE: allergic rxn

Hepatitis B immune globlin
Dosage/Range: Newborns of HBsAg-Positive Mothers IM 0.5 mL.
Onset /Peak/ Duration: Onset of immunity is rapid. Duration is up to 3 months.
Indication: Provides passive immunization to hepatitis B following exposure.
Contraindications: hypersensitivity to previous hepatitis immune globulin, to preservatives, or other additives (may contain thimerisol, neomycin, and/or egg protein).
Nursing Considerations: Assess for fever >39.5, dyspnea, hives, urticaria, severe lethargy or weakness, convulsions, or swelling of eyes, face, or inside of nose.
AE: allergic rxn

(Vitamin K) Phytonadione
Dosage/Range: 0.5-1 mg IM, within 1 hr of birth, may repeat in 6-8 hrs if needed.
Onset /Peak/ Duration: 1- 2 hours/ Normal PT achieved 12 to 14 hours.
Indication: Prevention of hemorrhagic disease of the newborn.
Contraindications: Use cautiously with impaired liver function.
Nursing Considerations: Monitor for frank and occult bleeding (guaiac stools, Hematest urine, and emesis). Monitor pulse and blood pressure frequently; Apply pressure to all venipuncture sites for at least 5 min; avoid unnecessary IM injections.
AE: pain at site, hyperbilirubinemia if dose is too large, kernicterus, rash

Psychopharmacology Study Guide

ANTIDEPRESSANTS

Antidepressants Atypical (Selective (*serotonin, dopamine, norepinephrine*) Reuptake Inhibitors)

- SSRIs
  - Prozac, Celexa, Paxil, Zoloft, Luvox, Lexepro.
  - **Mnemonic**: *Professors Can Produce Zillions of Little Lessons*
- S(N/D)RIs:
  - Wellbutrin, Effexor, Remeron, Duloxetine.
  - **Mnemonic:** *WE(i)RD!*
- Side Affects for atypical antidepressants
  - Potential for change in libido, appetite and weight (up or down), sleep patterns, heart rhythms.
  - Potential for diarrhea, N/V, anxiety, dry mouth, confusion, headache (especially during dose changes for about 3 weeks)
- Goofy Side Effects Story for Atypical Antidepressants *(SSRIs, SNRIs, SDRIs)*
  - The atypical girl was heartbroken and depressed after her boyfriend left her. She couldn't eat, she couldn't sleep. She was so upset that she felt sick to her stomach all the time, causing horrible diarrhea. She was very confused about why her boyfriend would leave her, but he truth was, her boyfriend left because of her low libido...it seems she always "had a headache." She wanted to please her boyfriend, but every time she thought about sex she got nervous, felt dizzy and broke out into a sweat. Her hands would shake so bad that she couldn't even hold a glass of water and take a drink...talk about having a dry mouth!

Antidepressants Traditional (TCAs/QCAs - Tricyclic and Quatracyclic antidepressants)

- These end in *tyline* or *amine* except Amoxapine, Doxepine and Maprotiline. You just have to remember those 3. There are no other drugs in other groups that end with'tyline' or 'amine' (EXCEPT diphenhydramine/Benadryl).
- Side Affects
  - **Narrow therapeutic window and an overdose can kill you!!!**
  - If someone is suicidal, the doc will only prescribe a few days or a weeks worth of these at a time to prevent an overdose!
  - Grand mal seizure and hyperthermia (cooks the brain).
  - Potential for: decrease in libido, decrease in all blood cell production, changes in HR and rhythm, constipation, difficulty in urinating, orthostatic dizziness, weight gain, muscle twitches
- Goofy Side Effects Story for Typical Antidepressants
  - A very traditional man became depressed when his dog B.C. ran away. He ran through the neighborhood, and worked up quite a sweat. His heart raced, and as he searched for his dog, he realized that for the first time in years he wasn't thinking about sex. This realization stopped him dead in his tracks, and his heart slowed. As he stood there, mouth dry and muscles twitching from the exertion, he saw B.C. trying to urinate on a fat lady's lawn. He ran to his dog and scooped him up, dizzy with happiness. He danced around the yard with graceful rhythm, until he stepped in a pile of dog poo. "BC", he exclaimed. "I thought you were constipated!" He flailed around the yard trying to get the poo off his shoe as the fat lady watched from her window. She was convinced the traditional man who was flailing about on the lawn was having a seizure or a stroke.

  **B.C. = blood cells (decrease in white and red blood cell production)*

Psychopharmacology Study Guide

MAOIs (Monoamine oxidase inhibitors)

- Marplan, Nardil, Parnate. They sound like alien names to me and that is how I remembered them.
- Side Affects
  - **Lots of drug and food interactions!!!**
  - Avoid food and drugs containing Tryptophan or Tyramine. These substances can lead to malignant hypertension.
  - Don't eat or drink anything that you would if you were on a fancy vacation! Wine, beer, aged cheese, chicken liver, chocolate, bananas, soy sauce, meat tenderizers, salami, bologna, pickled fish or caffeine.
- Side Effects Goofiness
  - My plan is to not die at the party where they serve fancy food.

    •my plan = Marplan

    •not die = Nardil

    •party = Parnate

ANXIOLYTICS

Benzodiazepines

- Most of these end with "am".
- Librium (Chlordiazepoxide) doesn't, and is used to "liberate" alcoholics from their addiction.
- Tranxene doesn't.
- Important to remember:
  - Xanax (Alprazolam) -most habit forming
  - Valium (Diazepam) falls into this group
- Side Affects
  - Potential for dependence
  - Stopping abruptly can increase anxiety, HA, loss of appetite and in extreme cases: *seizures*
  - Do not use with alcohol
- Goofy Side Effects Story for Benzos
  - Benzo the clown, like most clowns, was very tolerant of small children. Though, truth be told, they made him extremely tired. One day, he decided to stop seeing the children completely. "I'm done with this headache" he said. But once he got home he realized he missed the kids and he stayed up all night thinking about them. The next day he skipped breakfast, which made him feel dizzy, but he didn't care. He ran so fast to see the kids that he got dizzy, fell down, hit his head and had a seizure.

Nonbenzodiazepines

- There are 2 that end with "am"s (Triazolam/Halcion and Temazepam/Restoril) and it is OK to learn them with the benzodiazepines since there really isn't much difference.
- I think that the brand names are easier to remember:
  - Restoril, Halcion, Buspar, and Desyrel
  - **Mnemonic:** *Anxious on buses? Bring bunnies because nobunnys(nonbenzodiazapines) will restore (Restoril) the desire (Desyrel) to hallucinate (Halcyon) on buses (Buspar).*

Atypical Anxiolytics

- Sonata, Ambien, Lunestra
- Think of a woman who takes Ambien and falls asleep to Frank Sinatra (Sonata) while the Lunar moon (Lunestra) shines through the window.

Psychopharmacology Study Guide

Other Anxiolytics
- This is just a weird combination of drugs.
- There are 3 beta blockers: Atenolol, Inderal, and Catapres.
- Then Atarax/Vistaril and Benadryl (most often used for allergic reactions).
- **Mnemonic:** *All Inquisitive Cats Attack Birds*

ANTIPSYCHOTICS

Atypical antipsychotics
- There are 6 of these and this mnemonic may help you remember them.

  All (Abilify)
  Good (Geodon)
  Zoos (Zyprexa)
  Save (Seroquel)
  Rare (Risperdal)
  Cats (Clozaril)
- Side effects: Weight gain and diabetes (also see end of traditional antipsychotics as these two groups share those S/As)

Rare cats
get fat.
Too much sugar
makes them huger.

Traditional antipsychotics
- There are a lot of these so there is a little song to help!
- (Sing it to the tune of "The William Tell Overture" also known as the theme song from "The Lone Ranger")

Loxitane, Trilafon, and Thorazine,
Serentil, Mellaril, and Stelazine,
If you're poor and have psychosis try them all
And Moban and Haloperidol!

- These drugs are cheaper than the atypicals but are not used much because the S/As are more pronounced.
- Both antipsychotic groups share these side effects
- Side effects:: think muscle control problems such as tremors, rigidity, contraction, dystonia, loss of facial expression, stooped posture, shuffling gait-pseudo parkinsonism, Tardive Dyskenesia (irreversible); also neuroleptic malignant syndrome where your temperature goes way up and your brain cooks to death.
- Goofy Side Effects Story for Traditional Antipsychotics
  - Bob was a single guy who could not control his muscle-building obsession. He really wanted a girlfriend, so he decided to try some other hobbies in hopes of meeting someone with skin problems just like his. His dream girl wasn't the typical type. He liked them big and he liked them diabetic! So, he went to a few speed-dating meetings, but they only made him restless, even when they played shuffle board. His favorite activities were poker (he has a great poker face), and limbo (his stopped posture made him a natural). After weeks of speed-dating, he finally met a girl at the Tardive, a dive bar near his house. The sad part of this tale is that she had neuroleptic malignant syndrome and died on their wedding night. Bob eventually wrote a screen play about the romance and is now back to contracting his muscles.

Psychopharmacology Study Guide

MOOD STABILIZERS/ANTICONVULSANTS

Traditional

- Lithium products: (this is easy since they all have 'lith' in them!)
    - Eskalith, Eskalith CR, Lithane, Lithobid, Lithium Citrate

- Side effects: Weight gain, drowsiness, weakness, nausea, fatigue, hand tremor, increase in thirst and urination, hypothyroidism, enlarged thyroid
- Lithium can be toxic and has a narrow therapeutic window. (0.6 – 1.2mmol Li+/liter and over 1.5mmol Li+/liter can kill you)
- Signs of Li+ toxicity are: N/V, drowsiness, slurred speech, blurred vision, confusion, muscle twitching, irregular heart beat, SEIZURES, coma
- Goofy Side Effects for Lithium
    - The fairy princess Lithium was the fairest, most delicate princess in all the land. One day she dared to argue with her future mother-in-law, the great Queen Eskalith. In retaliation, the queen cursed the princess, causing her to have an uncontrollable weakness for ice cream. In just a few weeks she gained a ton of weight. As a result, she just lied around all day feeling constantly tired. One day, her fiance Prince Thyroid came for a visit and saw her in this enlarged state. It made him nauseous to look at her. His hand tremored as he reached out to take her hand. He didn't really want to touch her, so he gave her a glass of water for her thirst instead.

Atypical

- Not so easy since there are a lot of them! However! Here is ANOTHER little song to help you remember them: (To be sung to the tune of "Jingle Bells")

Depakote, Depakene, Keppra all the way,
Moods unstable? Having fits?
These drugs will make your day!

Tegretol, Lamictal, Neurontin, Gabatril,
Trileptal and Topamax,
They're all Atypical!

ANTI-OBSESSIVE/COMPULSIVE MEDS

- There are just 2 of them!!!
    - Luvox: which I am sure you remember from the SSRI's!
    - Anafranil: which is less expensive!

PSYCHOSTIMULANTS

- Think of drugs to treat ADHD:
    - Ritalin/Concerta-methylphenidate
    - Dexedrine/Adderall-Dextroamphetamine
    - Strattera: non stimulant SNRI
    - Provigil/Modafinil

Deglin, Judith Hopfer, and April Hazard Vallerand. *Davis's Drug Guide for Nurses, with Resource Kit CD-ROM (Davis's Drug Guide for Nurses)*. Philadelphia: F A Davis Co, 2009. Print.

Varcarolis, E. M., Carson, V. B., & Shoemaker, N. C. (2006). *Foundations of psychiatric mental health nursing: a clinical approach* (5th ed.). St. Louis: Elsevier Saunders.

Bipolar Disorder

- Diagnosis based on 2 sources of data: The current clinical picture (depression or mania) and a clear history of both manic and depressive episodes. A key thing to ask is if they have ever had a time in their life when they didn't need much sleep.
- Depressive episodes may range from minor to major depressive syndromes
- Manic episodes typically are described as full blown or less intense manic episodes, referred to as hypomania

Common Disorders that may cause Mania

- Brain tumors
- CNS syphilis
- Delirium (due to various causes)
- Encephalitis
- Influenza
- Metabolic changes associated with hemodialysis
- Multiple sclerosis

Drugs that may cause Mania

- Amphetamines
- Bromides
- Cocaine
- Antidepressants
- Isoniazid
- Steroids

Classification Schemes; Bipolar I & II

- Multiple episodes including depressive episodes common in both
- Bipolar I (0.04%-1.6%)
  - Fits more classic description of bipolar illness with clearly recognized episodes of depression and mania
  - Hx of at least 1 manic episode in lifetime
  - Manic episode of at least 7 days of severe sx of elated mood or irritability & major impairment
- Bipolar II (0.5%)
  - Presents with hx of obvious major depressive episodes & at least 1 hypo-manic episode
  - Manic phases are often less intense, unrecognized and thus unreported by patient
  - More common in women-typically more depressive episodes & more severe depression

Other Gender Differences in Bipolar Disorder

- Women more likely to experience mixed mania and rapid cycling (4 or more episodes per yr.) that tends to be more depressive then manic
- Women are often misdiagnosed and given inappropriate meds
- Men and women differ in how they present with mania
- When inquiring about manic episodes patient often denies any.

– Best way to diagnose is to witness a hypomanic episode clinically or to carefully inquire about the history - In particular, if hypomanic episodes are suspected, the most important question to ask is: *"Have you every had a period of time when you didn't need as much sleep?"* A decrease need for sleep and a lack of daytime fatigue are red flags for hypomania. The pt will not be TIRED with little sleep.

Typical Bipolar vs. Rapid Cyclinig Bipolar Disorders

- In the typical BP patient, depressive and manic episodes last for several weeks or months, often with periods of normal mood occurring between periods of depression and mania.
- When there are two or more episodes of both depression and mania (e.g., depression-mania-depression-mania) within a year – referred to as "rapid cycling". Sometimes rapid cyclers can dramatically switch moods from week to week or even day to day.

Dysphoric Mania (or Mixed Mania)

- Diagnostic term which describes patients that have concurrent manic and depressive symptoms (e.g., increased activity, pressured speech, suicidal ideas, and feelings of worthlessness). Pt is irritated and agitated...Belinda!
- The subclassifications of Bipolar I and Bipolar II, typical vs. rapid cycling, and dysphoric mania are important because they have different treatment implications.

Target Symptoms

- Vary depending on the current phase of the illness

Clinical Features of Mania

- A pronounced and persistent mood of euphoria (elevated or expansive mood) or irritability and at least 3 of the following:
  - Grandiosity or elevated self-esteem
  - Decreased need for sleep
  - Rapid, pressured speech (often these people are hard, if not impossible to interrupt)
  - Racing thoughts
  - Distractibility
  - Increased activity or psychomotor agitation
  - Behavior that reflects expansiveness (lacking restraint in emotional expression, will get right up in your face!) and poor judgment, such as increased sexual promiscuity, gambling, buying sprees, giving away money, etc.
  - Flight of ideas (sound got lost here, so look this up!)
  - Sometimes have psychotic features including delusions (usually grandiose or paranoid) and command hallucinations may be present – may give rise to self-injury, suicide and danger to client's safety

Medications Used to Treat Bipolar Illness

- Treatment of Bipolar illness has two goals: Reduction of current symptoms and prevention of relapse
- Episodes are invariably recurring and thus prophylactic treatment is important
- Research indicates that failure to treat leads to relapse and to progressively worsening condition
- Subsequent episodes tend to become more and more severe & can, at times, become treatment refractory

Medications Used

- Lithium is primary...it stabilizes mood, can prevent relapse (or lessen intensity of subsequent episodes) if tx is on an ongoing basis. Lithium seems to be somewhat more effective in preventing relapse of mania rather than depression

Medication Regimen for Mania

- Other drugs are used as adjunctive or alternatives
- If patient quite agitated, out of control or psychotic the initial plan is to begin treatment with both a mood stabilizer and an antipsychotic medication.
- The atypical anti-psychotics seem to improve behavioral control more rapidly

Atypical Antipsychotics (All Good Zoos Save Rare Cats)

- Risperidone (Risperdal); Olanzapine (Zyprexa); Quetiapine (Seroquel); Ziprasidone (Geodon); Aripiprazole (Abilify)

Mood Stabilizers/Anticonvulsants: Atypicals

- Carbamazepine; Divalproex sodium; Valproic Na/Valproic acid; Gabapentin; Lamotrigine; Levetiracetam; Oxcarbazepine; Tiagabine HCl; Topiramate
- With most mood stabilizers the patient may require 10 days to show a clinical response so an antipsychotic is used on a short term basis. Once the mood is stabilized, the antipsychotic may be phased out. Alternatively, high potency benzodiazepines can be used in place of antipsychotics (e.g. clonazepam [Klonopin])
- *Treatment with lithium* is initiated after necessary lab tests are conducted; Generally starting dose is 600-900mgm/day given in divided doses.
  - Therapeutic and toxic range are very close to one another – thus it is necessary to gradually increase the dose while carefully monitoring blood levels. Most patients must reach a level between 1.0 and 1.2 mEq.L.
  - Not infrequently the level may need to be higher to obtain symptomatic improvement (1.2 to 1.6), but on these higher levels, side effects are more common and adherence is poor.
  - On occasion, patients may need and tolerate blood levels up to 2.0 mEq/L, however there is higher risk of toxicity at such doses. Generally, daily doses range from 1200-3000 mgm.
  - Once mood is adequately stabilized, the dose can be lowered somewhat (0.8 – 1.0 mEq/L) for maintenance treatment

If Presenting Phase is a Depressive Episode

- Antidepressants alone in the treatment of bipolar depression can cause significant problems, by provoking a rapid shift into mania (as well as increasing frequency of episodes; i.e., causing cycle acceleration).
- The treatment of choice therefore is to use a mood stabilizer in combination with an antidepressant (e.g., imipramine (Tofranil); amitriptyline (Elavil).
- There are also 2 mood stabilizers that contain antidepressant properties that may be effective (lamotrigine [Lamictal] and divalproex [Depakote-SR]).

Side Effects of Lithium and Signs of Toxicity

- Side Effects: Nausea, diarrhea, vomiting, find hand tremor, sedation, muscular weakness, polyuria, polydypsia, edema, weight gain, and a dry mouth

- Adverse Effects from chronic use: Leukocytosis (reversible if discontinued), hypothroidism and goiter, acne, psoriasis, teratogenesis (first trimester, although risk is low) and kidney damage.
- Signs of Toxicity: Lethargy, ataxia, slurred speech, tinnitus, severe nausea/vomiting, tremor, arrhythmias, hypotension, seizures, shock, delirium, coma and even death. Since the toxic range is near to the therapeutic range, blood levels and adverse effects must be monitored closely

Nursing Considerations in Mania

- Patient safety first (may need one-to-one in manic phase)
- Basic needs a priority
- Medication adherence
- Monitor for side effects, adverse effects and toxicity
- Patient education
- Outpatient support groups and self-help groups

Key Points in Patient Education

- Lithium is a medication that treats your current emotional problem and will also be helpful in preventing relapse. So it will be important to continue with treatment after the current episode is resolved
- Since the therapeutic and toxic ranges are so close, we must monitor your blood level closely. This will be done more frequently at first and every several months thereafter. Never increase your dose without first consulting with your health care provider.
- Lithium and other mood stabilizers *are not addictive*
- Many side effects can be reduced/minimized by taking divided doses or may subside as treatment progresses
- Bipolar disorders often run in families. Any relatives that have pronounced mood swings should be alerted to the possibility of a treatable condition and the need for professional evaluation (the yield on this maneuver is high, since medical awareness of bipolar disorder is still low, especially with milder forms, and family history is impressively often positive for this disorder)
- You and your family need to be aware that this is a biological disorder, not a moral defect or a character flaw. When severe, you may not always be able to control your behavior, necessitating that practical steps be taken to protect all concerned from poor judgment during episodes
- Many self-help groups have been developed to provide support for bipolar patients and their families. In this community the local mental health association can help you find groups in your area (Mental Health Association of Sacramento County (MHASC.org) – (916) 366-4600) also Sacramento County Family Alliance for the Mentally Ill – (916) 874-9416

Cyclothymic Disorder

- Characterized by mood swing that alternates between mania and depression
- Milder than mania
- Mood swings have occured for at least 2 years without symptom remission for 2 months
- Can be a precurser to mania
- Constantly need attention, can lead to poor interpersonal relations (especially at work)

Delirium and Dementia

Identify the expected psychobiological changes that occur with aging
- Cognitive: Decrease in processing speed, impaired explicit memory recall
- Sensory: decreased auditory and visual discrimination (GET THE GLASSES AND HEARING AID!)
- Psychological/Emotional: changes in self-concept r/t los

Discuss ageism and elder abuse in the U.S.
- Neglect (48%): failure to provide necessities
- Psychological Abuse (35%): conduct that causes mental anguish ("If you don't stop peeing on the cat I'm going to put you in a home!")
- Financial Exploitation (30%): Misappropriation of assets
- Physical/Sexual Abuse (25%): hitting, burning, non-consensual sexual contact

- The abused = Risk factors for abuse: female, 80+, isolated, combative, hx of troubled past relationship, cognitive impairment
- The abuser = substance abuse, psychological disorders, previous hx of family violence, financially dependent on the victim
- Signs of Abuse
  - Home: falling apart house, lots of people using house, drug activity, stinky
  - Financial: irregular pattern, buying inappropriate items, bills not paid, new "best friend."
  - Physical: bruises, burns, inadequate food, unkempt
  - Elder: fearful, depressed, anxiety, isolation
  - Caregiver: excessive concern with cost, verbal abuse, doesn't let elder speak for themselves (see "abuser")

Describe biological, psychological, and sociocultural theories on aging.
- Erickson: Integrity vs. Despair; recognize life accomplishments to achieve acceptance and satisfaction
- Butler's Life Review: Reminiscence of life experiences to arrive at some degree of closure
- Stability of Personality: Changes in personality and psychological crisis are not universal expectations; elders can develop new responses to change
- Disengagement Theory: Task of old age is to let go
- Activity Theory: Use it or lose it
- Family/Transgenerational: The family unit functions to support entry into and exit from the family

Compare and contrast the clinical picture of delirium with dementia. *already on study guide*

Describe 3 delirium syndromes common in older patients.
- Sundown: fatigue increases as daylight decreases, ability to orient is compromised leading to fear/anxiety
- Sunrise: confusion and grogginess occur in the early AM; result of sleeplessness or meds
- Relocation: disorientation increases in new environment

List 9 nursing interventions for the patient with a cognitive impairment.
- Address underlying cause
- Always check to see if they have their hearing aid, glasses. QUESTION ON TEST ABOUT THIS!
- Always evaluate their meds for possible reactions, side effects, toxic doses. Know which meds are your anti-cholinergics b/c these cause blurred vision, urinary retention, confusion, etc.... MAYBE A QUESTION ABOUT THIS
- Make sure well rested, hydrated, safe, nourished
- Assign consistent staff
- Assess need for 1:1 (see chart)
- Use distraction, offer attention to personal interests
- Use antianxiety meds and antipsychotics carefully
- Communicate to reorient/reassure (stuff we learned in Gero)
- Institute fall precautions (room near nurses station, orient to call light, have family sit with pt, 1:1 prn)

Distinguish between delirium, dementia and depression. *already on study guide*

List the DSM-IV criteria for dementia

- Memory Impairment! Impairment ability to either learn new information or recall previously learned info.
- 1+ cognitive disturbances: apraxia, aphasia, agnosia, disturbed executive functioning
    - apraxia = cannot perform activity even though no motor impairment
    - aphasia = can't find the words, progresses to muteness
    - agnosia = doesn't recognize people or objects; sensory not impaired
    - disturbed executive functioning = cannot plan, organize, sequence, reason

Understand the use of the MMSE in the dx of dementia

The MMSE is only a small part of the dx for dementia. A LOT of things are done to determine this dx.

List the sequential steps for the management of an agitated patient. *(see handout for more detail)*

1. Ensure immediate safety of the pt
2. Assess and Intervene for possible causes (physical or physiological needs such as pain, hunger, missing glasses, medication reaction)
3. If behavior persists, then do one of these things:
    1. Environment management: move closer to nurses station, put in chair in hallway, check lighting, familiarize pt to surroundings and personal belongings in the room
    2. Behavioral management: frequent reorientation and supportive communication, routine ambulation and toileting q 3 hrs, diversionary activities, stagger visits
    3. Request consultation: psych consult and/or Geriatric CNS
4. If behavior persists, consider the use of restraints and/or meds
    1. Use least-restrictive restraint (i.e. a lap hugger or wedge cushion)
    2. Meds are antipsychotics (Haldol at low dose). Avoid narcs and long-acting benzos. Start low, go slow.
5. If behavior persists, use a special care attendant (a "sitter")

List the 4 questions on the CAM

1. Acute Onset/Fluctuating Course: Is there a history of acute change in mental status with evidence of fluctuation in the degree of symptoms?
2. Inattention: Does the pt have difficulty focusing attention...being easily distracted or failing to focus on the discussion or sustain an effort?
3. Disorganized Speech: Is the patient's speech disorganized or incoherent...rambling or irrelevant conversation, unclear or illogical flow of ideas, unpredictable switching of subjects?
4. Altered Level of Consciousness: Is the pt's level of alertness either hyperalert or hypoalert?

Know the 4 stages of Alzheimers

- 1st stage
    - "He forgets which bills are paid"
    - "He loses items more often"
    - "She's more withdrawn and disinterested"
- 2nd stage
    - "She doesn't know what to do or who to call in an emergency."
    - "During the night he got out of bed, drove off, got lost, and died of exposure"
    - "She calls me right after we visit, wanting to know when we'll be stopping by."
- 3rd stage
    - "Mom is fearful and won't leave me alone while I'm cooking."
    - "She accuses me of hiding things"
    - "Dad doesn't remember mom's name and is unaware of holidays."
- 4th stage
    - "Mom has lost almost all verbal abilities."
    - "Grandma needs complete help with walking and will be bed-bound soon."
    - "Gramps needs help with all his ADLs."

Depression

Introduction

- Ranges in emotion are part of the human condition...all of us as healthy people experience a range of emotions all day long. Affect should be animated, should change frequently. What we notice the most is when people are flat.

- Continuum of emotional responses
  Note that there is such a thing as Chronic Sorrow...a nurse did some research on this. Grief/sorrow that lasts longer than 1 year...Dr. V says that it's normal to set aside grief or issues aside when you can't deal with them at that time...this is "suppression of emotions". As you get down to delayed grief and depression reaction...these are more maladaptive responses. Sadness and depression are a fluid kind of experience, it's not all-or-nothing.

- At least 10-15 million affected by mood disorders at any one time.

- Of the 30,000 annual suicides, approximately 16,000 associated with depressive disorders. THIS IS A MEDICAL EMERGENCY!

- Fewer than half of those with mood disorders receive help. If you are functional to some extent, you are at risk for not getting the help and treatment you need.

Epidemiology

- 1 in 4 persons will experience some type of mood disorder in their lifetime
- Major depressive disorder is most common mood disorder, with a lifetime prevalence of approximately 15%

- Major depression is two times more common among women. Dr. V thinks this is a misnomer, but she thinks its manifested differently in men (more agitated, sociopathic...this is Dr. V's opinion, no research to back this)

- Major depression is 1.5 - 2 times more common among 1st degree relatives with this disorder. GENETIC!

- Major depression as a recurring pattern: 50-60% can be expected to have a 2nd episode. Those who have a 2nd episode, have a 70% chance of having a 3rd episode. The chances of having an episode go up! This is why it is so important to get early treatment...you are more debilitative each time you have an episode. It's not always the case that someone stopped taking meds. Stress can exacerbate symptoms (voices, moods) and lead to person not taking meds...maybe the voices say "don't take that!". A person could identify early signs of when starting to deteriorate or starting to experiencing stress. Ask pt "what are your early signs of stress?" This is KEY!

  Every time someone comes into the hospital, don't want pt to feel they have done something wrong...this would cause more stress. Want them to come in as early as possible, stabilize meds and get them out as quickly as possible. Lot of drug-shifting going on in the acute setting...trying to figure out what works.

- Untreated episodes of major depression last 6-24 mos. A little aside: It is VERY difficult to get someone who is bipolar to recognize they have a problem d/t the periods of mania (they feel great!). Then when they get super manic they are out of touch with reality (psychotic). With depressed people, the work is in getting them moving and motivated to understand their illness and options. Don't let the depressed person sleep all day...get them up and out in the milieu. Once they start getting out in the milieu and out of their self-absorption...can do a lot of teaching and discussion so they can do some self-analysis.

- Common age of onset of depression is 18-44. Highest age of onset is the 18-24 age group. Research says depression is rising in younger age groups...but V asks if this is reliable? It's up to the consumer to decide if the research is viable.
- Rate of depression is rising in younger age groups, or is it just that we are able to better diagnose it? Is our world more stressful now? Is there something wrong with the family? Are there toxins in the environment? Hmmm....

PREDISPOSING FACTORS

Biological Correlates (two key ones are neurotransmitter and neuroendocrine)

- Neurotransmitter hypothesis: Variety of them involved - Serotonin; Nor-epinephrine; Gamma-aminobutyric acid (GABA); Acetylcholine; Dopamine. These are all dysregulated in mood disorders...reuptake problems, problems at the synaptic cleft. This is a trial-and-error process, you just try the drug and see how it works! You may see a pt getting worse after they were better for awhile...is it a drug effect?
- Neuroendocrine hypothesis: Biological rhythms - melatonin. Dr. V doesn't think we give enough attention to this. We should all get 20 mins of sun every day to help us maintain our biological rhythm! Get outside!
- Genetic hypothesis:
  - Life time risk in relatives is 20-24%, compared to 6% in general population.
  - Identical twin has a 2-4x risk than fraternal.
- Kindling: Early episodes precipitated by psychosocial stressors/crisis in premorbid individuals. This is a newer idea. You might see someone who is functioning quite well, but at age 18 when leaving home they have their first major episode. The stress/change is not enough for them to handle. Does not just apply to depression...this theory can apply to many illnesses.

Psychosocial Correlates (can help you tune in to areas where you need to gather more data)

- Aggression turned inward. Pt does not know how to express emotions readily, then the stress can build up internally leading to a major depressive episode. Especially attributed to women b/c it's not attractive for women to express anger emotions.
- Object loss. For men this tends to be a job loss, and for women it is more related to loss of family structure.
- Personality disorganization...maybe a personality disorder to some extent...an underlying personal structure that does things to undermine self.
- Cognitive theory. People have faulty ideas that are not part of reality. These people will have a hard time developing sustaining relationships.
- Learned helplessness-hopelessness. "I can't do this", person feels they have no control or ability and gives up.

Complicated/Unresolved Grief (Delayed Grief)

Assessment:

- Symptoms of grief and depression overlap. Everything about grief exhibits as depression. This is why you want to find out if the person has any underlying losses in the past year. It may not just be related to loss...could have an underlying depression as well. Once grief is addressed and still showing depression, then the dx will shift. Otherwise, it is unresolved grief. Most people do get through losses within a few months and go on with their lives.
- Excessive hostility & grief: could be that the person left them and they are now angry that they have to cope alone. It is not uncommon to have some hostility/anger at some point in the resolution of the grief...should get past this. If not, then concerned!
- Prolonged feelings of emptiness & numbness. This should pass within a few months to a year.
- Inability to weep or express emotions. "I do feel profound loss, but I have to put that aside right now." They DO have to address it at some point, b/c delayed grief is going to decrease their functioning.
- Low self-esteem "I can't function without Bob." You hear stuff like this a lot with delayed grief.
- Use of present tense instead of past in relation to loss

- Persistent dreams about the loss is very common. A lot of adults who lost their parents (and were overly attached) will have persistent dreams.
- Retention of clothing of the deceased, some people even keep the body in the house for weeks.
- Inability to visit grave b/c they can't face it.
- Projection of living memories onto an object held in place of the lost person.

ASSESSMENT OF MOOD DISORDER

Major Depression (if no symptoms of mania, then you have major depression)

- Characterized by one or more recurrent episodes of depression
- May range from mild to severe...a lifetime illness of remissions and exacerbations
- Presenting symptoms unique for each person. Ask your pts what their early signs are to hep them recognize when an episode is coming on. Maybe they stop making their bed, or can't sleep, or stop eating. Might start spending more time alone.
- Experiences current mood as a change (unlike self)..."I'm just not like myself anymore." This is a key finding!
- Depressed mood is the most common symptom. This is sometimes difficult for men to talk about and identify.
- Unable to enjoy life.
- Tearfulness and crying are fairly common, although some do not cry. This is individualized, so ask pt if this is one of their symptoms.
- Anxiety, experienced as a pervasive feeling of worry and fear with agitation. An anger in the voice may be present, may be jumpy. Kids likely to be angry b/c they don't understand why they are not like their peers.
- Sometimes persons will seek medical care for somatic complaints. There is almost a blame attached to this and not an understanding that the person is trying to seek out help but isn't sure how to do so...may be due to a cultural stigma of mental illness.
- Often have a concrete reason why their energy left them. "I got sick, my wife left me." "I lost my job." Pay attention to see how much they talk about this reason...may bring it up in group. There is an emotional response surrounding the concrete reason for the loss, so pay attention!
- When clients have somatic complaints, pay particular attention to mood and cognition.

Seasonal depression (SAD)

- Pretty common among older adults in LTCF, b/c they don't get outside much. Starting to administer artificial light in LTCFs to help. Also, some people live in areas where it is dark most of the time, you see higher rates of addiction and depression of people who live in these regions. Melatonin supplements can also help.

Postpartum depression

- Dr. V talked about Andrea Yeats...thinks she did not have PDD but was actually psychotic. Anyway, PPD is more common than we think. Assess the mothers on the OB unit for this! The huge change of motherhood can be a huge stressor for women.

Dysthymic Disorder

- Characterized by chronically depressed mood.
- Milder than major depression. DD is a precurser to diagnosing someone for major depression.
- Down in dumps most of day, on more days than not, and lasts <u>for at least 2 years</u>. Person is functional!

- When depressed, at least two of the following symptoms are present...
    - Poor appetite or overeating; Insomnia or hypersomnia; Low energy or fatigue; Low self-esteem; Poor concentration or difficulty making decisions; Sometimes have double depression (also have MDD...periods of mood-swings and non functionality)

Risk for Suicide

Not characterized as a disorder, but you are at higher risk if you have:

– Depressive disorders; Schizophrenia; Substance use disorder; Personality disorder; Panic disorder; Organic mental disorder

Epidemiology of Suicide

- 8th leading cause of death in U.S.A. 3rd among 15-24 year olds. Highest rate of suicide is among white men > 85 yrs (men more likely to do so when spouse dies or can no longer be functional)
- Firearms most common method (men tend to use more volatile methods than women. Women tend to use overdoses, car exhaust in the garage).
- High rates among: Native Americans and Alaskan Natives...addiction rates are highest among these groups also!

THEORETICAL PERSPECTIVES

- Psychobiological:
    - Loss of love (people get profoundly depressed...maybe they even killed the person...ouch!) The homicidal, suicidal shift can go either way...hard for them to see the difference between the two.
    - Narcissistic injury. Person has perceived notion they have been profoundly hurt in some way
    - Overwhelming moods (see in rapid cycler bipolars)
    - Identify with a suicide victim
    - Group suicides (ex: Plano Tx)...suicide pacts on the internet
- Biochemical-Genetic Theories
    - Runs in families – ex: Hemingways (interaction of alcohol and depression). May even think it is part of the family tradition...can get ingrained socioculturally into family members.
    - Lower levels of 5-HT/serotonin Higher 5-HT-2 in brain and platelets (may lead to biological markers)

Assessment

- Look for clues, both verbal and non verbal. Dr. V gave example of the pt who came up to nurses station while she was getting meds and reminiscing about his life. She'd never heard him do that before, but she was mutli-tasking so didn't think too much of it at the time. Intuitively, she thought something wasn't right, so she later went and checked on him...the door was partially shut and he came walking out of the bathroom with a wrapped up wire in his hand...he gave it to her and said "I was thinking of killing myself." Usually the mood is more elevated b/c they have more energy to commit suicide...so notice ANY mood/behavior changes in your depressed patients.
- State of despair & loneliness
- Any change from usual behavior (You feel uneasy but often cannot pinpoint what it is) -Behavioral; Somatic &/or Emotional

Dissection of Suicide Plan

- Helps to determine degree of suicide risk
- Evaluate specificity of details (if they have a plan to hang themselves, do they have a rope?)
- Lethality of proposed method (how many Xanax do they actually have?)
- Availability of means (do they have the gun in their possession?)

High Risk Factors

- Social isolation (no support system)
- Severe life events (lots of losses, stress or change)
- Suicide by imitation (15-24 yr. olds)
- Low self-esteem in vulnerable adolescents (ex: discounting their own contributions/opinions, talking about not measuring up to peers)

Assessment Tools: SAD PERSONS Scale (pg. 478)

Sex **A**ge **D**epression **P**revious attempt **E**thanol use **R**ational thinking loss **S**ocial support lacking **O**rganized Plan **N**o spouse **S**ickness

Health Care Worker Self-assessment

- Anxiety, irritation, avoidance, denial are all common.

Client Assessment

- Risk and protective factors; Personal and family history
- Other health problems, demographics
- Determine level of risk and assess for major change to peaceful mood
- If outpatient, then supports must be in place...also a contract!

Risk Factors

- Suicide ideation with intent
- Co-occurring disorders
- Recent isolation; Recent major stress
- Panic attacks
- Impulsivity; Aggressiveness
- Access to firearms

* Lethal plan
* Hx childhood abuse/family suicide
* Hopelessness
* Shame/humiliation
* Loss of cognitive function
* Substance abuse

Protective Factors

Sense of responsibility (fam; spouse); Pregnancy; Religious beliefs; Satisfaction with life; Positive social support; Effective coping skills; Effective problem-solving skills; Intact reality testing

Planning

- Determine priority for care (is it the suicidal ideation? maybe they need to find ways to build a social support system, or determine their prodromal symptoms)
- Manage other health problems
- Activate resources
- Continue ongoing assessment
- Evaluate experience of loss and grief

Intervention

- Involve a variety of services and providers...need to tell pt they can talk to anyone on the unit.
- Match client needs to services
- Treat person as an individual
- **Primary Intervention:** Provide support, education, information
- **Secondary Intervention:** Treatment of acute crisis (does not have to be inpatient, can be outpatient, could include going to support group); Work with client ambivalence (client may be indecisive and this can be frustrating for the nurse. Assess their level of understanding and concern for this, intervention may be to have fewer options.)
- **Tertiary Intervention:** Work with family/friends of person who has committed suicide; Interventions with person who has attempted suicide- minimizing trauma is important (don't let them get hurt)

Hospitalized Suicidal Patient

- Suicide precautions: arms length, one-to-one (step down to staff line-of-site, step down accompanied by staff off unit) restraints if absolutely necessary, records/assessments every 15 mins. Make contract with patient! It gives them power and responsability (increases internal LOC)

Outside the Hospital

- Garner support of family/SO/friends
- Social support: at least 3 contacts they can talk to if they feel depressed
- Appropriate treatment maintained: medication, ECT, other
- Key supports should be given primary providers contact info.
- Appts in place for ongoing evaluation
- Family, SO, and friends should be alerted to signs and symptoms and change from morose to carefree or from sad to happy or "worry free"
- Record-keeping important for rationale as to why to hospitalize, or rationale not to hospitalize.
- Limited supply of medications (2-3 days worth at a time). SSRIs not much of a problem, but benzos/alcohol/ sedatives could be used to overdose.
- Provide list with #'s of support people and crisis lines for family and patient
- Latest research suggests replacing contract with pt. not to kill self, with contract in which pt. agrees to notify staff if feels suicidal, a sense of hopelessness or despair.

Therapeutic Techniques for All Settings

- Establishment of interpersonal relationship...the sense of hope that we impart to pts has a huge impact on pt's own sense of hope. Don't be glib, but carry a sense of hope to the pt "Let's work on this together", "I think that we can perhaps establish some ways that you can work better for yourself out there in the community."
- Encouragement of realistic problem solving
- Reaffirm hope

Crisis Management for Suicidal Persons

- Remain calm. If person tells you they are contemplating suicide, call police!
- Deal directly with topic of suicide "Do you have thoughts of killing yourself?" Be confident and up front with it!
- Encourage problem solving and positive actions
- Encourage person to get assistance
- UCLA – Suicide Prevention. Important to let client know these things: crisis is temporary, unbearable pain can be survived, help is available, you are not alone. Client may have tunnel vision and feel totally alone.

Crisis Management for Suicidal Persons in the Community

- Relieve isolation
- Remove all weapons
- Encourage alternative expression of anger
- Avoid final decision for suicide during crisis
- Reestablish social ties
- Relieve extreme anxiety & sleep loss

Survivors of Completed Suicide

- Intervention initiated within 24-72 hours after suicide
- Often must grieve without the usual informal social supports
- Stigmatized and cut off
- Confused feelings of pain, anger and guilt
- Few seek counseling
- May experience symptoms of PTS reactions
- Initiate post traumatic loss debriefing can help to precipitate an adaptive grief process
- Stages of debriefing: Introductory, Fact (talk openly about every detail, go to grave, make it real so no hidden pieces), Life review, Feeling (express the feelings fully), Reaction, Learning, Closure

Diagnoses Examples

- **NANDA:** Dysfunctional grieving, Powerlessness, Spiritual distress, Hopelessness
- **DSM IV:** Dysthymic disorder, Major depressive disorder
- **Outcome identification:** The patient will be emotionally responsive and return to a pre-illness level of functioning

- Planning Implementation: Counseling, Therapeutic use of self
- **Critical pathway:** Facilitating expression of feelings, Facilitating self-esteem, Cognitive restructuring, Group interventions, Family interventions, Milieu therapy, Promoting physical activity, Self-care activities
- Somatic interventions: ECT: electroconvulsive therapy; Phototherapy for melatonin issues; Psychopharmacology

Electroconvulsive Therapy (ECT)

- Can achieve higher than 90% remission rate in 1-2 weeks
- Useful for people who don't respond to antidepressants (20-30%)
- Long-term results are mixed; however, there is some indication that it is an effective treatment for selected clients

How Does ECT Work?

- It's believed that ECT works by using an electrical shock to cause a seizure. This seizure releases selective neurotransmitters (especially GABA in the occipital cortex) in the brain. The release of these chemicals improves communication between brain cells.
- The neuroendocrine hypothesis, (from human studies), argues that the affective disorders result from a deficiency of a mood-modifying peptide (antidepressin) from the hypothalamus.
- Convulsive therapy stimulates the production and release of antidepressin.

Indications for ECT

- Need for rapid effective response in a suicidal and homicidal client
- Client is extremely agitated, stuporous or has marked psychomotor retardation
- Risks of other treatments greater
- History of poor drug response &/or positive response to ECT
- Client's request
- For clients with major depression and bipolar disorder with delusions (guilt, somatic or infidelity)
- Also helpful in manic clients resistant to lithium and antipsychotic meds, and in rapid cyclers.
- Known to be effective in catatonia, schizoaffective, pregnant psychotic clients, & some clients with Parkinson's

Course of ECT Treatment

- 6-12 treatments, 2-3 times a week
- Special care to clients with a history of MI, CVA, Cerebrovascular lesions
- Informed consent for voluntary. For involuntary: kin- or court-ordered.
- General anesthesia and muscle-paralyzing agents prevent grand mal seizure
- Bilateral side effects include: confusion, disorientation and short-term memory loss, most everyone gets HA.
- Post treatment may require frequent orientation
- Clients often complain of memory deficits for the first few weeks, but the memory usually returns
- Headache common for 8-24 hours after treatment

- Not a permanent cure for depression – supplemented with TCAs or lithium decreases the relapse rate
- Maintenance ECT: Once a week to once a month; May also help decrease relapse rates in those who tend to relapse. Some pt may get a "tune up" once a year.

Psychopharmacology Antidepressants

- **Tricyclics (TCAs):** Enhance neurotransmission of selected neurotransmitters. Block their reuptake at presynaptic neuron; Inhibit their metabolism & subsequent deactivation; Enhance the activity of receptors.
- TCA Client Teaching
    - 7-28 days for mood elevation
    - Reinforce frequently
    - Drowsiness, dizziness and hypotension usually subside after a few weeks
    - Be careful driving, operating heavy machinery
    - Alcohol can block effects
    - Full dose at bedtime to avoid side effects
    - If forgets bedtime dose or 1 a day dose, take within 3 hrs or wait until next day
    - Do not stop meds abruptly: nausea, altered heartbeat, nightmares, and cold sweats in 2-4 days
- **SSRI's:** Inhibit reuptake of serotonin; Permit serotonin to act for an extended period at synaptic site. They have fewer side effects (such as anticholinergic); Examples: Prozac, Lexepro, Paxil, Zoloft
- **MAOI's: Monoamine Oxidase Inhibitors:** Prevent inactivation of certain brain amines, such as norepinephrine, serotonin, dopamine, and tyramine. Therefore, an increase of these amines available for synaptic release in the brain. Increase of tyramine poses a problem...Can lead to high blood pressure, hypertensive crisis, and later, to CVA, so must reduce intake. Avoid foods and drugs that contain it (i.e., avocados, figs, bananas, fermented foods, almost all cheeses, beer and chianti)
- **Novel Antidepressants-** Bupropion (Wellbutrin or Zyban): Active serotonin (5 HT2) receptor antagonist; Binds to the serotonin transmitter (inhibits serotonin reuptake)

IN CLOSING, your pts with MDD and DD need...

- Health teaching re: Prodromal symptoms
- Case management includes managing needs in community
- Health promotion and health maintenance to de-stress and have healthier lifestyle
- Differentiation of: Symptoms of grief vs. depression; Interventions - grief vs. depression
- Evaluation

Dissociative and Personality Disorders

List and define five dissociative symptoms

- Numbness: not in the book, and didn't watch lecture. (sorry guys!)
- Detachment: An interpersonal and intrapersonal dissociation from affective expression. Therefore, the individual appears cold, aloof, and distant. This behavior is thought to be learned and is viewed as defensive.
- Derealization: The false perception by a person that his or her environment has changed. For example, everything seems bigger or smaller, or familiar objects seem strange.
- Depersonalization: A phenomenon whereby a person experiences a sense of unreality of or estrangement from self. For example, one may feel that one's extremities have changed or that one is in a dream or seeing oneself from a distance.
- Dissociative amnesia: Inability to recall important personal information, often of a traumatic or stressful nature. May be localized to certain events in a certain period or selective (able to remember some but not all events in a period)

Identify five traumatic events that could precipitate PTSD.

- War
- Victim of crime
- Sexual assault
- Physical abuse
- Nursing school final exams

Describe the technique of cognitive restructuring.

- Cognitive restructuring or "reframing" has been found to be positively correlated with greater positive affect and higher self-esteem.
- It includes recasting irrational beliefs and replacing worried self statements "I can't pass this class" with more positive statements, "If I choose to study 24 hours a day I will pass."
- It can be used to reduce stress by changing the individual's perception of stress.
- Essentially, it is reassessing a situation....the desired result is to restructure a disturbing event or experience into one that is less disturbing and in which we have a sense of control.
- Cognitive distortions often include overgeneralizations and "should" statements.
- This technique is often done along with progressive relaxation.

Define dissociative amnesia, fugue, and Dissociative Identity Disorder

- Dissociative amnesia
  - Inability to recall important personal information, often of a traumatic or stressful nature.
  - May be localized to certain events in a certain period or selective (able to remember some but not all events in a period)
- Dissociative fugue
  - A sudden, unexplained travel away from the customary locale and inability to recall one's identity and information about some or all of of the past.
  - In rare cases, the person assumes a whole new identiy.
  - During fugue state, person tends to lead simple life. Doesn't call attention to himself.
  - After a few weeks or months, they remember their former identities and become amnesiac about their time in the fugue state.
  - Usually precipitated by a traumatic event.
- Dissociative Identity Disorder
  - Presence of two or more distinct personalities states that recurrently take control of behavior.

List the 7 most challenging behaviors seen in patients with personality disorders and therapeutic nursing interventions for each.

- Manipulation (pt tells you you're the best nurse ever when she asks for special treatment)
  - Say "I've noticed that when you compliment me, you want something from me. When you do that, I wonder if I can trust you." SET LIMITS
- Impulsiveness (pt striking others)
  - Say "I am going to ask you to agree to sitting 5 feet away from the group members until you have better control of your impulses. I want to help you be safe here."

- Splitting (pt blaming you for everything, you are evil and bad because you won't let him off the uit for lunch, but another nurse named "Omar" will...often used to manipulate staff)
  - Say "Omar and I will talk about it and we will let you know what we decide. If you think you are going to get mad and cut on yourself, then you need to stay here in my presence until I have Omar join us." SET LIMITS
- Devaluing others (pt says they don't want to go to group with all those "losers")
  - Say "Hmmmm.....I guess if you go to a meeting with people you think are losers, you risk feeling like a loser, too. But if you don't go, you risk feeling alone or like an outsider."
- Suspiciousnes (pt says "what do you mean by that? Are you calling me crazy?)
  - Say "I was talking to the group as a whole, my comment wasn't meant for you. Do you wonder if I think you are crazy?"
- Blaming others (pt complains about night staff not doing their job and blaming them for his headache)
  - Say "I am uncomfortable when you disparage others. I believe you are working on clear and direct communication while you are here, and I hope you can express any frustration you are feeling directly to the night shift staff."
- Demanding (pt makes lots of demands)
  - Say "I wonder if you'd be willing to work on asking for things in a different manner. I know I don't feel like helping you when I'm asked in this way, and I imagine that might be true for other people in your life as well."
- Helplessness (pt says they can't do something on their own, even when they can)
  - Say ... ooops, the notes aren't on the slide. What do you say?

Understand the 7 diagnostic features of all personality disorders
- Inflexible and maladaptive response to stress
  - For example, an engineer is able to organize complex details at work. However, when this same compulsion carries over to other parts of life it may be too rigid or limited to allow personal or social functioning. This rigid behavior serves the function of controlling deep anxiety in the person.
- Limited occupational/social functioning
  - I think this is pretty self explanatory.
- Significant interpersonal conflict
- The ability to elicit frustration in others
  - Intense emotional upheaval and hostility lead to frequent interpersonal conflict. Their inability to take responsibility for their actions creates strong negative emotions in others. They cannot trust otehrs and are constantly fearful of being hurt.
  - These people have an uncanny ability to merge personal boundaries with others and "get under their skin." This process is often unconscious and the result is bad.
- Limited insight
- A tendency to try to change his/her environment rather than his/her behavior
  - This person does not take responsibility for their behavior.
- Difficulty accepting the consequences of his/her behavior.

Discuss theories about the developement of personality disorders
- Biological Determinants
  - It is proposed that certain traits are present at birth. PDs may represent an extreme variation of a natural tendency resulting from genetic alterations and/or unfavorable environmental conditions. These personality traits have been identified as being potentially inherited: novelty seeking, harm avoidance, reward dependence, persistence, neuroticism versus emotional stability, introversion versus extroversion, conscientiousness versus undependability, antagonism versus agreeableness, closedness versus openness to experiences.
  - Family and twin studies suggest genetic factors of linkages between PD and other mental illnesses. Schizotypal PD is often seen in people with first-degree relatives who have shizophrenia.
  - There is a definite genetic influence in antisocial PD: biological children of parents with antisocial PD have a higher risk for having it
  - Individuals with borderline PD often have family members with mood or impulse control disorders.
  - Some people with PD have a history of repeated psycholigical, sexual, physical trauma during childhood. Thus, the neurobiological research related to chronic stress may relate to PD.

- Structural brain changes
- Neurotransmitter imbalances, especially serotonin

- Psychosocial factors
  - Learning theory says that the child developed maladaptive responses based on modeling or reinforcement.
  - Cognitive theory excessive anxiety is caused by a distortion in thinking that is amenable to correction.
  - Psychoanalytic theory focuses on the uses of primitive defense mechanisms.
  - People with paranoid PD had excessively critical parents who may have role-modeled projection of anger and resentment.
  - People with schizoid PID may have suffered from emotional isolation b/c parents were indifferent or detached.
  - People with antisocial PD have histories that may reveal excessively harsh punishment and encouragement of aggression.
  - People with borderline PD have a consistent evidence of childhood trauma (sexual abuse/physical abuse and significant parental conflict or loss). This early distress is associated with the fear of abandonment.
  - People with histrionic PD may have had excessive family reinforcement of attention-seeking behavior.
  - People with narcissistic PD may have had parents that were neglectful or inconsistent in rewards and punishments.
  - People with avoidant PD may have had overprotective parents. As with dependent PD, there may have been parental overprotection or excessive clinging to the child, which interferes with normal development and separation.
  - People with obsessive-compulsive PD may have copied the behavior from authoritarian parents, but there may also be issues of unconscious guilt or shame involved.
  - Separation-individuation
  - Enmeshmant vs abandonment
  - Identity integration vs. identity diffusion

Defense Mechanisms used by PD pt

The defense mechanisms used by the PD person are repression, suppression, regression, undoing, splitting.

- Repression = the exclusion of unpleasant or unwanted experiences, emotions or ideas from conscious awareness; considered the first line of psychological defense.
- Suppression = the conscious removal from awareness of disturbing situations or feelings; the only defense mechanism that operates on a conscious level
- Regression = In the face of overwhelming anxiety, the return to an earlier and more comforting way of behaving
- Undoing = an act or behavior unconsciously designed to make up for or negate a previous act or behavior
- Splitting = a primitive defense mechanism in which the person sees self or others as all good or all bad, failing to integrate the positive and negative qualities of the self and others into a cohesive whole.

Define the three clusters of Axis II diagnoses

- CLUSTER A: these people are described as "odd or eccentric."
  - Avoid interpersonal relationships
  - Have unusual beliefs
  - May be indifferent to the reactions of others to their views
  - Seldom seek psychiatric treatment
    - *Paranoid* buzz words: distrust, suspicious, preoccupied, bears grudges, questions fidelity of partner
    - *Shizoid* buzz words: detachment, restricted range, no close relationships, no interest in sex, no pleasure, no close friends, indifferent, emotional coldness, detachment or flattened affect.
    - *Schizotypal* buzz words: discomfort with and reduced capacity for social relationships, cognitive or perceptual distortions, eccentric, ideas of reference, odd beliefs, bodily illusions, odd speech, suspicious, lack of close friends, social anxiety
- CLUSTER B: these people are "dramatic, emotional, or erratic."
  - Seek out interpersonal relationships but can't retain them b/c of excessive demands and emotional instability
  - Manipulative; may seem charming but are really trying to use you for their own benefit
  - Display a sense of entitlement, deny negative feelings of others, put on needs first
  - Many receive psychiatric care voluntarily or involuntarily b/c they broke the law

- *Antosocial* buzz words: consistent disregard, psychopath, sociopath, conduct disorder as child, no remorse, tell lies, destructive, illegal, no insight, do not volunarily seek care
- *Borderline* buzz words: instability in affect, identiy and relationships; seek relationships to avoid feeling abandoned; drive others away; demands, impulsive uncontrolled anger; use splitting as a defense; one of most common seen in psych treatment settings; psychosis-like symptoms, chronic depression or self-destructive behavior; hx of dramatic suicide gestures; significant risk of suicide
- *Histrionic* buzz words: attention seeking, impulsive, melodramatic, flirtatious, provocative, partner feels smothered, no insight, seeks tx for depression or other comorbid condition, demands "the best of everything", very critical.

- CLUSTER C: these people are "anxious or fearful"
  - feel insecure or inadequate
  - depend on others for reasurrance
  - isolate themselves for fear of rejection
  - come into pysch care for tx of anxiety r/t fear of relationships or loss of relationships
    - *Avoidant* buzz words; social inhibition, avoids contact, want relationships but are preoccupied with fear of rejection, appear timid, low self-esteem, poor self-care, often mistreated, clingy.
    - *Dependent* buzz words: extreme dependency, no decisions, seeks reasurrance, submissiveness, vulnerable to abuse, belief of incompetence, fear they cannot survive on their own, seek tx for anxiety or mood disorders, most frequently seen PD in clinical setting, can occur in pt with medical disability
    - *Obsessive-Compulsive* buzz words; perfectionism, orderliness, control, preoccupied with details, can't complete task, have affection for friends/family, fearful of imminent catastrophe, rehearse over and over how they will respond in social situations.

Communicating with a pt with personality disorder

Communicating with the pt with a personality disorder (General Info)

- People with PD are impulsive, aggressive, manipulative and even psychotic during times of stress.
- They are more difficult to engage in treatment because they have a problem with trust.
- Difficult to develop a therapeutic relationship
- Because the pt with PD lacks the ability to trust, they will need to have a sense of control over what is happening to them. Giving realistic choices may enhance compliance (for example, you may let them choose which group activity to do).
- Open-ended statements such as "Tell me what happened."
- Maintain non-judgmental attitude
- See pg 294 for a dialogue between pt and nurse
- Milieu therapy
  - Community meetings, coping skills group and socializing groups are helpful
  - Staff should remain calm and united to deal with emotional issues that arise
  - Limit setting and confrontation bout negative behavior is better accepted by the pt if the staff first employs empathic mirroring.
  - Showing empathy can decrease aggressive outbursts

Basic Communication Interventions for Various Types of Behavior

- Communication Interventions for Manipulative Behavior
  - Discuss concerns about behavior with pt
  - Identify undesirable patient behavior (with pt input if appropriate)
  - Discuss with patient (when appropriate) what is desirable behavior in a given situation
  - Establish consequences
  - Communicate established behavioral expectations and consequences to patient in language that is easily understood and nonpunitive.
  - Refrain from arguing or bargaining with patient about established behavioral expectations and consequences
- Communication Interventions for Aggressive Behavior
  - Encourage pt to seek assistance from staff during periods of increasing tension
  - Provide reassurance to pt that staff will intervene to prevent pt from losing control
  - Assist pt in identifying sources of anger
  - ID consequences of inappropriate expression of anger
- Communication Interventions for Impulsive Behavior
  - Teach pt to cue himself to "stop and think" before acting impulsively
  - Provide positive reinforcement for successful outcomes
  - Encourage pt to self-reward for successful outcomes
  - Encourage problem-solving skills
- Communication Interventions for Paranoid Behavior
  - Use a non-judgmental, respectful and neutral approach
  - Be honest and consistent
  - Use clear and simple language
  - Explain to client what you are going to do before you do it
  - Do not do things in front of client that can be misinterpreted...laughing, whispering, talking quietly when client can see but not hear what you are saying
  - Be nondefensive if attacked
  - Provide verbal and physical limits when client's hostile behavior escalates
  - Set limits in a clear, matter-of-fact way, using a calm tone.
- Advanced Practice Interventions
  - Dialectical Behavior Therapy is a structured, long-term approach that provides significant teaching for clients along with a support system for therapists. The pt receives individual therapy, group skills training and telephone access to therapist.
    - set realistic goals
    - use clear action words

The Odd or Eccentric Cluster (Cluster A)

- Communicating with *Paranoid Personality* Disorder Pt
  - They will be distrustful and suspicious
  - They will anticipate hostility, be hypervigilant, may provoke hostile responses by initiating a "counter attack."
  - They are difficult to interview b/c they are reluctant to share information
  - Very anxious about being harmed
  - Don't be too nice or friendly
  - Clear and straightforward explanations of tests and procedures prior
  - Simple, clear language. Avoid ambiguity
  - Project a neutral but kind affect
  - Warn pt about any side effects of medications or any delays in treatment
  - Written plan may help encourage participation
- Communicating with *Schizotypal* Personality Disorder Pt
  - This person will have odd beliefs, magical thinking or perceptual distortions
  - Their speech may be difficult to follow d/t a personalized style with vague associations
  - Cannot understand interpersonal cues and so will not relate to others appropriately
  - Pt may be unwilling to discuss symptoms, so careful dx assessment is needed to uncover any other medical or psychological symptoms that need tx (i.e. suicidal thoughts)
- Communicating with *Schizoid* Personality Disorder Pt
  - They are emotionally detached, will not seek out or enjoy close relationships
  - Will be indifferent to praise or criticism from others
  - Avoid being too nice or friendly
  - Do not try to re-socialize the pt
  - Pt may not want to discuss symptoms, so a thorough dx assessment is needed

The Dramatic, Emotional or Erratic Cluster (cluster B)

- Communicating with *Borderline* Personality Disorder Pt
  - This person has instability in affect, identity, relationships
  - This person desperately seeks relationships to avoid feeling abandoned
  - They use the defense of splitting
  - Significant risk of suicide
  - Set realistic goals, use clear action words
  - Set clear and consistent boundaries and limits
  - Clear and straightforward communication
  - When behavior problems arise, calmly review therapeutic goals and boundaries
- Communicating with *Antisocial* Personality Disorder Pt
  - This person has consistent disregard for others (previously called psychopath or sociopath)
  - This person will repeatedly tell lies and do other destructive things with no insight into predictable consequences
  - Set clear and realistic limits to prevent or reduce effects of manipulation
  - Be aware that this pt may use guilt to get what they want. do not let yourself be manipulated because they've made you feel guilty
- Communicating with *Narcissistic* Personality Disorder Pt
  - Primary feature is arrogance and grandiose view of self-importance
  - Lack of empathy for others
  - Feel intense shame and fear of abandonment if they are "bad"
  - Remain neutral
  - Avoid power struggles, do not become defensive in response to disparaging remarks
  - Convey unassuming self-confidence
- Communicating with *Histrionic* Personality Disorder Pt
  - Has emotion attention-seeking behavior (has to be center of attention)
  - This person demands "the best of everything" and can be very critical.
  - Keep all communication and interactions professional (client will probably flirt with you or be very flattering)
  - Encourage and model the use of concrete and descriptive language (do not use vague or impressionistic language)

The Anxious, Fearful Cluster (Cluster C)

- Communicating with the ***Avoidant*** Personality Disorder Pt
  - This person will be socially inhibited
  - They want to have close relationships but fear rejection
  - Will be clingy if they do develop a relationship
  - A friendly, gentle, reassuring approach is best.
- Communicating with the ***Dependent*** Personality Disorder Pt
  - This person will have extreme dependency in a close relationship
  - Will have difficulty making independent decisions
  - Will constantly be seeking reassurance
  - Set limits in a way that does not make pt feel punished
  - Strong countertransference often develops d/t extreme clinginess
- Communicating with the ***OCD*** Personality Disorder PT
  - This person is a perfectionist
  - Will be very preoccupied with details and rules, may not be able to accomplish tasks
  - Guard against engaging in power struggles
  - This person has a high need for control
  - Understand that they will use intellectualization, rationalization and reaction formation as common defense mechanisms

Diagnosis and Care Planning (communication focus only)

- Risk for Injury
  - Encourage pt to express feelings r/t stress and tension instead of engaging in self-injurious behavior
  - Discuss alternative ways for pt to meet demands of the current stressful situation
  - Secure a verbal or written no-harm contract
  - Use a matter-of-fact approach when self-mutilation occurs
    - Neutral approach prevents blaming which increases anxiety
    - After treating wound, discuss what happened right before + thoughts and feelings the pt had before they self-mutilated
  - Set and maintain limits on acceptable behavior
  - Use a non-punitive approach when setting and enforcing limits
- Chronic Low-Self Esteem
  - Maintain a neutral, calm and respectful manner (may be always be easy!)
    - Helps pt see himself as respected even when behavior is not appropriate
  - ID with pt realistic areas of strength and weakness
  - Focus questions in a positive and active light to help client focus on the present and look to the future "What could you do differently now," or "What have you learned from the experience?"
  - Give honest feedback regarding observations of client's strengths and areas that need additional skill
  - Do not flatter or be dishonest. This can undermine trust.
  - Discuss plans for future to minimize dwelling on the past and negative thoughts.
- Impaired Social Interaction
  - Explain expected behaviors, limits and responsibilities in a respectful, neutral manner
  - Set limits on manipulative behaviors (arguing, begging, flattery, seductiveness, guilt, clinging, etc...)
  - Expand limits by clarifying expectations for client in a number of settings. This can reduce power struggles and confrontation.
  - Monitor your own thoughts and feelings consistently b/c of strong countertransference reactions.
- Ineffective Coping
  - Be clear with client as to the unit policies
  - Give brief concrete reasons for the rules (if asked), then move on.
  - Be clear about consequences.
  - Be consistent with approach in all interactions to enhance feelings of security and provide structure.
  - A clear written plan of care helps minimize manipulations and can encourage cooperation
  - Do not share personal information with the pt. This opens up areas for manipulation and undermines professional boundaries.

Alcohol and Other Drug Use/Abuse/Dependence

DEFINITIONS (we look at each of these in regards to primary, secondary and tertiary treatment)

- **USE**: Refers to non-therapeutic consumption of psychoactive drugs. For example, drinking moderately at a party when you have to drive home (sipping each drink over an hour - 1½ oz. per...this is b/c alcohol reaches its peak in about an hour...so you don't want to drink 3-4 drinks quickly then you are over the unsafe level of alcohol in the blood at 0.8). Alcohol is absorbed primarily from the stomach, so eat some food with your drink. Mix the alcohol with other substances to mix the drink (not straight shot).
- **ABUSE:** Abuse refers to the consumption of psychoactive drug(s) with biological, psychological, social, environmental and/or legal consequences (American Psychiatric Association, 2000).For example, a patient is admitted with a diagnosis of a compound fracture of the left ulna resulting from an accident caused by driving under the influence. Other examples include, drinking or even occasional consumption of substances, such as marijuana, in people who have a history of major depression. Even smoking if you have COPD is abuse. Using psychoactive drugs increases the risk of exacerbating an existing depressive state or of precipitating a depressive episode. FYI: Alcohol causes the most health problems besides cigarettes!
- **SUBSTANCE DEPENDENCE**: Dr. V says this is a neurobiological illness that has a genetic underpinning. A maladaptive pattern of substance use, leading to clinically significant impairment or distress, as manifested by three (or more) of the following, occurring at any time in the same 12-month period:
  - (1) Tolerance, as defined by either of the following (d/t body handling the drug more efficiently):
    - (a) A need for markedly increased amounts of the substance to achieve intoxication or desired effect
    - (b) Markedly diminished effect with continued use of the same amount of the substance. If this changes and you only need a little drug/alcohol to get the effect this means there is pretty bad liver damage. Fatty liver then hepatitis then cirrhosis...bad news.
  - (2) Withdrawal, as manifested by either of the following (occurs when taking a substance for at least a week):
    - (a) The characteristic withdrawal syndrome for the substance
    - (b) The same (or closely related) substance is taken to relieve or avoid withdrawal symptoms
  - (3) The substance is often taken in larger amounts or over a longer period than was intended. If you only asked one question and they answered that this is occurring (a loss of control), is a classic symptom of addiction.
  - (4) There is a persistent desire or unsuccessful efforts to cut down or control substance use (more loss of control)
  - (5) A great deal of time is spent in activities necessary to obtain the substance (e.g., visiting multiple doctors or driving long distances), use the substance (e.g., chain-smoking), or recover from its effects.
  - (6) Important social, occupational, or recreational activities are given up or reduced because of substance use.
  - (7) The substance use is continued despite knowledge of having a persistent or recurrent physical or psychological problem that is likely to have been caused or exacerbated by the substance (e.g., current cocaine use despite recognition of cocaine-induced depression or continued drinking despite recognition that an ulcer was made worse by alcohol consumption)...remember Tracy E from Fat City?
- **CHEMICAL DEPENDENCE:**
- **ADDICTION**: a broad term used to cover a variety of activities (gambling, shopping, alcohol, drugs)
- **PREVENTION** refers to health care activities related to interventions aimed at persons who currently do not have the disease or are in the early stages of the disease rather than the treatment of disease. Prevention activities include reduction of risk; promotion of health behaviors that prevent occurrence of disease and reduce harm and early detection and treatment to prevent the development of additional consequences of the disease. Dr. V is very interested in focusing on folks who are at risk for addiction.

FACTORS THAT INFLUENCE ATTITUDES

- Family background (if I have an alcoholic father this affects my attitude toward alcoholics. It is important to be forgiving of the addicts and have compassion)
- Early experiences (if you live in an environment where there is a lot of abuse/dependence, this can affect attitude)
- Other life experiences
- Clinical experiences

Incidence of AOD problems

- USA is one of the world leaders in AOD problems (more money to spend on drugs, more leisure time)
- Approximately 10 million people reported heavy alcohol use in the past month (5%)
- Approximately 15% of drinkers progress to alcoholism
- 36% reported using illicit drugs sometime in their lives
- Key is the fact that over 40% of hospital admissions are related to AOD abuse
- Adolescent substance abuse
- Deaths US Per Day: 1000 Smoking; 300 Alcohol; 150 Second Hand Smoke; 100 Other Drugs
- Risk Factors for Substance Abuse and Addiction
  - Family History – Genetic predisposition (ask about family history!)
  - Pre-existing mental illness (a lot of times people self-treat, especially bi-polar folks)
  - Poverty, Peer Pressure (peer pressure a big issue for kids who have trouble fitting in)
  - Parental drug use, parental attitudes
  - Divorce, parental rejection,family instability (we are now intervening with kids earlier to help them deal with behaviors and gain some control...think of the adolescent/child unit at Sutter Psych)
  - Historical/Social factors: example the sexual revolution, historical trends, signs of the time, new drugs, new methods of use

Historical Perspective

- Mind-altering drugs have been used by humans since before recorded history
- The earliest psychoactive drugs were alcohol, opium, marijuana, coca and psychedelic mushrooms
- Ancient cultures saw wine as a gift from god, Osiris gave ETOH to the Egyptians as did Dionysus to the Greeks, and Jewish peoples have long used wine in religious celebrations.
- Heavy drinking was recognized as a problem by the Egyptians in 1500 BC where hieroglyphics advise moderation
- 6,000 years ago the Sumerians living in what is now Iran used opium calling it the "joy plant" using it for pain relief, diarrhea, and euphoria
- The Chinese emperor Shen_Nung in 2737 BC wrote about Cannabis and its medicinal uses
- Eight centuries ago the Inca prized the use of coca leaves more than silver and gold, nobility carrying their precious supply in ornate bags
- Coffee (caffeine was originally found in Ethiopia about 600 AD, is called the wine of Islam. Coffee is to Arabia what Tea is to China
- Alcohol was forbidden by the Koran, after the 6th century opium was acceptable sub. to control pain & treat grief
- Khat (a stimulant) was also a permissible substitute, was used during long prayers to help people stay awake
- In the middle ages other psychedelics were discovered such as plants which contained belladonna, henbane, mandrake root and jimson weed. These drugs caused a disorientation and delirium. They were often used by medicine men and women accused of witch craft.
- During the Renaissance and Enlightenment Tobacco use, distilled alcohol, and opium smoking spread. Governments controlled trade for economic gain
- Nineteenth Century saw refinements with the synthesis of heroin from opium, new synthetic drugs, more wide spread use, government control, and criminality
- Twentieth Century wider distribution, better refining, newer synthetics, wide spread illegal use
- Today and Tomorrow
  - After a decline in the 1980's the use of illegal drugs in the 1990's has increased, especially marijuana, methamphetamines, MDMA, LSD,and heroin. Despite these increases in use of illicit drugs, Alcohol and Tobacco remain the most dangerous drugs of use and abuse
- Potency
  - **Drugs are more dangerous today because we know how to refine them to make them more potent, grow them to increase the content of the psychoactive substances, and because *we have new and improved ways to deliver them more quickly to the brain***
- Improved Delivery
  - Opium poppy became opium, than morphine, than the syringe was invented, and heroin was developed. Heroin was first manufactured to create a substance that could kill pain, without the problems of tolerance and addiction

- Heroin actually crosses the blood brain barrier more efficiently, is not as good a pain killer (shorter half life), but because it's absorption in the brain is so fast it causes more euphoria resulting in compulsive heroin use – addiction.
- Cocaine was first chewed limiting it absorption
- Cocaine was than processed into a white powder that was sniffed (1970's)
- Cocaine was further refined in the 1980's to a rock that was than cooked, and the vapor's smoked. This development directly lead to the cocaine epidemic of the 1980's
- The marijuana of the 1960s was far less potent than the marijuana grown today Better growing methods as given us plants that are 14 times more potent
- Cigarettes first became an addiction problem after the development of the cigarette rolling machine which resulted in using increased amounts, and greater distribution

Psychoactive Drugs

- Classification
  - Uppers: stimulants, such as cocaine, amphetamines, Ritalin, caffeine and nicotine
  - Downers: depressants such as opioids, sedative-hypnotics and alcohol
  - Inhalants: Organic solvents, volatile nitrites, nitrous oxide
  - All arounders: Psychedelics, marijuana, MDMA, LSD,
  - Psychiatric Medications: anti depressants, anti psychotics, anti anxiety drugs
- Etiology of AOD dependence
  - Complex
  - Unique configuration of factors within each person
  - Progress in our understanding
- Neurobiological: Nerve Cells and Neurotransmitters
  - Understanding the precise ways messages are transmitted by the nerve cells and how neurotransmitters work has changed the way we view and treat addiction.
  - Neurobiobehavioral
    - Highly regarded area of theory and study; also very complex
    - Role of neurotransmitters (play a strong role in relapse...meds are available to help deal with cravings)
    - New information
      - Neural sensitization
      - Learned changes in the emotional brain
      - Failure in the frontal/prefrontal cortex (decisions are made by emotional part of brain)
  - Loss of control – key feature in all addictions
  - Brain chemistry changes same across addictions
  - Priming-action of drug to induce craving (binge-drinking is a way people prime their addiction)
  - Repeated exposure→Kindling (kindling their addiction earlier...they may also have a genetic predisposition)
  - Initiation of addictive process
  - Emotional brain-limbic system
  - Activation of brain's "pleasure pathway (medial forebrain bundle) – dopamine is the transmitter...it is artificially enhanced by the addictive process. This is why they become dysphoric in the recovery stage...it takes a long time for the dopamine levels to readjust in the body.
  - Neural response to drug exposure is rapid with rebound below baseline before returning to it
  - All addictive drugs increase dopamine activity within the limbic system
  - Environmental stimuli (cues) associated with drug seeking provide a powerful stimulus for activating learned neurochemical patterns (it's a combination of environment and limbic system)
- Psychological (work in concert with neurobiological to bring on the problem earlier)
  - Oral stage of development
  - Linked with psychological traits such as depression, anxiety, antisocial personality disorder, and dependent personality
  - Human tendency to seek pleasure and avoid pain
  - Negative childhood experiences, e.g., physical and sexual abuse associated with low self-esteem and difficulty expressing emotions. You have to deal with the abuse issues in order to have lasting recovery from addiction.

- Sociocultural
  - Background
  - Nationality and ethnicity
  - Gender differences (women are at higher risk b/c our alcohol goes directly to our organs and causes increased damage earlier..it is not metabolized the same way as in men)
  - Community vulnerabilities (advertising is one way communities are vulnerable to abuse, also drug-dealing, poverty)
- Dynamics of AOD dependency
  - Use of defense mechanisms
    - Denial (I can quit anytime, I don't have a problem)
    - Rationalization (If you wouldn't get so mad at me I wouldn't drink)
    - Projection
  - Omnipotence (need example)
  - Dependence(need example)
  - Crisis creation (create crisis to take the heat off themselves)
  - Diversion strategies (will divert the problem to your anger regarding the situation, trying to take the attention away from the abuse problem)
  - Victim stance (I'm doing the best I can, and no one is supporting me!)
  - Offensive stance (They start to pick on things you're not doing so great..and making that the issue to put others on the defensive...this takes attention away from the abuser's behavior.)
- Specific characteristics of abuse or dependence, physical effects, behavioral changes, and medical consequences (SEE HANDOUT!...major ones are CNS depressants, opioids and stimulants--biggest problem wit stimulants is suicidal ideation.) KNOW S/S OF WITHDRAWAL!!! 2 hr mark in stream.
- Depressants
- Alcohol (prototype)
- Barbiturates
- Benzodiazepines
- Alcohol (see handout)
- Key characteristics
- Withdrawal
- Special considerations
- Key points in alcohol withdrawal syndrome
- Mild withdrawal
- (see handout)
- Key points in alcohol w/d syndrome (cont.)
- Moderate withdrawal
- Key points in alcohol w/d syndrome (cont.)
- Severe withdrawal: more of a concern...by the time they get to the ER, they are often in severe withdrawal from depressants. They have all symptoms of moderate withdrawal, plus hallucinations, seizures...DTs is the big concern. Need to do a really good interview b/c if they progress to DTs, it is irreversible...it has to run its course. It occurs in about 20% of chronic alcoholics. Treat the withdrawal b/f it reaches DTs, they won't get them. It is a medical emergency! 5% of people who go into DTs actually die. They are thrashing about...have to be strapped down. Delirious, screaming. Dr. V gave an example of a pt on the M/S floor with the DTs. If she had known he was an alcoholic, she could have prevented it...seizure precautions, on a depressant such as librium or valium and reducing the amount over several days. Monitor this via vital signs...(if BP dropping too fast this is too high of a dose...if going up then not getting enough).

Addressing alcohol withdrawal syndrome

- Assessment is key
  - Last drink
  - Current drinking pattern
  - Amount currently consumed
  - Gather above data on all other psychoactive drugs consumed
  - History of w/d including shakes, seizures, hallucinations

Assessment of alcohol withdrawal (cont'd)

- Detoxification
  - Compatible medication
  - Stabilizing (loading) dose
  - Gradually taper dose over several days (usually 3-5)
  - Carefully monitor v/s (every 15 minutes while awake)
  - V/S dictate detoxification regime

Detoxification

- Follow w/d protocol for your setting
- Examples are chlordiazepoxide (Librium), clonazepam (Klonopin), diazepam (Valium)
- Phenobarbital effective-when physical dep. On alc & sed/hyp

Stimulants

- Amphetamines
- Cocaine, crack, free base
- Nicotine

Opioids (opiates, narcotics)

- Heroin
- Morphine
- Meperidine
- Codeine
- Opium
- Methadone

Hallucinogens

- Marijuana
- Phencyclidine

Other psychoactive drugs

- Inhalants (gases, solvents, aerosols, nitrites)
- MDMA – Methylenedioxymethaphetamine (aka: Ecstasy, XTC, E, Adam, etc.
- Inhalants
  - 896,000 Americans have used inhalants
  - They are quick acting, readily available, and cheap
  - Inhalants cause disorientation, hallucinations, and intoxication similar to being drunk
  - Neurological damage can include hearing and visual impairment, loss of coordination and memory, and learning disabilities (can damage more quickly than other substances)
  - The low status of inhalants as a drug problem compound the difficulty of getting users into treatment
  - Warning signs for inhalant use
    - Chemical odor on body or cloths
  - Red, glassy, or watery eyes, dilated pupils
  - Slow thick, or slurred speech
  - Staggering gait, disorientations, and lack of coordination
- GHB – Gamma-hydroxybutyric acid (aka: liquid Ecstacy, scoop, goop, etc)
- Club drinks: Adrenalin Rush, Stamina, Dark Dog, Red Bull

Time-related symptoms of alcohol withdrawal syndrome

-minor withdrawal symptoms: insomnia, tremulousness, mild anxiety, GI upset, headache, diaphoresis, palpitations, anorexia, 6-12 hours after cessation

Alcohol Hallucinosis: Visual, auditory, or tactile hallucinations (12-24 hrs) generally resolve within 48 horus.

Withdrawal seizures: Generalized tonic-clonic seizures. 24-48 hours after drinking

Alcohol withdrawal delirium (delirium tremens): hallucinations (predominately visual), disorientation, tachycardia, hypertension, low-grade fever, agitation, diaphoresis...48-72 hours (peak at 5 days).

Social and family problems

- Isolation
- Abuse/neglect
- Stigma
- Secrets
- Codependency (easy to spot...taking responsibility for other people when they should be taking responsibility for themselves...enabling is the same thing)

Culture (cultural groups...see book for examples)

- Varying manifestations of problems
- Dictates definitions

Developmental issues

- Stage of development influences intervention approaches (look at what is developmentally motivating)
- Specific examples

Nursing process

- Guides thinking and direction of the nurse
- Prevents errors by its systematic nature
- Assessment (see handout)
- Screening: Pyramid approach or cut to the chase (see handout). WIll cut to the chase in the ER b/c you need to treat immediately. Use pyramid in Med/Surg.
- Screening: CAGE, MAST, etc.
    - CAGE is used when you suspect they have a problem. Answer YES is a red flag.
    - Cut Down: have you ever had someone suggest you need to cut down on your drinking?
    - Annoyed: Have people been annoying you about stopping your abuse?
    - Guilty: Have you ever felt guilty for behaviors related to drinking?
    - Eye Opener: Do you need something to get going?
- Screening: Breathalyzer and urine drug screen
- Level of prevention (look at your level of prevention and move forward...that's what she said?)
- Maslow's hierarchy of needs...this is why you have to cut to the chase in the ER. Treat the withdrawal and deal with addiction issues later when crisis has passed.
- Assessing status of drug use...need to know if they are going to go into withdrawal or may be suicidal.
- Assessing for alcohol, depressant use...withdrawal is very dangerous!

- Outcome goals for alcohol/depressant use:
    - **Short-term:** Stabilize w/ depressant drugs; develop trust; meet needs; address presenting problems
        - Sometimes they give the depressant to help mask the symptoms of withdrawal...sometimes people will seek detoxification as a form of abuse (b/c they get drugs to detox). You give Ativan to those people so you can see breakthrough symptoms (Ativan is short-acting). This will enable you to see if they are really in withdrawal. Also, don't want to give elderly anything that will accumulate, and Ativan won't accumulate b/c it is short-acting.
    - **Long-term:** Pursues treatment and recovery; addresses needs of long-term recovery. Dr. V said there will be relapses during long-term treatment...this is to expected.
- Planning
    - Determine resources...may not be in an alcohol-specific setting, so determine the resources that are available.
    - Collaborate with client and family...b/c systems theory says that the system doesn't want change...the way the family operates can push pt back into using again, so family needs to get straightened out as well.
- Implementation
    - Operationalization of plan – concrete activities. Put plan into action.
- Evaluation
    - Identified goals (did you get them to contemplate their situation? did they state that they have a problem? etc...)
- Treatment of CNS depressant withdrawal
    - Assess severity
    - Monitor v/s longer period of time
    - Collaborate with MD or NP or Clinical Nurse Specialist with addictions expertise
    - If appropriate, begin detoxification regimen
    - Treatment of CNS depressant w/d (cont)
    - Continue to monitor
    - Refer to long-term treatment
        - Self-help groups
        - Residential treatment
        - Outpatient treatment

Pharmacologic treatment for chemical dependency

- Antabuse therapy (inhibits the metabolism of alcohol, to yield the toxic product acetaldehyde). It is aversion therapy! If you use alcohol you get very sick/vomit. Pt has to be motivated to take the Antabuse...maybe their environment has a lot of drinking so it's going to be hard for them to abstain.
- Pharmacologic treatment for craving
  - Cocaine: Norpramin (desipramine); Tegretol (carbamazepine); need to be in support program while taking this.
  - Alcohol: ReVia (Naltrexone) – competitive antagonist at a morphine-like (mu opioid) receptor in the brain; blocks receptors & reduces craving : Acamprosate (Campral) – stimulates brain receptors for glutamate and indirectly modify dopamine activity in the limbic system
  - Heroin
    - Dolophine (Methadone) – mimics morphine at opiate receptors
    - LAAM – longer acting than methadone
    - ReVia (Naltrexone)
    - Subutex and Suboxone - sublingual (buprenorphine)...this drug is also for alcoholics...it is able to be prescribed now by general practitioners...NPs are trying to get permission to prescribe this to increase # of people treated.
- Pharmacology for Nicotine Dependency (need a triple tx: Wellbutrin/antidepressant, support group, nicotine patch)
  - Bupropion – Zyban (Wellbutrin)
  - Dose 150 – 300 mgs QD start one week before quit date, no make up missed dose
  - Antidepressant and dopamine stimulation
  - SE – dry mouth, insomnia, HA, rhinitis, rash, shakiness
  - Contraindications – seizure, allergic,Anorexia, MAO inhibitors, hx severe head trauma, active addiction alcohol or other drugs
  - Reduces withdrawal symptoms of irritability, frustration, anger, anxiety, difficulty with concentration, restlessness,depressed mood, craving
  - May use in conjunction with nicotine patch
  - Often used after previous quit attempts
- Other treatment modalities for addictions
  - Motivational interviewing
  - Solution focused therapy
  - Assertiveness training (Dr. V thinks this is super important...it is a process of learning skills to be assertive. This can decrease a person's stress, improve self-confidence and self-awareness.)
  - Relapse prevention
  - Group therapy
- Goals of long-term recovery
  - Longer periods of abstinence
  - Seek healthy coping with stress
  - Assume responsibility for behavior
  - Engage drug-free social support system
- Prevention strategies
  - Family strategies: open honest communication; flexibility; level of prevention
  - Community strategies: zoning; networking; monitoring youth; community education
  - Local and state governments
  - Federal government
- Criminal justice system
- International scene
- Integrated approach
- Apply nursing process to case study (see case study)

Immunity

Stem cells can form:

- lymphocytes (T, B and large granular lymphocytes). 30% of WBC are lymphocytes
  - Cytotoxic T cells fight off viruses and cancer
  - Helper T cells coordinate the immune response
  - B cells make antibodies
- polymorphonuclear cells (neutrophils, basophils and eosinophils)
- mast cells
- megakarocytes that produce platelets

B-Cells: Trained in the bone marrow
Make antibodies
Each B Lymphocyte makes only one shape of antibody
Plasma cell is a type of B-Cell that secretes antibodies
Memory cells are long-lived, inactive cells that are activated at subsequent exposure to an antigen. They are a key component of long-term Immunity

PMNs (Polymorphonuclear cells)

When mature, WBCs are PMNs. When immature, the nucleus is just a band, so they are called Band Cells. If you see a lot of bands, then you know the infection is new.

- 60% of all WBCs are neutrophils. They are the first to arrive in bacterial infections and then they call the others to join via chemotaxis. They also activate complement.
- Eosinophis are not very numerous…important in allergic responses and in parasitic infections.
- Basophils and Mast cells. Mast cells release histamine as part of the allergic response. Note that narcotics cause histamine release, but this is not mediated by antibodies…it is a side effect, not an allergic reaction.

CBC Differential

- RCB 4-5 million/cu. Mm (H&H)
- WBC 5000-10,000 cu. Mm
  - Neutrophils 50-60% (range from immature band cells to mature PMNs)
  - Lymphocytes 20-40%
  - Monocytes 2-6%
  - Eosinophils 1-4%
  - Basophils 1%
- Platelets 150,000 to 300,000/cu mm.

What to do about abnormal lab values:

ANC: -Normal absolute neutrophil count is 60% of the total WBC (about 2500-7000 cells/microliter)

-Below 500 there is a great risk for infection, and often few S&S. If your pt is below 500, then they would be on neutropenic precautions, including IV antibiotics for the fever.

-Above 1000, there is not a significant risk for infection (note that the NCLEX still thinks there is)

-So, for example…a week after chemo a pt's ANC is 200/microliter. What interventions will you do?

- Use alcohol-based hand wash
- Prohibit fresh flowers in the room
- Triple wash fruits and veggies
- No fresh unpeeled fruits

Complement has many functions in the inflammatory response.

- Increased vascular permeability causes fluid to leave the vessel travel through the interstial area and trough the lymphatics. Maybe bacteria will be washed into the lymph system too.
- Smooth muscles contract in blood vessels and airways.
- Mast cells degranulate, releasing substances like histamine.
- Complexes of antigen-ab are trapped in the lymph node. The WBC responding to the antigen is cloned up in the nursery for making new WBC (the germinal center). This causes the lymph node to swell.
- Sticks to the bacteria, making phagocytosis easier.
- Neutrophils are activated and called into the area.
- Holes are poked in the walls of microbes. The microbes being under increased hdrostatic pressure, explode.
- Foreign cells are lysed too.

Platelets

Note that platelets don't just clot. They also release substances that increase permeability and activate complement allowing for chemotaxis of WBC.

Lymph Nodes

When lymph nodes are removed, pts are at higher risk for infection. Pts with mastectomy are at risk for infection on the side of the mastectomy, so you would never start an IV line on that arm. You would also want to watch for edema on that arm as it is very likely. Elevation is helpful and note that this is not an arterial problem, so no need to check pulses. It is a venous problem!

When bad things happen to the 1st line of defense (the epithelium)
Respiratory epithelium are damaged by smoking. It paralyzes the cilia, which means that all that gunk you breathe in gets dumped in the lungs.

Gastrointestinal defenses are designed to keep pathogens at bay. Lysozymes in secretions, rapid pH changes (2 in stomach to 8 in small intestine), normal flora, flow, peristalsis, secretions, exfolation…all work to keep the microbes from causing harm.

What is the clinical significance of:

- Bypassing the top part of the GI tract with a feeding tube? You want to be sure to change bags out daily and not hang more than about 4 hours of food.
- What if you give an H2 blocker? Stomach not so acidic, more likely to get infection with aspiration? (not just chemical pneumonitis which is bad enough).
- GI Surgery… it is important to decontaminate gut before GI surgery. In emergency with no time, the peritoneal cavity can get contaminated, so you would give antibiotics like Flagyl post op. When you give lots of broad spectrum Abx, you wipe out normal flora and can get overgrowth, for example with clostridium difficile.

Genitourinary defenses
Females are at higher risk for UTI due to a shorter urethra. Males have the benefit of antimicrobial seminal fluid. Both males and females have acidic urine and the bladder mucosa secretes mucus, IgA and ysozymes. Both have peristalsis, valves and macrophages.

The clinical significance of this:

- Inserting a Foley has a high risk of UTI
- Better to do an in-and-out cath multiple times a day.
- Residual urine increases the risk of UTI
- Infections can tract up to the kidneys…very serious!

2nd line of defense, nonspecific defenses:

- Inflammation
  - Can be caused by pathogens (cellulites), thermal (cold test tube on arm), radiation (sunburn) and chemical (aspiration of gastric juices into lungs)
  - The hallmark features of inflammation are:
    - Red (vasodilation)
    - Hot (vasodilation)
    - Swollen (leaky capillaries)
    - Painful (chemical response, also swollen tissue stims nerves)

Oral care every 4 hours on ventilator!

- Pathophysiology of inflammation: When the vessels vasodilate, the neutrophils arrive via chemotaxis. They get into the tissue because the vessels have increased permeability. (see A&P notes for more)
- Therapies include drugs, heat & cold, elevation
  - There are three general classes of drugs commonly used in the treatment of rheumatoid arthritis: non-steroidal anti-inflammatory agents (NSAIDs), corticosteroids, and remittive agents or disease modifying anti-rheumatic drugs (DMARDs). NSAIDs and corticosteroids have a short onset of action while DMARDs can take several weeks or months to demonstrate a clinical effect. DMARDs include methotrexate, leflunomide (Arava™), etanercept (Enbrel™), infliximab (Remicade™), adalimumab (Humira™), anakinra (Kineret™), antimalarials, gold salts, sulfasalazine, d-penicillamine, cyclosporin A, cyclophosphamide and azathioprine. Because cartilage damage and bony erosions frequently occur within the first two years of disease, rheumatologists now move more aggressively to a DMARD agent.
  - Heat & Cold: Heat increases superficial blood flow. Use heat for muscle spasm, stiff joints, superficial thrombophlebitis. Cold vasoconstricts, decreases swelling, decreases metabolism, slows nerve conduction. Use cold after a trauma, either intermittently or continuous (some studies show continuous is better)
- Phagocytosis
  - This is the domain of the neutrophils and macrophages.
  - Pus is basically dead neutrophils that responded to bacterial infection.
    - Pustules are involved in an acne bacterial infection
    - Vesicles are blisters and present in herpes virus.
- Fever
  - Temp is regulated by the thermostat in the hypothalamus
  - Metabolism creates heat
  - Perfusion and diaphoresis dissipate heat
  - Increased temp with pyrogenic factors (infection) or injury to the hypothalamus (head injury or brain attack) or inability to dissipate (heat stroke)
  - 37-degree is normal. We start treating/culturing around 38.5. At 40-degrees, thermoregulation is impaired. 41-degrees is lethal! A slight fever is beneficial because it interferes with bacterial growth.
- Interferon
  - Protects adjacent cells from infection or cancer
  - Improves immune response
  - Is suppressed by high dose steroids.

The 3rd Line of Defense: Acquired Immunity

- B & T Lymphocytes
  - Lymphocytes are "trained" in the bone marrow (B cells) or the thymus (T cells). As lymphocytes mature, the DNA that codes for cell surface receptors is sliced and diced so that (when expressed into RNA and ultimately protein) each cell makes a different shape of receptor. Cells with receptors that will fight off the bad guys and not hurt one's own tissue are further developed and sent out into the circulation. Those receptors with the potential to interact and destroy native (self) tissue are destroyed. Well, not always. If they get out into the body, later in life they can get activated and will then attack one's normal tissue (thus causing an autoimmune disease).
- Lymphocyte function
  - B cells make antibodies.
  - Cytotoxic T-cells destroy non-self expressing cells (cancer, transplant, virally infected cells).
  - Helper Ts help!
- Immunizations (see A&P notes for more)

Hypersensitivity

- Allergies (Type I)
- Autoimmune (Type II)
- Immune Complex (Type III)
- Delayed hypersensitivity

<u>Type I Hypersensitivity</u>

This is the allergic response. It is a rapid response to an antigen against which the individual has pre-existing IgE antibodies. IgE is present in very low levels in most people and it has a half life in the serum of only 2-3 days. However, if it is bound to high-affinity receptors, then its half-life is about 3 weeks. The high-affinity receptors are found on mast cells and basophils.

<u>Type II Hypersensitivity (Autoimmunity)</u>

This type is caused by specific antibodies (IgM or IgG) binding to cells or tissue antigens. Except in cases of autoimmunity, the target cell is foreign to the host…so this is usually only seen in blood transfusion pts and people with certain autoimmune diseases.

Some problems with physiology similar to autoimmune disease:

- Transfusion reaction: Normal gut Ab cross react with blood of different type.
- Hemolytic disease of newborn: Rh- mom makes Ab against Rh+ baby
- Transplant graft rejection
- Some drug reactions: drug binds to RBC, Ab binds to drug, RBC lysed.

<u>Type III Hypersensitivity (Immune Compelx)</u>

This type is mediated mainly by IgG antibodies. It is now thought that this form of hypersensitivity has a lot in common with Type I, except that the antibody involved is IgG and therefore not bound to mast cells. The IgG soaks up Ag and forms complexes while it waits for mast-cell attachment…these large complexes are not easily cleared by the spleen or liver and they tend to lodge in areas of high BP, blood flow turbulence, and in joints where inflammation is set up.

The Arthus reaction is the name given to a local type III hypersensitivity reaction. It is easy to demonstrate experimentally by subcutaneous injection of any soluble antigen for which the host has a significant IgG titre. Because the FcgammaRIII is a low affinity receptor and because the threshold for activation via this receptor is considerably higher than for the IgE receptor the reaction is slow compared with a type I reaction, typically maximal at 4-8hrs, and consequently more diffuse. The condition extrinsic allergic alveolitis occurs when inhaled antigen complexes with specific IgG in the alveoli, triggering a type III reaction in the lung, for example in 'pigeon fanciers lung' where the antigen is pigeon proteins inhaled via dried faeces. Complement is not required for the Arthus reaction, but may modify the symptoms.

Generalized or systemic reactions
The presence of sufficient quantities of soluble antigen in circulation to produce a condition of antigen excess leads to the formation of small antigen-antibody complexes which are soluble and poorly cleared. In the normal animal these complexes fix complement but experiments in animals genetically deficient in C3 or C4 have shown that complement is not required for pathology to be observed following antibody-antigen complex challenge. The major pathology is due to complex deposition which seems to be exacerbated by increased vascular permeability caused by mast cell activation via FcgammaRIII as above. The deposited immune complexes trigger neutrophils to discharge their granule contents with consequent damage to the surrounding endothelium and basement membranes. The complexes may be deposited in a variety of sites such as skin, kidney and joints. Common examples of generalised type III reactions are post-infection complications such as arthritis and glomerulonephritis.

Delayed Hypersensitivity
Diseases related to delayed hypersensitivity include TB, Rheumatoid Arthritis, Type 1 DM, Multiple Sclerosis, contact dermatitis, sacoidosis and talc-related disease.

Tx: Avoid the allergen, suppress the immune system, stimulate SNS, desensitize

Talc is difficult for the body to clear and it sets up a glanulomatous reaction (similar to delayed hypersensitivity). Talc has thus been replaced with corn starch in many patient care areas (though in my hospital we don't use any talc or corn starch at all...nothing that could potentially be inhaled).

Nervous System

Central Nervous System

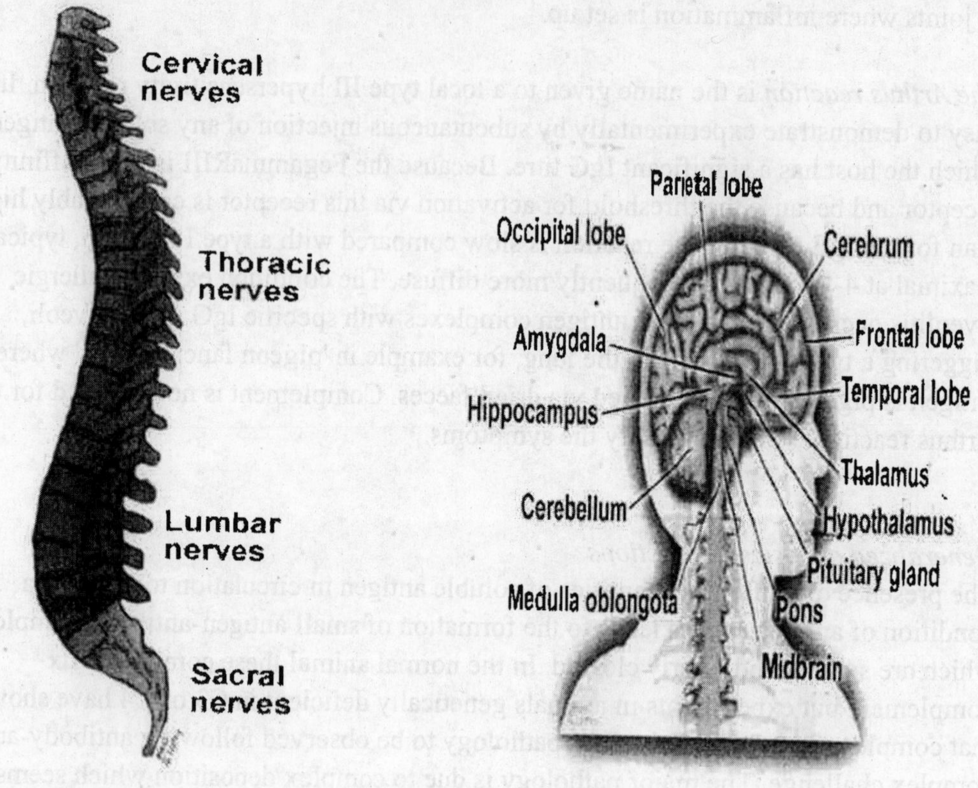

Nerve Tissue in CNS

Glial Cells- allow for nervous tissue to perform

- Astrocytes- structural support
- Microglia- attack microbes, remove waste
- Ependymal-cover surfaces, line cavities
- Oligodendrites-hold fibers together to make lipid insulation-MYELIN

Nerve Tissue in PNS

Glial Cells- Schwann cells make up myelin in the PNS

Neurons

- **Sensory Neurons** are known as **Afferent Neurons**
  - Carry messages from the skin and sensory organs to the brain and spinal cord
- **Motor Neuron** are known as **Efferent Neurons**
  - Carry messages from away from the brain and spinal cord

Neurotransmitters

- Used to send signals across the synapse to the next cell in line
  - **Acetylcholine-** in CNS and PNS (excite or inhibit the next cell)
  - **Norepinephrine-** in CNS and PNS (excite or inhibit the next cell)
  - **Epinephrine-** in CNS and PNS (excite or inhibit the next cell)
  - **Serotonin-** in CNS (generally inhibit)
  - **Endorphins-** in CNS (generally inhibit)

Acetylcholinesterase: is an enzyme which breaks down acetylcholine, to ensure that the neurotransmitter will not continually bind to the receiving cell

Nerve Impulse Conduction

- Dendrites carry sensory information to the cell body
- The cell body takes that information and generates an action potential
- The action potential (resting, depolarized, depolarized) travel down the axon of the nerve cell to the terminal junction or synapse
- The speed along the axon is determined by the presence of myelin and the diameter of the axon
- Myelin is lipid insulation sheath- formed by the Oligodendrites in the CNS, and Schwann Cells, in the PNS
- Myelinated axons are white, therefore called, White Matter.
- Unmyelinated axons are grey, therefore called, Grey Matter.

Outside View of Brain

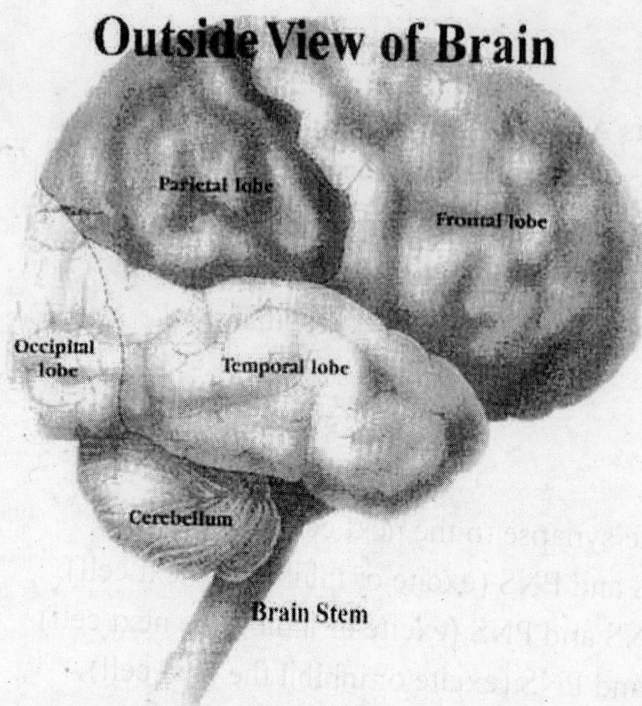

The Brain – The Cerebrum

- **Cerebrum**
  - Reasoning/intellect
  - Personality/mood
  - Interaction
  - Multiple Lobes
  - **Left hemisphere**
    - Controls right side body
  - **Right hemisphere**
    - Controls left side body

Lobes:

- **Frontal** – motor control of speech/vision, intellect, memory, Broca, high reasoning, planning, judgment
- **Temporal** – Wernicke's, interprets visual and auditory input, memory, language, meaning
- **Parietal** – spatial orientation, size, shape of input, touch, pressure, pain, taste, temp
- **Occipital** – eye reflexes, object recognition

The Brain - Diencephalon

- **Thalamus- Pineal Body- Hypothalamus**
- Temperature control
- Water metabolism
- Pituitary
- Hunger
- Physical response to emotions (crying etc.)
- Sleep/Wake cycle

Cerebellum

- Coordination
- Balance
- Muscle synergy

Brainstem

- Controls breathing, reflexes, swallowing
- **Includes the:**
  - **Midbrain**
  - **Pons**
  - **Medulla Oblongata**

The Spinal Cord

- Protected by membranes and cerebrospinal fluid
- Connects the brain to the Peripheral Nervous System and vice versa
- Relays information and also controls some reflexes.
- 1/2 - 1/4 inch in diameter
- About 44 cm long,
- Conveys sensory (afferent) impulses along dorsal roots nearer to the visual spine
- Conveys motor (efferent) impulses along ventral roots.

Diagnostic Tests for Nervous System

- **MRI** –safe for pregnant women
  - For tumors/masses - **No Metal! No pacers!**
- **Cerebral Angiogram** – visualization if cerebral blood vessels for aneurysms, vascularity of tumors, to inject medications, treat blood clots, or administer chemotherapy
  - NPO 4-8 hours, check for iodine and shell fish allergies
  - Check for anticoagulant therapy – potential bleeding
  - pregnancy
- **CT** –to detect stokes/bleeds/tumors, contrast media may be used
  - NPO 4-8 hours, check for iodine and shell fish allergies
- **EEG** –non-invasive to assess electrical activity of the brain, to identify seizure activity, sleep disorders, and behavioral changes
  - hold anticonvulsants and CNS depressants prior to study
- **Positron Emission Tomography (PET) and Single-Photon Emission Computed Tomography (SPECT)**

– Three dimensional head images

– Glucose based tracers injected, initiates metabolic activity (hot spots seen)

– Tumor activity, response to treatments, presence of dementia

– Check for history of DM- tracer is short acting broken down as sugar, not excreted

- **Lumbar Puncture- CSF analyzed to determine constituents,**

  – **Multiple Sclerosis, Syphilis, Infections, Malignancies**

  – In 'cannonball " position for the procedure

  – CSF is colorless, clear, no blood, no bacteria, glucose 40-80, and protein 16-45 normal.

  Anything else is ABNORMAL!

Collecting Data for the Client with Nervous System Disorder

Cranial Nerves

- I– Olfactory – smell?
- II– Optic – vision?
- III, IV, VI– Oculomotor, trochlear, abducens – ptosis, cardinal fields, PERRLA?
- V– Trigeminal – blink response?
- VII– Facial – raise eyebrows?
- VIII– Acoustic – hearing?
- VIX, X– Glossopharangeal, Vagus – gag reflex?
- XI– Spinal – turn head?

XII – Hypoglossal – tongue midline?

Motor Function

- Grip, Pedal strength
- Shoulder shrug with resistance
- Leg raise with resistance
- Coordination tests
- Compare symmetry and equality
- Watch for clonus, tremors, twitching

Sensory Function

- Touch discrimination with closed eyes
- Stereognosis – identify object in hand
- Graphesthesia – identify letter drawn in hand
- 2 point discrimination
- DTR's
- Abdominal reflex
- Babinski – fanned toes abnormal/ curved normal
- Normal reflex = 2+
- No reflex = 0
- Hyperactive = 4+

Assessment of LOC

- RESTLESSNESS –First sign of altered LOC
- Are they alert, oriented x 4, conscious?
- Confused? Irritable?
- Lethargic, obtunded, (reduction of alertness) stuporous, (daze) comatose?
- Is it delirium or dementia

Glasgow Coma Scale (GCS)

- Neurological function and LOC
- Reported as a number
- GCS to determine LOC for head injuries, cerebral infarctions, encephalitis
- Best score is 15
- Less than 7 = severe head injury and coma
- 9-12 = moderate head injury
- Greater than 13 minor head trauma

Glasgow Coma Score		
Eye Opening (E)	**Verbal Response (V)**	**Motor Response (M)**
4=Spontaneous 3=To voice 2=To pain 1=None	5=Normal conversation 4=Disoriented conversation 3=Words, but not coherent 2=No words......only sounds 1=None	6=Normal 5=Localizes to pain 4=Withdraws to pain 3=Decorticate posture 2=Decerebrate 1=None
		Total = E+V+M

Increased Intracranial Pressure

- Manifestations
  - Altered vital signs
    - Cushing's triad (Cushing's response),
    - Increase in Systolic Blood Pressure
    - Bradycardia -Slow bounding pulse
    - Alteration in respiratory pattern
  - Change in body temperature
  - Headache
  - Projectile vomiting
- Manifestations
  - Motor functioning
    - Hemiparesis
    - Hemiplegia
    - Posturing
      - Decorticate – supine, flexed arms, extended legs, plantar flexion of feet
      - Decerebrate – supine arms extended, rotated outward, hands flexed adducted
  - Difficulty speaking
  - Blurred vision

- Diplopia

Fatal Complications

- Hydrocephalus
- Cerebral edema
- Permanent brain damage
- Brain herniation
  - Shifting of brain
  - Compression of brain/brainstem
  - Do not do lumbar puncture to prevent brain herniation from pressure change.
- Brain death

Cessation of cerebral blood flow/vital functions

Lab Tests

Blood glucose

Arterial blood gases

Toxicology screening

Metabolic screening

Serum Creatinine and BUN

Liver function test

Complete blood count

NO LUMBAR PUNCTURE !!!!!!

X-ray, CT, MRI,PET

Surgical Intervention

- Shunt
- Skull Boring

Medications:

- **Osmotic diuretics** - Mannitol (Osmitrol)- to reduce acute cerebral edema
    - Monitor fluid and urinary output
- **Corticosteroids**- Dexamethasone (Decadron)- reduce cerebral edema
    - Use with caution in presence of DM, HTN, Glaucoma, and Renal Impairment
- **Anticonvulsants**- Phenytoin (Dilantin)- Prophylactic, to prevent seizures
    - Check for medication interactions
- **Barbiturates** – Phenobarb (Nembutol)
    - used to induce a barbiturate coma to decrease cerebral edema
    - Analgesic- Fentanyl (Sublimaze) (Opioid)
        - For control of pain and restlessness
        - Mechanical ventilations

Nursing Considerations

- Monitor neuro status & VS q 1-2 hours
- Maintain airway
- HOB <30 degrees
- Prevent valsalva, (forceful attempted exhalation against a closed airway)

- Decrease stimuli
- Fluid restrictions
- Closely Monitor I/O
- Check glucose levels
- Avoid coughing/sneezing/bending/straining/blowing nose

Meningitis

- Inflammation or the meninges, the membrane which protects the brain and the spinal cord
- VIRAL, or aseptic, the most common form and resolves without treatment
  - Related to viral is illness such as mumps, measles, herpes, or mosquito-borne West Nile Virus
- BACTERIAL, or septic is contagious infection, high mortality rate
  - Prognosis depend on how quickly care is initiated
  - Bacterial-based infections, otitis media, pneumonia, sinusitis- micro-organisms such Neisseria meningitidis, Sterptococcus pneumonia, and Heamophilus influenza
  - Invasive procedure, skull fractures, penetrating head wounds (Direct access to CSF
- Data
  - Constant headache
  - Nuchal rigidity (Stiff Neck)
  - Photophobia
  - Fever, chills, tachycardia
  - N & V
  - Altered LOC, restlessness
  - Positive Kernig's sign (resistance and pain with extension of leg from a flexed position
  - Positive Brudzinski's sign (flexion of extremities, flexion of neck)
  - Seizures
  - Red macular Rash

- **Labs and Diagnostics**
- Urine, throat, and blood cultures
- CBC- possible elevated WBC count
- Lumbar puncture
  - CSF analysis – most definitive diagnostic procedure
    - Appearance of CSF – cloudy
    - Elevated WBC
    - Elevated protein
    - Decreased glucose (bacterial)
    - Elevated CSF pressure
- **Medications**
- **Ceftriaxone (Rocephin) or Cefotaxime (Claforan)** effective abx's until till C&S results are available
- **Phenytoin (Dialantin)**- anticonvulsant to prevent seizures
- **Acetaminophen (Tylenol), Ibuprofen (Motrin),** for head ache and fever, opioids mask level in consciousness
- **Ciprofloxacin (Cipro)**- given to those in close contact with the client

- **Nursing Considerations**
  - Isolate client
  - Isolation Droplet Precautions
  - Fever reduction- cooling blanket
  - Provide quiet environment
  - Minimize bright lights to decrease photosensitivity
  - Bed rest, HOB elevated 30 degrees
  - Safety for seizure precautions
  - Monitor IV fluids
  - I&O

SEIZURES

- Abrupt, abnormal and uncontrolled electrical discharges of neurons within the brain, which can cause alteration in LOC, motor/sensory ability
- Three Categories
    - Generalized- loss of consciousness, involves both cerebral hemispheres
        - Tonic phase- 15-20 sec- muscle stiffening, cessation of breathing, dilated pupils, cyanosis
        - Clonic phase- 1-2 min- rhythmic jerking of extremities, irregular respirations, biting of tongue or cheek, bowel and bladder incontinence
        - Postictal- may last for several hours, unconsciousness may last for 30 minutes, wakes confused and disoriented, fatigued, sore muscles, weakness, many clients have no memory of incident
    - Absence Seizures
        - Most common in children
        - Loss of consciousness for a few sec, blank- starring gaze
    - Partial or focal/local- loss of consciousness, begins in one hemisphere
        - **Complex partial seizures**
        - Associated with automatism (lip smacking or picking at clothes)
        - **Simple partial seizures**.
            - maintain consciousness
            - Unusual sensations, flushing abnormal extremities movement, pain and offensive smell
    - Unclassified, idiopathic
        - Do not fit in any category, these type of seizures account of half of all seizure disoders
- Risk Factors
    - Genetic
    - Acute febrile state
    - Head trauma, cerebral edema, brain tumor
    - Infection, metabolic disorder, F&E imbalance

- Acute withdrawal from ETOH, drugs
- Cessation of antiepileptic medications
- Triggers
  - Increased physical activity
  - Excessive stress
  - Fatigue
  - ETOH, Drugs
  - Caffeine
  - Flashing lights
  - Chemicals

Labs and Diagnostics

- ETOH and drug tests
- EEG- to identify origin of seizure activity
- MRI, CT, CSF analysis, to rule out tumors or infections

Medications

Antiepileptic Drugs-to prevent further seizure activity

- **Phenytoin (Dilantin)**- may cause sedation, cognitive impairment, bleeding gums, interfere with Vit D metabolism
- **Carbamazepine (Tegretol)**- may cause diplopia, leucopenia, thrombocytopenia, dermatitis, fluid retention
- **Valporic Acid (Depakote)**- GI effects, hepatotoxicity, thromocytopenia
- **Lamotigine (Lamictal)**- skin rash, toxicity if taken with other antiepileptics

Benzodiazepines

- **Diazepam (Valium), Lorazapam (Ativan)**- may cause respiratory depression, resuscitation may be required, administer O2

Nursing Considerations

During Seizure -SAFETY

- Do not attempt to restrain client
- Protect head
- Move furniture out of the way
- Turn client's head to the side to prevent aspiration
- Do not insert any object in mouth
- Document length of seizure , loc, apnea or cyanosis

Post Seizure

- Maintain side-lying position
- Check V/S
- Check for injuries
- Perform Neuro check
- Allow time for client to rest
- Calm client, may need reorientation
- Institute seizure precautions: bed in lowest position, padding of side rails, suction ready and available at bed side

Client Education

- Advise client that treatment is not a cure
- Monitor seizure frequency
- Take prescribed medications on time every day
- Do not stop medications
- Report side effect to prescriber
- Follow up for serum drug levels
- Avoid pregnancy as some medications may cause birth defects

Status Epilepticus

- Prolonged seizure activity, longer than 30 min
- May cause loss of brain function, death

Parkinson's Disease

- Caused by deficiency of dopamine as substantia nigra of brain and it atrophies
- Dopamine is responsible for voluntary motor function
- Acetylcholine is no longer inhibited which results in constant excitement of motor neurons aka all the signs and symptoms.
- Progressive degenerative, difficult to perform ADL's
- Bradykinesia, (extreme slowness in movements) akinesia, (impaired, loss of voluntary muscle movement), tremors, muscle rigidity, difficulty chewing and swallowing, primary symptoms
- More common in men
- Genetic
- Onset usually age 40 – 70
- Cognitive impairment, dementia, pill-rolling of fingers
- No definitive diagnostic procedure available, rule out other disease processes

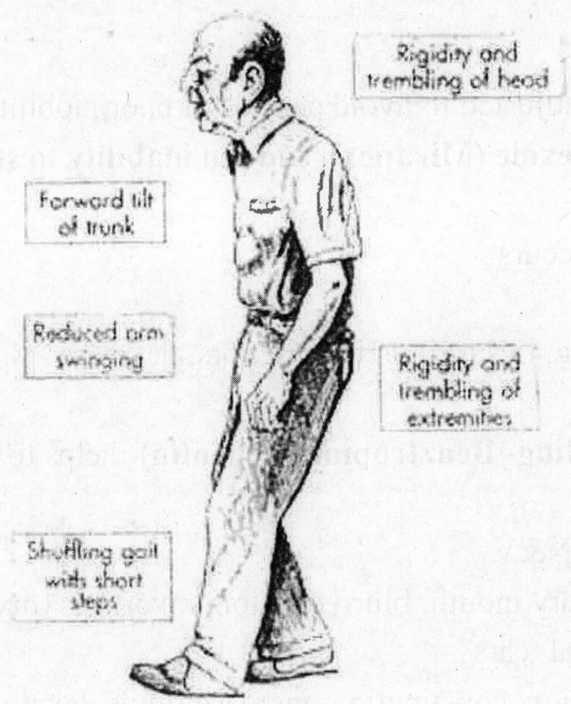

▪

Medications

- **Dopaminergics- Levodopa (Dopar), first line medication for the treatment of PD-** converts to dopamine in the brain
  - N&V, administer with food,
  - Orthostatic hypotension, Monitor BP-slow to change position
  - CV stimulation- Monitor V/S, tachycardia, palpitations, irregular heart beat
  - Dyskinesia, head bobbing, tics, grimacing, tremors, decrease medication
  - May experience hallucinations, treat with antipsychotics
  - **Caridopa (Sinmet)-** smaller dose to make the same amount available to the brain
  - N&V, administer with food,
  - Orthostatic hypotension, Monitor BP-slow to change position
  - CV stimulation- Monitor V/S, tachycardia, palpitations, irregular heart beat

- **Medication tolerance**- adjusted to avoid periods of poor mobility

- **Dopamine Agonists- Pramipexole (Mirapex)- sudden inability to stay awake**
  - Advise provider if this occurs
  - Orthostatic Hypotension
  - Dyskinesia, head bobbing, tics, grimacing, tremors, decrease medication
- **Anticholinergics- Central acting- Benztropine (Cogentin)**- helps to control tremors
  - Take with food to avoid N&V
  - Anticholinergic effects, dry mouth, blurred vision, mydriasis (dry eye), hard candy, artificial tears
  - Urinary hesitancy, retention, constipation- increase fluids, laxatives and stool softeners
  - Antihistamine effects, sedation and drowsiness, avoid strenuous activities
- **Anti-virals , Amantadine (Symmetrel)**- CNS effects, confusion, dizziness, restlessness, avoid activities which require attention
  - Anticholinergic effects- see above
  - Discoloration of skin- will subside when medication is discontinued

Client Education

- Effects of medication may take several weeks
- Report side effects
- Avoid high protein meals and snacks, can reduce effectiveness of medication
- Rehabilitation/ROM
- Nutrition
- Speech therapy
- Nutrition therapy
- Fall Risk reduction
- Constipation
- Incontinence
- Encourage ADL's and self care

Alzheimer's Disease

- Non reversible type of dementia (multiple cognitive deficits that impair memory and can affect language, motor skills, and abstract thinking)
- Severe physical decline occurs along with deterioration of cognitive functions
- Amyloid proteins plaques, and neurofibrillary tangles found within brain on autopsy
- Framework is based on early, mid, and late stage

Medications

- Temporarily slows the course of the disease, but does not work for all client's
- **Donepezil (Aricept)**
    - Prevents breakdown of acetylcholine, increase amount available, as a result increases nerve impulses

Nursing considerations

- Provide safe environment
- Monitor for cognitive status, memory, judgment, and personality changes
- Encourage client and family to participate in AD support group
- Check client's for skin breakdown
- Keep structured environment
- Use calendar to assist with orientation
- Provide memory training
- Promote consistency in placing items used in the same location
- Validation therapy, acknowledge client's feeling
- Don't argue with client
- Promote self-care when possible
- Reduce agitation, calm voice, redirect statements, provide diversion
- Promote toileting schedule

Cerebrovascular Accident

- Disruption in blood flow secondary to ischemia, hemorrhage, or embolism
- Affects 700,000 people in the U.S. per year
- Third leading cause of death in the U.S.
- Most frequent cause of chronic neurologic disability
- Risk factors include drug abuse, HTN, diabetes,hyperlipidemia, age, smoking, oral contraceptives, obesity, African American, sickle cell
- CT and MRI diagnostic as well as CNS/PNS deficits
- Ischemic
    - Thrombus – blood clot
    - Emboli – traveling blood clot
- Hemorrhagic
    - Blood vessel ruptures
- Speech Deficits
    - Expressive aphasia - know what you want to say but can't say what you want to
    - Anomic aphasia – mix up words - substitution
    - Receptive aphasia – can't make sense of words/letters
    - Global aphasia – cannot speak, read, write, understand
    - Dysarthria – difficulty articulating words/sounds due to damage to muscles involved in speech
    - Dysphagia – difficulty swallowing due to damage to muscles involved

Visual Deficits

- Due to parietal and/or temporal lobe damage
- Diplopia – double vision
- Hemianopsia – loss of half visual field either right or left side on one or both eyes
- Sensory-Perceptual Deficits

- Agnosia – recognition loss
- Apraxia – loss of coordination
- Unilateral neglect – unaware of 1 side of the body
- Increased risk for injury
- in chewing and swallowing

Stroke – Diagnostic Tests

Diagnostic Tests

- CT scan/MRI
- Cerebral arteriogram
- Doppler ultrasound
- PET scan
- Lumbar puncture
- Hemiparesis
- Hemiplegia

Interventions

- **Thrombolytics** for ischemic stroke – **Activase-** 3-6 hours of onset of symptoms to dissolve embolism
- **Anticoagulants- Heparin, Levonox, Coumadin,** for embolic CVA to prevent additional emboli
- **Antiplatelets- ASA, Tilicid, Plavix-** for client's with thrombotic CVA, watch for bleeding
- **Gabapentin,** given for paresthetic pain of affected side
- Rehabilitation ASAP – use it or lose it
- ROM / Turning

- Swallowing evaluation
- Alternate communication strategies
- Side to side scan for loss of visual field
- Community resources
- Special equipment
- Nutrition needs
- Teach ADL's
  - Clothing affected side first

Transient Ischemic Attacks (TIA)

- Temporary reduction in cerebral blood flow
- Reversible neurologic deficits
  - Several minutes to 24 hours
- Warning sign of an impending or future stroke
- Carotid doppler to check for plaque build-up
- Endarterectomy treatment
- DVT prevention / Coumadin therapy

Spinal Cord Injuries

- Trauma most common cause
- Alcohol, age, drugs, gender, lifestyle risk factors
- Motor and sensory at level of injury and below is affected
- Paraplegia – lower spine
- Tetraplegia- Quadraplegia -cervical spine

- Spinal Shock – most dangerous period following spinal cord injury

Therapy and Interventions

- Acute phase – ABC's + immobilization + ventilation
- Stabilization (Halo)
- Steroids to reduce further damage
- Assist with quad cough (push up from xiphoid)
- Bladder and bowel training
- Catheters
- Peg Tubes
- Specialty devices for transfer/transport
- **Autonomic Dysreflexia**
    - Potentially life threatening condition which can be considered a medical emergency requiring immediate attention.
- Sweating, pounding headache, tingling sensation on the face and neck, blotchy skin around the neck and goose bumps.
- Vasoconstriction and dilation and systolic hypertension
    - Check bowel and bladder, Cholinergics- Urecholine to reduce spastic bladder, Stool softeners, bulk forming laxative for bowel motility
    - Control BP, antihypertensive medications
    - Muscle Relaxants- Baclofen (Lioresal)
    - Check that body is anatomically correct position
    - Elevate head
    - Check integrity of skin, prone to decubiti

Multiple Sclerosis

- Chronic degenerative disease
  - Damages Myelin sheath surrounding the axons of CNS.
  - Myelin sheaths make up the white matter in CNS.
  - Multiple Sclerosis destroys the sheath of the spinal cord, brain and optic nerve and replaces it with plaque. AKA demyelination
  - Unknown etiology – autoimmune? Permanent disability

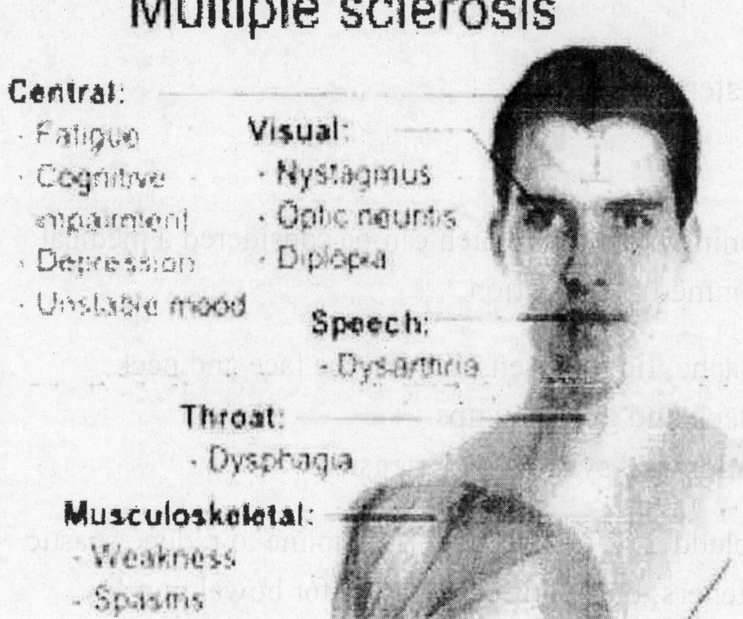

- **Medications**
  - **Immunosuppressant therapy**- Azathioprine (Imuran), Cyclosporin (Sandimmune)- watch for S&S of infection, monitor for HTN and renal dysfunction

- **Stool Softeners**- Colace
- **Steroids**- to reduce inflammation during exacerbation periods. Prednisone (Deltasone)- monitor for risk of infections, GI bleeding , Cushing's Syndrome
- **Anti-cholinergics**- Propantheline (Pro-Banthine)- for bladder dysfunction
- **Anti-Spasmodics**- Baclofen (Lioresal)- observe for weakness

Nursing care

- Supportive care
- Perform tasks in AM– set priorities
- Avoid illness – good nutrition and increased fluids
- Encourage involvement in support groups
- Encourage use of assistive devices to aid ambulation
- Adhere to medication regime

Amyotrophic Lateral Sclerosis (ALS) Lou Gerhrig's Disease

- Degenerative neurological disorder of both the lower and upper motor neurons
- Results in death of motor neurons
- Progressive paralysis, muscle wasting
  - Cause respiratory paralysis and death in 3-5 years after diagnosis
  - No known cure
- Risk Factors
  - Men between the age of 40- 70
- Physical Findings
  - Muscle weakness, atrophy
  - Stumbling
  - Dysphagia- difficulty swallowing
  - Dysarthia- stammering, stuttering speech, due to muscle weakness

- **Labs and Diagnostic Tests**
  - Creatine Kinase- CK-BB levels increases (denotes cerebral disruption)
  - Electromyography (EMG)- results in reduction of motor units of peripheral nerves
  - Muscle Biopsy, reduction of motor units in peripheral nerves and atrophic muscle fibers
- **Medications**
  - Rizole (Rilutek)- slows deterioration of motor neurons
    - Can add 2-3 months to lifespan
  - Baclofen (Lioresal)- to decrease spasticity

Nursing Considerations

- Utilize energy conservation methods
- Address the client's interest in advance directive
- Supportive care
- Promote ADL's as long as client is able to do so
- Family support, and hospice referrals

Myasthenia Gravis

- Chronic progressive disorder of PNS causing muscle weakness
- Autoimmune disease, destroys acetylcholine receptors
- Characterized by periods of exacerbation and remission
- Improves with rest
- Eventually leads to a complete paralysis of all muscles
- Tensilon test- Baseline assessment of cranial nerves, (temporary improvement in muscle strength lasting about 5 minutes
- **Medications:**
  - Anticholinesterase Agents- first line in therapy- given 4 times per day

- Watch for periods of weakness, use with caution with history or asthma or cardiac arrhythmias
- Neostigmine , Pyridostigmine – to increase muscle strength, prolongs acetylcholine
- Immunosuppressants-Imuron- given during exacerbation phase to decrease production of antibodies- watch for S&S of infection
- Corticosteroids- Prednisone- first drug of choice if Imuron ineffective
- NSAIDS

Guillain Barre Syndrome

- Acute destruction of the myelin sheath of peripheral nerves due to a virus, vaccination, surgery, URI, GI Flu
- Acute progressive muscle weakness, initially ascending
- Recovery is usually in descending order
- Muscle become flaccid
- Crawling sensation on skin
- Cranial nerve symptoms- diplopia, facial weakness, dysphagia, disarthria
- Decreased to absent tendon reflexes
- Autonomic dysfunction- alteration in BP, dysrhythmias
- Respiratory compromise

Labs and Diagnostic Test

- **EMG**- decreases in motor neuron in peripheral nerves
- **CBC**- Leukocytosis
- **Lumbar Puncture**- definitive test for GBS- increase in protein with out increase in cell count

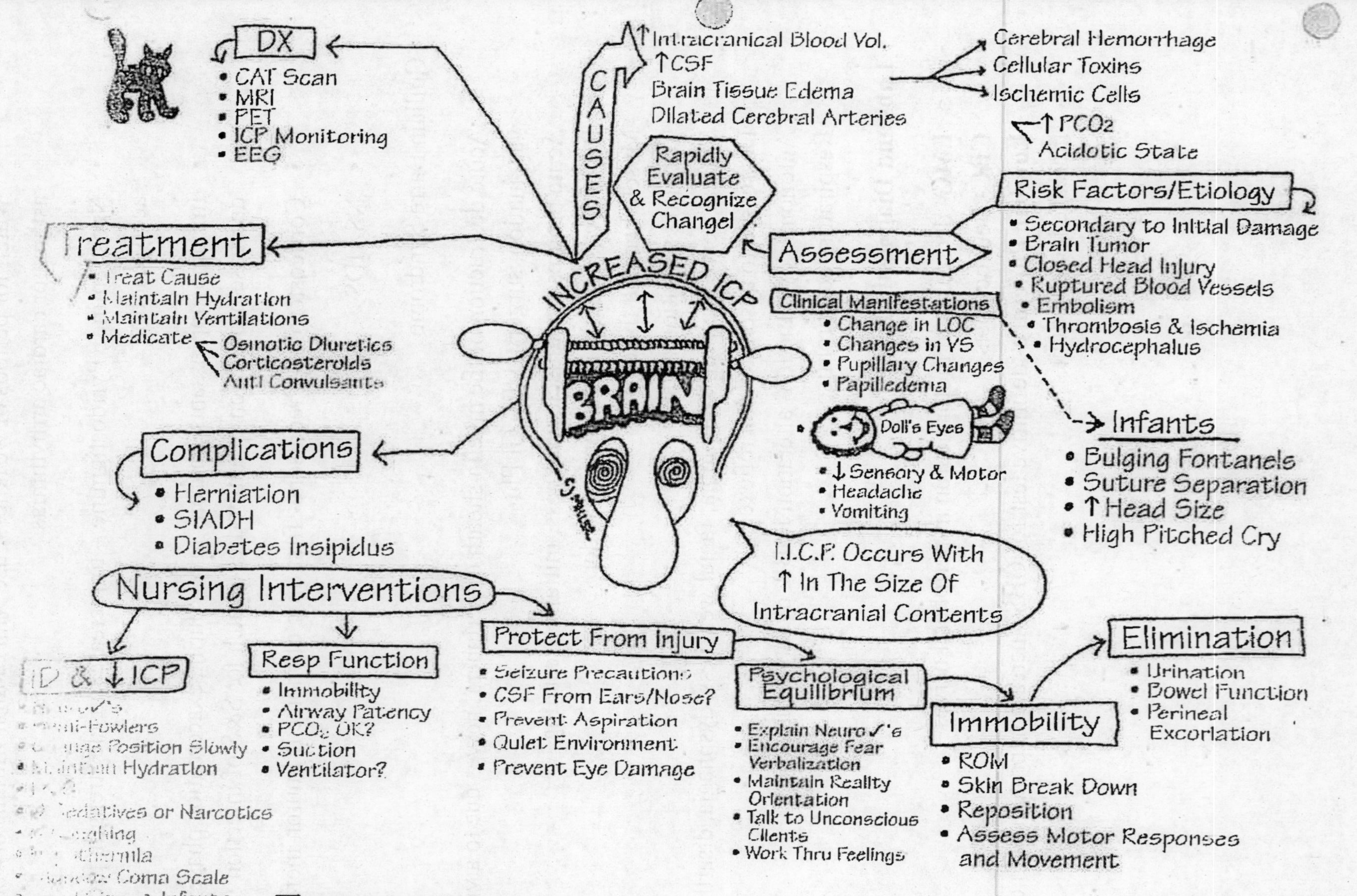

INCREASED ICP
BRAIN
CAUSES
↑ Intracranical Blood Vol.
↑ CSF
Brain Tissue Edema
Dilated Cerebral Arteries
Cerebral Hemorrhage
Cellular Toxins
Ischemic Cells
↑ PCO2
Acidotic State
Rapidly Evaluate & Recognize Changel
DX
• CAT Scan
• MRI
• PET
• ICP Monitoring
• EEG
Treatment
• Treat Cause
• Maintain Hydration
• Maintain Ventilations
• Medicate
Osmotic Diuretics
Corticosteroids
Anti Convulsants
Assessment
Risk Factors/Etiology
• Secondary to Initial Damage
• Brain Tumor
• Closed Head Injury
• Ruptured Blood Vessels
• Embolism
• Thrombosis & Ischemia
• Hydrocephalus
Clinical Manifestations
• Change in LOC
• Changes in VS
• Pupillary Changes
• Papilledema
• Doll's Eyes
• ↓ Sensory & Motor
• Headache
• Vomiting
Infants
• Bulging Fontanels
• Suture Separation
• ↑ Head Size
• High Pitched Cry
Complications
• Herniation
• SIADH
• Diabetes Insipidus
I.I.C.P. Occurs With ↑ In The Size Of Intracranial Contents
Nursing Interventions
ID & ↓ ICP
Resp Function
• Immobility
• Airway Patency
• PCO2 OK?
• Suction
• Ventilator?
Protect From Injury
• Seizure Precautions
• CSF From Ears/Nose?
• Prevent Aspiration
• Quiet Environment
• Prevent Eye Damage
Psychological Equilibrium
• Explain Neuro ✓'s
• Encourage Fear Verbalization
• Maintain Reality Orientation
• Talk to Unconscious Clients
• Work Thru Feelings
Immobility
• ROM
• Skin Break Down
• Reposition
• Assess Motor Responses and Movement
Elimination
• Urination
• Bowel Function
• Perineal Excoriation

INCREASED INTRACRANIAL PRESSURE (IICP)

(Symptoms Of IICP Are Opposite Of Shock)

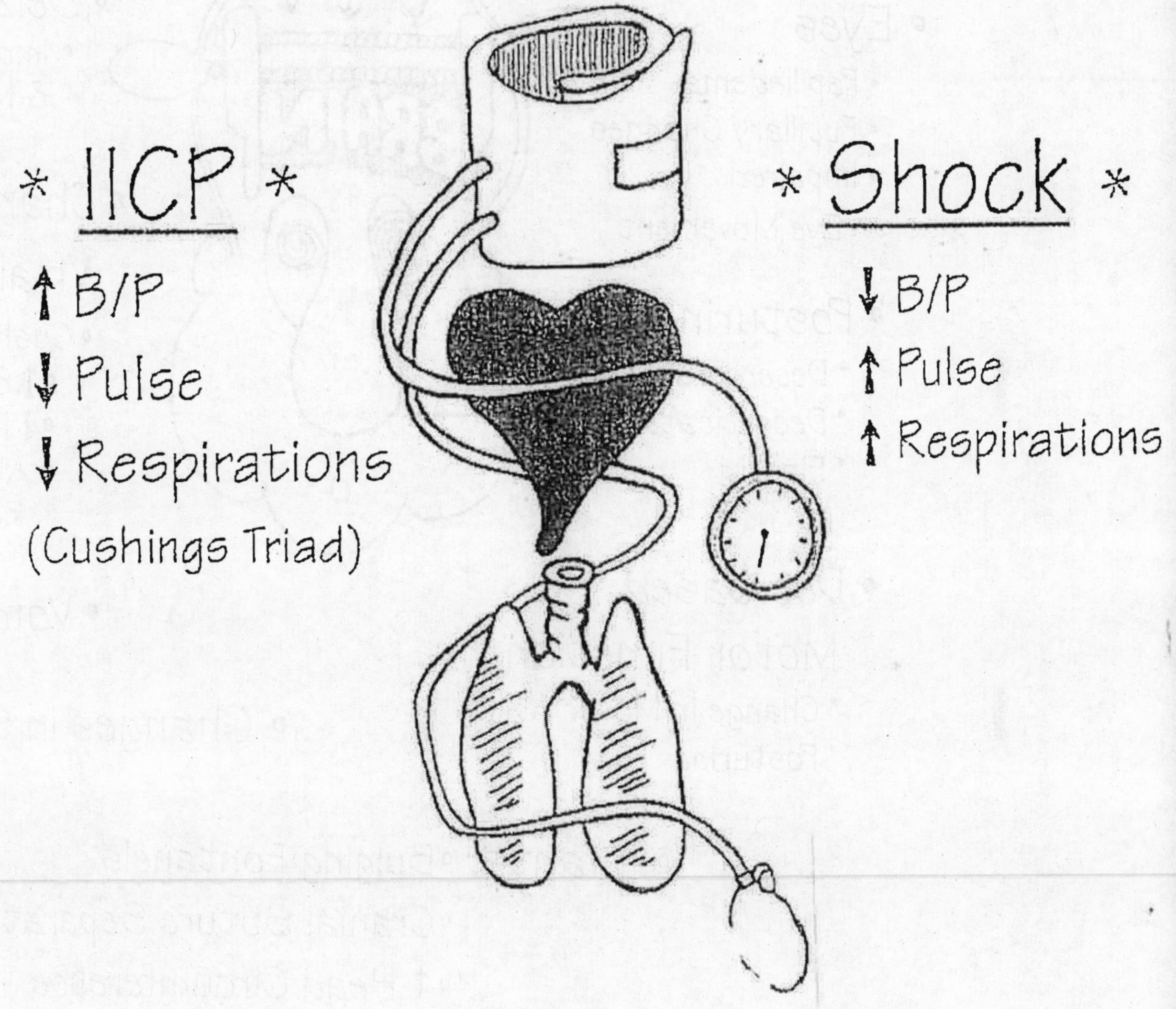

INCREASED INTRACRANIAL PRESSUR

- Changes in LOC
- Eyes
  - Papilledema
  - Pupillary Changes
  - Impaired Eye Movement
- Posturing
  - Decerebrate
  - Decorticate
  - Flaccid
- Decreased Motor Function
  - Change in Motor Ability
  - Posturing
- Headache
- Seizures
  - Impaired Sensory & Motor Functior
- Changes in Vital Signs:
  - Cushing's Triad:
    - ↑ Systolic B/P
    - ↓ Pulse
    - Altered Resp Pattern
- Vomiting
- Changes in Speech

BRAIN

◎ Infants:
- Bulging Fontanels
- Cranial Suture Separation
- ↑ Head Circumference
- High Pitched Cry

PARKINSON'S DISEASE

- Onset usually gradual, after age 50. (Slowly progressive)

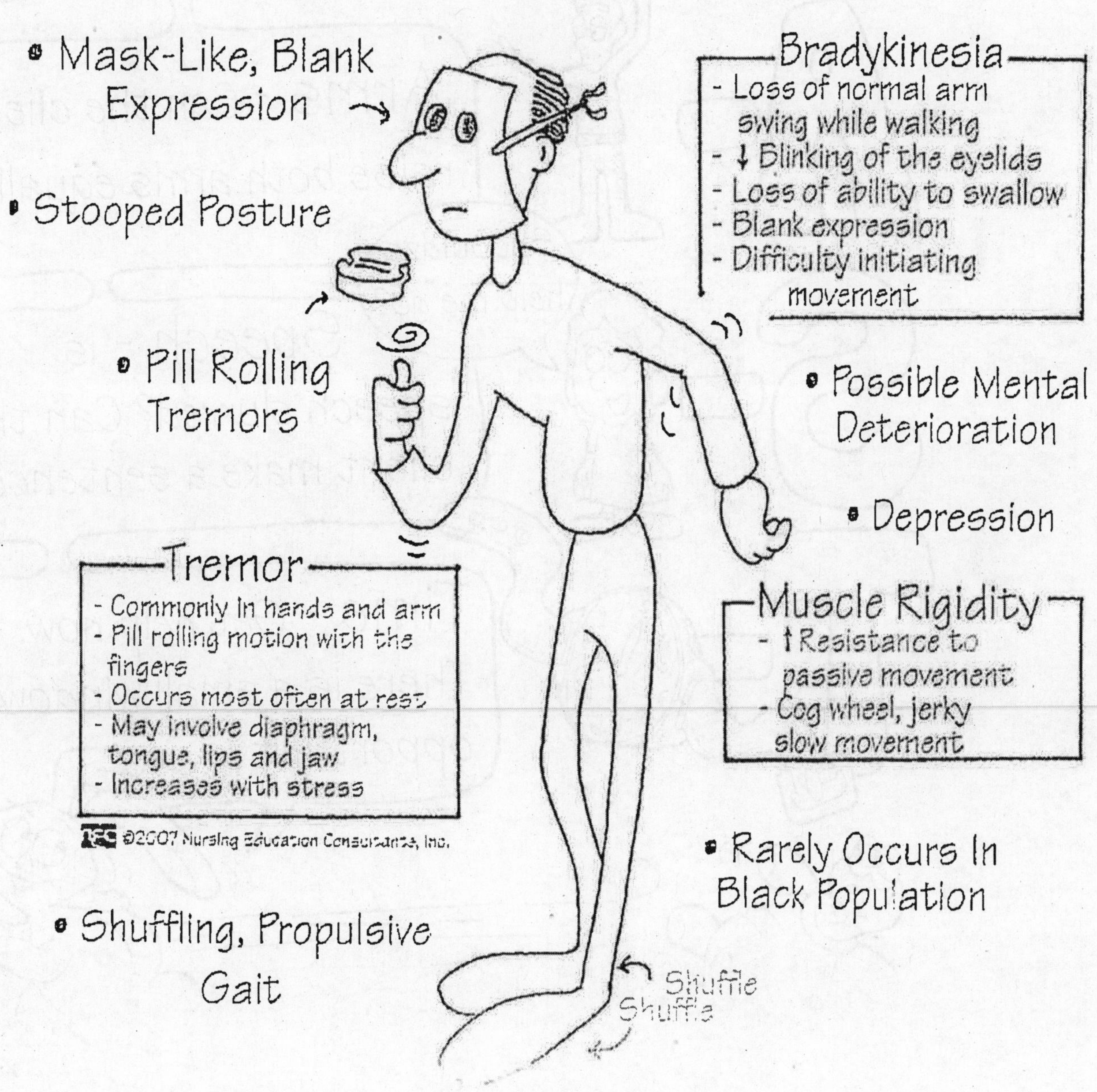

FAST Recognition Of A Strok

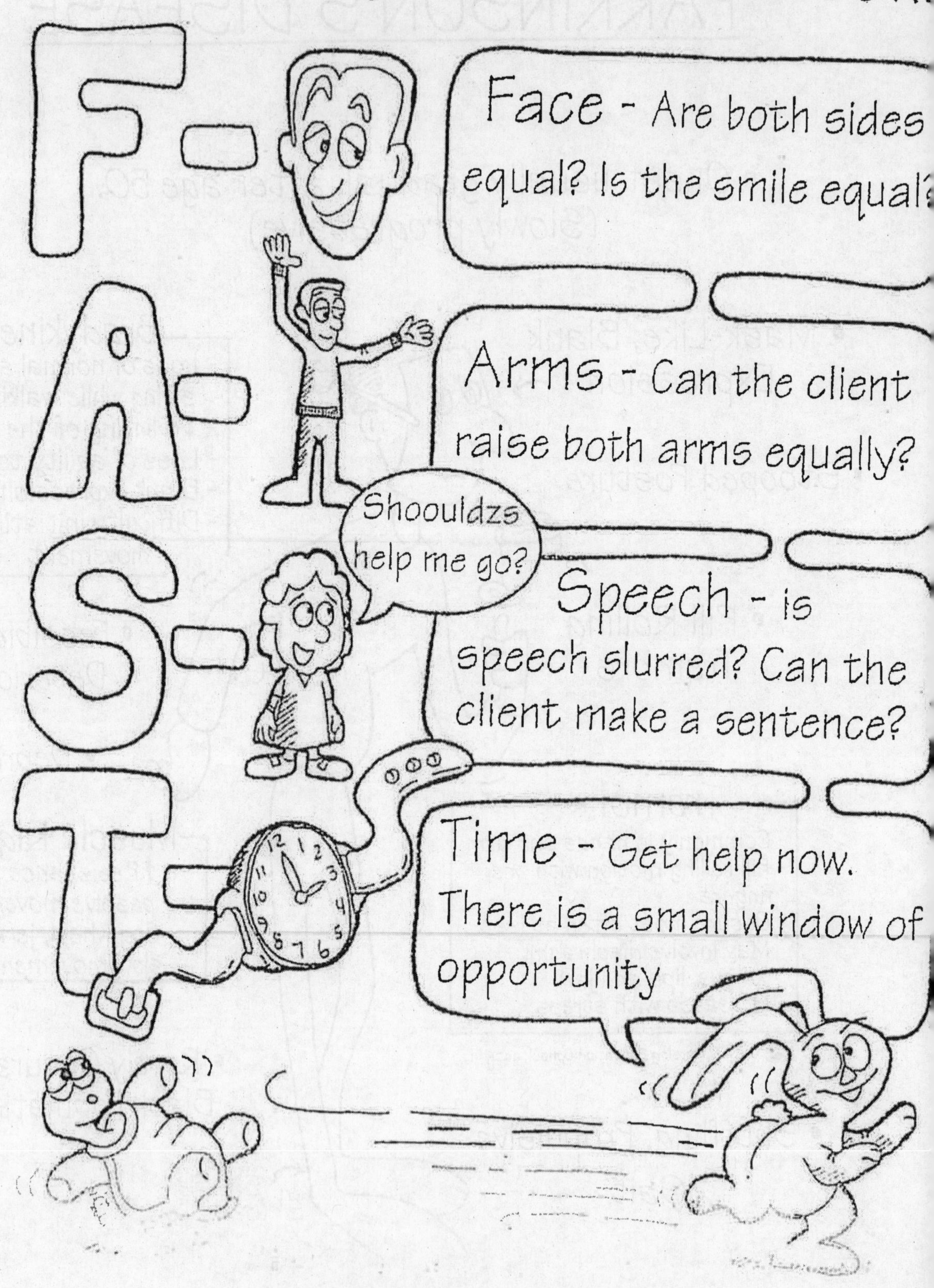

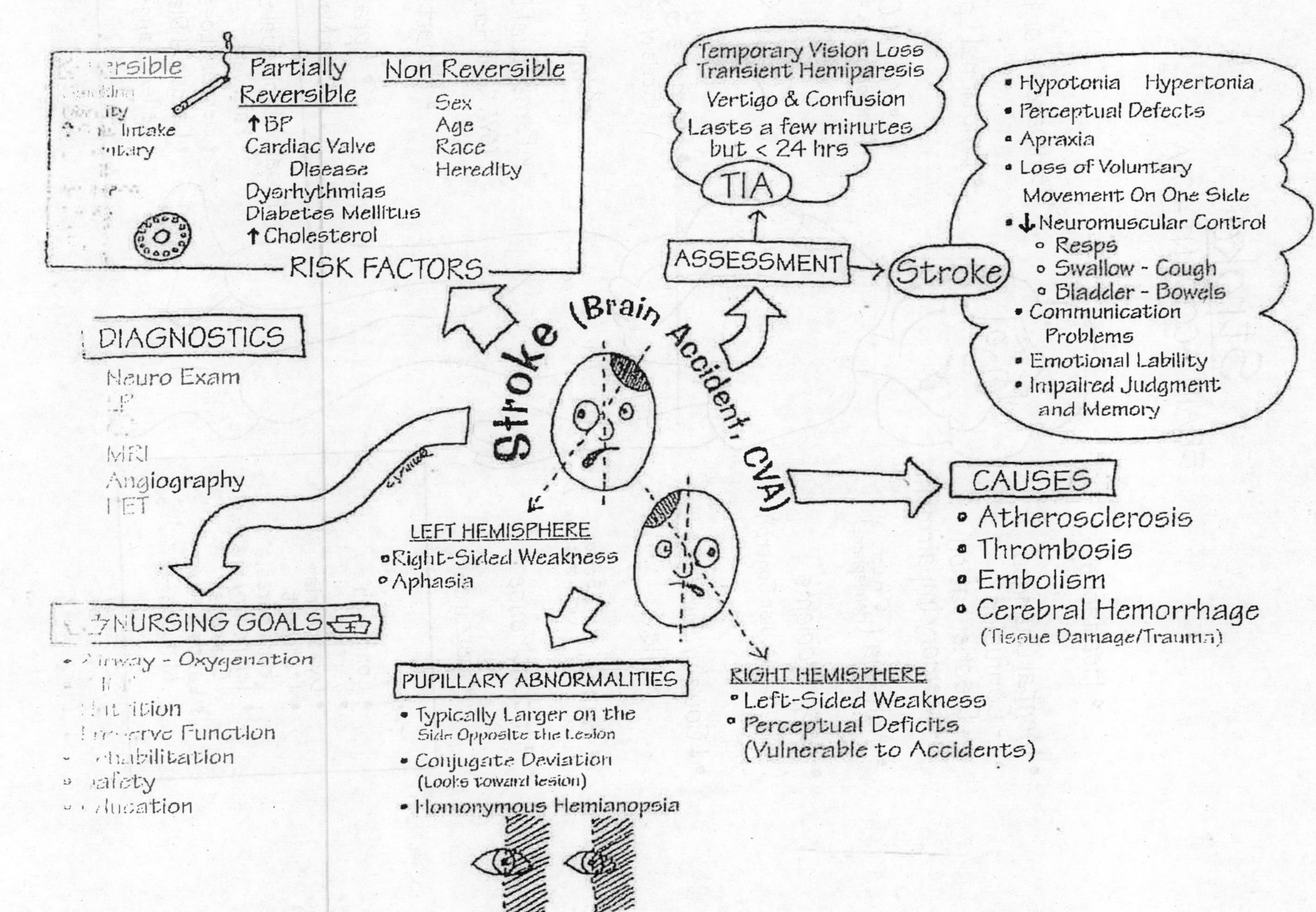

Partially Reversible
↑BP
Cardiac Valve Disease
Dysrhythmias
Diabetes Mellitus
↑Cholesterol
Non Reversible
Sex
Age
Race
Heredity
RISK FACTORS
DIAGNOSTICS
Neuro Exam
MRI
Angiography
NURSING GOALS
Oxygenation
Function
Rehabilitation
Stroke (Brain Accident, CVA)
Temporary Vision Loss
Transient Hemiparesis
Vertigo & Confusion
Lasts a few minutes but < 24 hrs
TIA
ASSESSMENT
Stroke
• Hypotonia Hypertonia
• Perceptual Defects
• Apraxia
• Loss of Voluntary Movement On One Side
• ↓ Neuromuscular Control
○ Resps
○ Swallow - Cough
○ Bladder - Bowels
• Communication Problems
• Emotional Lability
• Impaired Judgment and Memory
CAUSES
• Atherosclerosis
• Thrombosis
• Embolism
• Cerebral Hemorrhage (Tissue Damage/Trauma)
LEFT HEMISPHERE
• Right-Sided Weakness
• Aphasia
RIGHT HEMISPHERE
• Left-Sided Weakness
• Perceptual Deficits (Vulnerable to Accidents)
PUPILLARY ABNORMALITIES
• Typically Larger on the Side Opposite the Lesion
• Conjugate Deviation (Looks toward lesion)
• Homonymous Hemianopsia

Stroke

BRAIN ACCIDENT - CVA

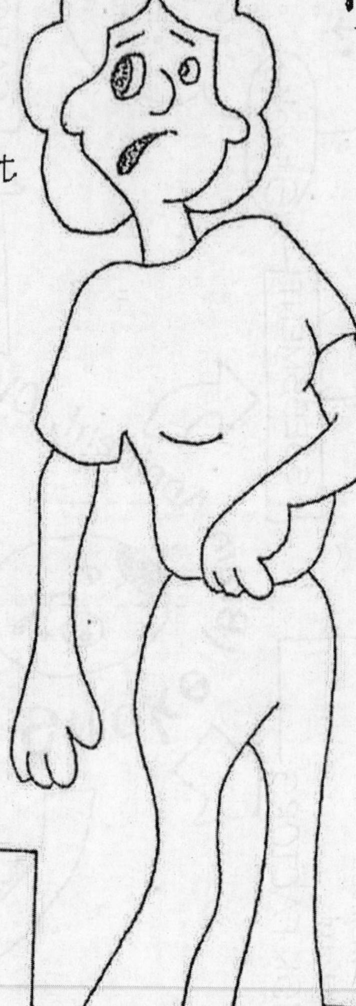

- Headache
- Mental Changes
  - Confusion
  - Disorientation
  - Memory Impairment
- Aphasia (CVA Left Hemisphere)
- Resp Problems (↓ Neuromuscular Control)
- ↓ Cough / Swallow Reflex
- Agnosia (↓ Sensory Interpretation)
- Incontinence
- Seizures

- Hemiparesis or Hemiplegia
- Emotional Lability
- Visual Changes (Homonymous Hemianopsia)

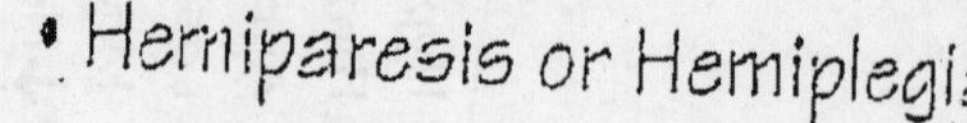
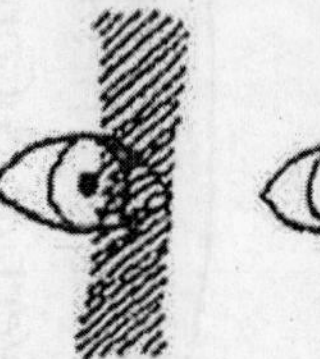
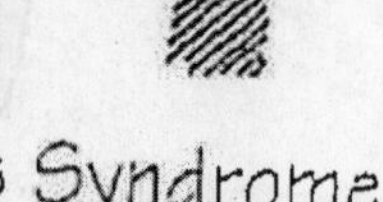

- Horner's Syndrome - Ptosis of Upper Lid
- Vomiting
- Perceptual Defects (CVA Right Hemisphere)
- Hypertension
- Apraxia (↓ Learned Movements)

TIA:
- Confusion
- Vertigo
- Dysarthria
- Transient Hemiparesis
- Temporary Vision Changes
- Lasts a Few Minutes→24 hrs.

Focal Neurological S & S:
- Paralysis
- Sensory Loss
- Language Disorder
- Reflex Changes

Care of the Client with Cancer

Definitions
- Neoplasm: abnormal mass with no useful purpose.
- Benign: harmless, unless space-occupying. If it is located near a vital structure it can be harmful.
- Malignant: harmful mass capable of invasion
- Cancer: refers to malignant neoplasms

Benign	Malignant
Slow growing, expansive	Proliferate rapidly
Localized	Infiltrative patterns, metastasize to nearby tissues
Encapsulated	No enclosing capsule
Rarely recur	May recur
Regular in shape	Irregular shape
Well differentiated	Poorly differentiated
Slight vascularity	Significant vascularity

Properties of Cancer
- Disease of the cell
- Mechanisms controlling growth is altered
- Invasive
- Spreads to surrounding tissues

Epidemiology
In 2007 there were 1.4M new cancer diagnoses. Approx. 10.1 million Americans are living with a history of cancer. Interestingly the incidence of cancer is increasing but perhaps this doesn't necessarily mean there is more cancer. It may just be an issue of diagnostic methods that are more precise, the increased use of screening exams, improved data collection procedures, more accurate reports and longer life spans.

Trends in Cancer
Median age of cancer diagnosis is 67 years. From 1995 - 2002 the incidence was stable in males and there was a 0.3% increase in females. Mortality rates for all cancers decreased 1.1% annually from 1999 - 2002

Risk Factors...
- Tobacco is the #1 cause of cancer-preventable death in the world. It is responsible for increased cancers of: lung, mouth and esophagus.
- Obesity
- Poor Diet (red & processed meat over plant foods)
- Inadequate Physical Activity (< 30 min./day)
- Drugs & chemicals
- Sexual activity (women who start sexual activity early and have multiple partners run the increased risk of cervical cancer d/t the potential for developing HPV which is often a precursor to cervical cancer.)
- Alcohol
- Age
- Genetic predisposition
- Immune dysfunction

Risk factors, cont'd
- Hormones
- Viruses
- Radiation

- UV-A & UV-B rays
- What about Stress? Stress & the relationship to neoplasms is still being investigated. We definitely know that ↑ stress compromises the immune system.

Note that hormones can be "feeders" for tumors...you will hear the term "estrogen dependent tumor". This is why women of child-bearing age who get breast cancer, uterine or ovarian cancer have a very grim prognostic outcome.

7 Warning Signs of Cancer "CAUTION"

- **C**hange in bowel or bladder habits
- **A** sore that does not heal
- **U**nusual bleeding or discharge
- **T**hickening or lump in breast or elsewhere
- **I**ndigestion or difficulty swallowing
- **O**bvious change in a wart or mole
- **N**agging cough or hoarseness

Pathophysiology (may add more here)

- Begins at the molecular level
- Cancer is many diseases (not sure what she means by this)
- Cells that are transformed, but are able to multiply and grow
- May begin with a mutation
- Change from normal to neoplastic cell is a process
- Occurs over many years

Carcinogenesis

Transformation of normal cells into cancer cells. It involves four stages: Initiation, promotion, malignant conversion and progression.

- Initiation occurs when a carcinogen damages DNA. This causes changes in the structure and function of the cell at the genetic or molecular level. This damage by be reversible or may lead to genetic mutation. The mutation may or may not lead to cancer.
- Promotion occurs with additional insults to the cell that results in further damage to the cell.
- Malignant conversion. If the insult continues, then malignant conversion occurs.
- Progression is when the cells are increasingly malignant in appearance and behavior, and develop into invasive cancer with metastasis to distant organs or system.
- Currently scientists are focusing on the underlying biology of the process of carcinogenesis. They have untaken the identification of ONCOGENES. Oncogenes are genes that when mutated or expressed at abnormally high levels contribute to converting a normal cell into a cancer cell. An oncogene is a gene that has sustained some genetic damage and thus produces a protein capable of cellular transformation. As a result of this research, scientists have begun developing better treatments. New chemotherapy drugs known as BIOTHERAPIES are becoming the standard in addition to surgery, chemotherapy and radiation.

Cell Differentiation

- Occurs in the embryonic phase & enables stem cells to become nephrons or hepatocytes or alveoli or neurons.
- Normal cells have well-organized structure, similar cellular components.
- Cancer cells come in variable sizes & shapes
- Notes: In a cancer cell, the nuclei may be abnormally large or there may be multiple nuclei. There may be an abnormal number of chromosomes or an abnormal arrangement of the chromosomes (aneuploidy). This finding is an unfavorable prognostic indicator.
  - Cancer cells have some properties that enable us to not only identify them, but treat them.
  - Benign masses are very well differentiated from normal tissue. The body encapsulates it off and prevents it from invading other tissues
  - Malignant masses are poorly differentiated from normal tissues and the body has difficulty recognizing that the malignant tissue is not its own.

Cancer Cell Properties

- Heterogeneity: There may be a number of variations of the malignant cell...won't all look the same and they'll mutate in different ways. This is caused by random mutations during tumor progression. One chemo may work on one type of cell...but may take other drugs to work on the other cell types. This is why they are now using combination chemotherapy. You use more than one drug, but can use lower doses of each one

- Cell membrane changes: Results in production of enzymes that actually allow and enable the cancer to spread and interact with the outside tissues and invade it.
- Tumor specific antigens on the cell surface: Some tumors express more of an antigen than is expressed by normal cells. These TSAs can be used as a dx tool such as prostate surface antigen (PSA). Basically, the antigens tell us the cancer is there before we would otherwise be able to find it. For example, when the PSA starts to rise we know the pt is at risk for cancer in the prostate. Embryonic antigen is another one that the cells often put out. For example, if a woman has been treated for ovarian cancer, she will get a yearly screen for this antigen. It tells us if the cancer is coming back.
- Functional changes: Cancers occupy space (when in the brain this is very dangerous, can lead to increased ICP!), and they also use up nutrients from the host. So, one of the things we see is weight loss b/c the cancer is drawing in all the nutrients the person is taking in. If the tumor is functioning it will do so abnormally as in the case of thyroid cancer (hyperthyroidism).
- Uncontrolled growth: Cancer cells have no inhibition of growth, and are almost always in a continuous process of cell-division. This continuous growth results in a term known as "doubling time." The doubling time of a malignant tumor can vary from weeks to months. This distinguishes slow-growing cancers like prostate cancer from rapidly growing cancers like breast cancer (breast cancer has a doubling time of 100 days.)
- Metastasis: Normal cells stick to other normal cells from which they arise. So for example normal breast tissue cells are not found anywhere else in the body...they all "stick together." Malignant cells do not stick to other cells and are more mobile than normal cells. So malignant cells have the ability to spread from the original site to distant organs. This of course, is called metastasis. This is a major characteristic of cancer cells and the reason why many cancer treatments do not succeed.
- Angiogenesis is the ability of the cancer to secrete substances that stimulate blood vessel growth and allow the tumor to create its own circulation and nutrient supply.
- Failure of apoptosis (apoptosis is cellular suicide): Normal cells have a code in them that tells them when to die...cancer cells don't have that, they live on and on and on. In addition, they never shrink or get phagocytized or digested by macrophages. They manage to avoid all those triggers that tell them to go off and die d/t their genetic damage/mutation.

Tumor Burden

- Metastatic tumors put severe stress on the affected person. We look at the size and mass of each tumor, and that tells us what your "tumor burden" is...how much it is affecting your system.
- Fewer metabolic resources are available for normal cells. So, the larger the mass or the greater the number of mass, the less chance you have of surviving that.
- When the total burden of the tumor approaches 1 kg, the tumor is potentially lethal. This is the "open and close" person in surgery. :-(

Immune system's job:

- Recognize a pathogen as foreign. A tumor cell is a type of pathogen.
- Mount a response to eliminate the pathogen.

Preventing Carcinogenesis

- Cancer cells arise continually. We are bombarded by these things every day and we fight them off!
- Immune cells recognize these cells and destroy them via T cells, Lymphocytes, Macrophages, Antigens
- The immune defenses are not always effective. The system may be unable to recognize cancer cells as foreign or to mount an immune response for several reasons.

Why does immune system fail?

- Immature system (infants)
- Old or weak immune system...can't fight cancer at the molecular level.
- Malnutrition
- Chronically ill (COPD, DM, RA, autoimmune diseases)
- Tumor burden may overwhelm it
- Cancer cells disguise themselves as normal cells
- Some cancer cells produce substances that shield them (i.e., fibrin)...especially neoplasms! The tumor necrosing factors and cytokines and WBC can't even get to the cancer cells.

- Interesting tidbit: the incidence of malignancy increases with the use of immunosuppresive drugs after organ transplant. Chemotherapy and radiation can also suppress the immune system.
- A malignant mass of 1cm or greater can overwhelm even a healthy immune system. Woah!

Carcinogens
- Radiation: natural sources, diagnostic or therapeutic sources
- Chemicals: tobacco/compute pack-years, occupational hazards, gasoline, high-tension lines
- Viruses: HPV, EBV & H-pylori (a bacteria that causes stomach ulcers...a set-up for gastric cancer)
- Other physical agents: (i.e., hormones, genetics)

Preventing Cancer (see notes)
- Prevention: Lifestyle behaviors that limit exposures
  - Smoking cessation, dietary habits, alcohol consumption, increasing physical activity, limiting sun exposure, modifying sexual practices and decreasing exposure to environmental carcinogens.
- Secondary prevention is also referred to as early detection: skin inspection, mammograms, pap smears, occult blood testing, endoscopy and chest x-rays. If caught early, premalignant lesions can be removed, arrested or reversed!
- The American Cancer Society estimates that 75% of all cancers in the US could be cured if all available screening tests and self examination methods were practiced routines.

Approaches to Cancer Prevention
- Education: Client's perception of susceptibility to developing cancer
- Regulation: Prohibiting sale of tobacco
- Host modification: Possible vaccines, chemoprevention to prevent or reverse carcinogenesis once cancer has been identified

Types of Cancers...
- Adenocarcinoma: arises from glandular tissues (includes cancers of the breast, lung, thyroid, colon, pancreas)
- Carcinoma: composed of epithelial cells, tissues lining organs (skin, uterus, breast, esophagus, mouth)
- Sarcoma: cancer of the connective tissue (cartilage, bone, muscle or fat)
- Lymphoma: originating from the lymphatic system
- Leukemia: malignant disease of the blood-forming organs
- Glioma: glial cells of the central nervous system (in the brain, typically very deadly)
- Melanoma: malignancy of the melanocytes
- Hepatomas: malignancies of the liver
- Carcinoma in situ: pre-invasive epithelial tumors with glandular or squamous cell origins (means it's confined and at an early stage...we can get rid of these!)

Staging Cancers
- Grading a cancer is to determine the malignancy
- Grade 1-4: deviate minimally from normal cells to very aberrant
- Staging a cancer is to determine the extent of the cancer
  - Stage 1= small cancer found only in the organ where it started
  - Stage 2= larger cancer that may or may not have spread to the lymph nodes
  - Stage 3= larger cancer that is also in lymph nodes
  - Stage 4= cancer in a different organ from where it started
- TNM
  - T – Primary Tumor (where is the primary tumor located, how big is it?)
  - N – Involvement of Lymph Nodes (number and location of lymph nodes involved)
  - M – Metastasis (the cancer has moved and invaded another tissue)

Plasias:
Hyperplasia=physiological proliferation...basically lots of cell growth
Metaplasia = cells look a "little different" due to cell type conversion....hard for immune system to recognize as foreign

Dysplasia = more poorly organized, maturational abnormality
Neoplasia = Cancer is the end result...few "normal" cells remain

Physiologic Effects of Cancer...

- Results of Obstruction or Pressure
  - Urine retention form prostate tumors
  - Intracranial pressure – gliomas (get horrible headaches, increased ICP and all the problems that causes)
  - Anoxia and necrosis of tissues...leads to organ function failure
  - Loss of organ function: liver, kidneys, lungs
- Hematologic Alterations
  - Abnormal function of blood cells
  - Loss of normal immune processes
  - Pancytopenia: lower counts of all indices of CBC (anemia of chronic disease)
  - GI tumors disrupt absorption of Vit B12 d/t loss of intrinsic factor (leads to pernicious anemia and get "megaloblastic anemia"..big fat RBCs that don't carry oxygen well!)
  - Growing tumors divert resources needed by bone marrow to produce RBCs
- Infection
  - Tumor invades and connects two incompatible organs (i.e., fistula between bowel & bladder)
  - Destroys viable tissue so metabolic processes are altered, tissue is easily infected
  - Tumors may become necrotic. When they do they leak toxins...can lead to necrotizing fasciitis.
  - Septicemia may result
- Anorexia – Cachexia Syndrome
  - Unexplained rapid weight loss can be 1st symptoms
  - Triggered by pain, infection, depression, or side effects of chemo (cause nausea and depression)
  - Neoplastic cells divert nutrition
  - Metabolic changes reduce client's appetite
  - Stress causes increased serum glucose, which also depresses appetite
  - Taste and smell are altered
  - Malignancy ↑ metabolic rate → catabolism
- Paraneoplastic Syndrome (tumor is secreting a hormone)
  - Endocrine: ectopic hormone production
  - Breast, ovarian, renal cancers cause ectopic parathyroid hormone sites leading to hypercalcemia (huge constipation is the presenting factor)
  - Oat cell (usually found in lung) may produce ectopic insulin, PTH, ADH and ACTH (SIADH is often caused by oat cell carcinoma)
  - Hematologic abnormalities: anemia, thrombocytopenia and coagulopathies
- Acute Pain
  - Well defined pattern, very malignant pain that is tough to treat
  - Common signs and symptoms
  - Identified with hyperactivity of autonomic system
- Chronic Pain
  - Lasts more than 6 months
  - Lacks objective manifestations
  - Results in personality changes
  - Loss of functional abilities. For example bone metastasis often occurs in the back and this is horrible back pain.
  - Disruption of lifestyle
- Physical Stress: Immune system mounts an all out assault on the foreign invader.
  - Chemical mediators (tumor necrosing factors, IgA...)
  - Hormones and enzymes
  - Blood cells
  - Antibodies
  - Proteins

- Inflammatory and immune responses
- Notes: these protective responses also mobilize fluid, electrolytes and nutritinal systems. This massive effort requires tremendous energy. If the neoplasm is small enough, the immune system can destroy it and a tumor will never manifest. A neoplasm of 1 cm is enough to overwhelm most immune systems; however, the body will continue to try to fight it until it reaches the stage of exhaustion and is no longer capable. This is why many pts present with fatigue, weight loss, anemia, dehydration and altered blood chemistries.

- Psychological Stress
  - Many see cancer as a death sentence. This is not true anymore...we have to help them work through this grief and see the hope that is there r/t new treatments.
  - Experience overwhelming grief
  - Some feel guilt, cancer is punishment for past behaviors
  - Feeling powerless / hopeless
  - Fear of the outcome, pain, death
  - Body image concerns
  - Sexual dysfunction, felt but unexpressed

Commonly Occurring Cancers

- **Breast Cancer**
  - Usually discovered by clinical mass or mammogram
  - Mass is hard, irregular, non-tender
  - Often in tail of breast (over by armpit)
  - There may be: nipple discharge, nipple retraction, dimpling or puckering of overlying skin, change in the size or texture of breast
- Breast Cancer Types
  - Non Invasive: carcinoma in situ is confined to ducts or lobules
  - Invasive: infiltrating cancerous cells penetrated tissue outside ducts or lobules
  - Inflammatory: swelling, erythema and invasion of dermal lymphatics
- Breast Cancer: Predicting Survival
  - Tumor size
  - Presence of lymph nodes
  - Presence of hormone receptors (negative is what you want)
  - 20% recur
- Breast Cancer: Treatment
  - Lumpectomy
  - Mastectomy
  - Breast reconstruction
  - Radiation: external beam (smaller dose than what was used in the past)
  - Chemotherapy: adjuvant & hormonal (need to shut down the estrogen to that cancer)

- **Colon & Rectal Cancer**
  - Majority are adenocarcinomas (solid mass cancers)
  - 40-50% are in the rectum
  - 20-35% are in sigmoid colon
  - 16% are in ascending colon
  - 8% are in transverse colon
- Signs of Colorectal Cancer
  - Changes in bowel habits; excessive flatulence
  - Blood in stool
  - Indigestion
  - Weight loss and fatigue
- Treatment for Colorectal Cancer
  - Surgery: colon resection with temp colostomy
  - Chemo therapy

- Radiation therapy
- Survival of Colorectal Cancer
  - Any metastases negatively impacts survival
  - Frequent follow up is needed after treatment
- **Prostate Cancer**
  - 95% are adenocarcinomas
- Causes of prostate cancer
  - Endogenous hormones
  - Possibly by some environmental factors
- Signs of prostate cancer
  - Frequent, painful urination, hematuria (BPH can be a precursor to cancer)
    - If a man has hematuria without pain we assume it is bladder cancer until proven otherwise.
  - See changes in bladder control around beginnings of Stage II
  - Bone, joint & back pain
  - Fatigue and weight loss
- Survival for prostate cancer:
  - Transitional zone involvement is less aggressive
  - Metastatic disease negatively impacts prognosis
  - Cancer is usually slow growing, so catch it early and take care of it!
- Treatment for prostate cancer
  - TURP (part of the prostate removed)
  - Prostatectomy (entire prostate removed)
  - Radiation: external beam
  - Chemotherapy
  - Watch and wait
  - Note: PSAs are routine at age 65 (tests for the prostate surface antigen)
- **Brain Cancer** (dangerous even if benign b/c they take up space)
  - Intracerebral tumors (spread out tentacles, and are hard to get to and treat without damaging brain tissue)
    - brain or neurons
    - blood vessels
    - connective tissues
  - Extracerebral tumors (easier to get to!)
    - meningiomas
    - acoustic nerve neuromas (deep inside the ear...we can get to these). First sign is dizziness!
    - pituitary tumors will cause radical changes in the endocrine system...ADH, aldosterone, TSH, oxytocin, etc. To get to this tumor you go through the nose...cool!
    - pineal gland tumors
  - Note that the classification for benign vs malignant is not differentiated in brain cancer because it is the surgical accessibility of the tumor that dictates prognosis and survivability: Astrocytomas are much more operable than glioblastomas...astrocytomas have a 50-70% survival rate and glioblastomas have 20% survivability.
- Brain Cancer: Early Signs & Symptoms
  - Headache
  - Seizures
  - Nausea
  - VOMITING (increased ICP causes vomiting)
- Brain Cancer: Late Signs & Symptoms
  - Impaired cognitive skills
  - Short term memory loss
  - Speech difficulties
  - Sensory and motor deficits
  - Visual changes
  - Personality changes
  - Dizziness that is persistent (especially acoustic neuromas)
  - Loss of sphincter control

- Brain Cancer: Treatment
  - Surgery: possible placement of chemotherapy wafers in the brain to target neoplasm
  - Radiation therapy
  - Laser therapy
  - Intraoperative hyperthermia (heating up the tumor to get it to shrink)
  - Chemo therapy (systemic)
  - Stereotactic therapy: gamma knife (a form of laser surgery)
  - Photodynamic therapy
- **Lung Cancer**
  - Types
    - Small cell (Oat cell) this one is very tough to treat!
    - Non small cell
    - Squamous cell
    - Adenocarcinomas
    - Mixed
  - Death Rates (see map...mostly in the southeast U.S.)
- Lung Cancer: Signs & Symptoms
  - Persistent cough that changes
  - Multiple respiratory ailments (constant bronchitis, PNAs). Lung cancer can "hide" behind infiltrate on CXR...so you need to repeat the CXR after the PNA is cleared up just to be sure there isn't a cancer there)
  - Dyspnea and wheezing
  - Clubbed fingernails (will also see on COPD, but it's really dramatic on lung cancer pt). This is a result of disease that causes you to be hypoxic. The body's response is to try to make more RBCs and you become polycythemic. So, if the kidneys are working and you can make EPO and the bone marrow responds to that, you will become polycythemic, and all those fat RBCs make the blood viscous and thick. When it gets to the tiny capillaries in the fingers, it gets stuck there, so the capillaries flatten out and enlarge to let those RBCs get through there...you get clubbing of the figners!
  - Hemoptysis
  - Weight loss, dysphagia and fatigue
- Lung Cancer: Survival
  - Best for carcinoma in situ
  - We find it early with CXR
  - Invasion of adjacent lymph nodes is worst prognosis
- Lung Cancer: Treatment
  - Surgery
  - Laser therapy (mostly debulks tumors)
  - Radiation therapy: external beam
  - Chemotherapy
- **Blood Cancers**
  - Multiple Myloma: The cells infiltrate the bone marrow and produce abnormal and excessive amounts of immunoglulin (myeloma protein). Accumulation of these cells in the marrow disrupts RBC, leukocyte and platelet production, which leads to anemias, increased vulnerability to infection and bleeding tendencies. In late stages, there is an increase in cytokine production which plays an important role in bone destruction. As a result, the patient often presents with bone or back pain. The bone cell destruction leads to hypercalcemia which can cause renal problems and failure along with GI problems (nausea and anorexia) and neurologic manifestations (confusion).
    - Immunocompromised
    - African Americans
    - Males
    - 70 yo
  - Multiple Myeloma S/S
    - Bone & joint pain with movement (back pain is very common!)
    - Hypercalcemia (causes GI problems and renal problems)

- Pathologic fractures – compression fractures
- Vertebral collapse
- Renal failure
- Anemia
- Coagulation disorders
- Peripheral neuropathy
- Confusion & altered mental status

- Treatment of Multiple Myoloma
  - There's no cure.
  - We can treat some symptoms, but 1/3 don't respond & die within weeks (how sad)
  - Chemotherapy
  - Corticosteroids
  - Immunotherapy
  - Bone marrow transplant
  - Radiation therapy
- Leukemia & Lymphoma
  - Cancers of the hematopoietic system
  - Proliferative cancers...not good!
  - Lymphoma - lymphoid tissue
- Leukemia (cancer of the bone marrow)
  - Leukemia:Risk Factors
    - Genetic factors: Especially in the chronic forms
    - Exposure to radiation & chemicals (benzenes, hydrocarbons)
    - Congenital abnormalities (Downs syndrome)
    - Primary immunodeficiency
  - Leukemia Pathophysiology
    - A control factor is missing:
      - Uncontrolled proliferation of leukocytes (WBCs) They are uncontrolled and do not mature. They are not effective as working as an immune-competent agent. Normal bone marrow is replaced by immature and undifferentiated leukocytes or blast cells.
      - Blast cell proliferation (precursors to leukocytes). Not effective in fighting disease, but can take over and replace the effective WBCs, at the same time depressing RBCs. These cells literally crowd out the bone marrow and cause cellular proliferation of the other cell lines to cease. "Blast Crisis" when the pt gets into this stage.
      - Massive accumulation of immature nonfunctional cells or blasts...leads to pancytopenia.
    - Acute leukemias include: difference is at the molecular level. Has to do which type of cell becomes proliferative
      - Acute lymphoblastic leukemia (ALL) See more often in children than adults
      - Acute myeloid leukemia (AML) See more often in adults than children

    - Acute Lymphocytic Leukemia
      - ALL is most common in children
      - Usually a result of radiation, chemicals, drugs or viruses.
      - S/S: malaise, fatigue, neutropenia, fever, bone pain, bleeding, bruising.
      - Also look for changes in CBC, look for lymph nodes that are swollen
      - Prognosis: complete remission 80-90% (yay!)
      - Treatment: BMT or stem cell transplantation, induction therapy with chemotherapy
    - Acute Myeloid Leukemia (the adult version)
      - AML Etiology: radiation, chemicals, drugs & viruses
      - S/S: anemia, malaise, fatigue, FUO, bone pain, thrombocytopenia, bleeding.
      - Prognosis: Patients over 70 are intolerant of chemo induction therapy. WBC >100,000 increases mortality.
      - Treatment: Induction therapy, monoclonal antibodies, BMT, stem cell transplant.
  - Chronic Leukemias
    - Chronic myeloid leukemia: starts off slower, can usually be treated pretty easily with chemo and BMT
    - Chronic lymphoblastic leukemia

- Both have a relatively slow course (15 years)
- CML enters a blast crisis that resembles ALL.
  - Median survival is <6 months
  - 85% die during blast crisis
- Leukemia: Manifestations
  - Severe infections (infections most people don't get if they are immunocompetent)
  - Anemia (Hgb are down in 7-8 range)..leads to fatigue, malaise, hypoxia, bleeding from gums, ecchymoses, petechiae, retinal hemorrhages.
  - Increased metabolic rate
  - Weakness, pallor, & weight loss
  - Headache, disorientation
  - Enlarged organs (spleen, liver)
  - Hyperuricemia (kidney stones)
  - Lymphadenopathy (non-tender, painless) and bone pain.
    - Supraclavicular painless lymph nodes are problematic...going to get biopsy of those guys.
- Lymphoma: Originates from the lymphatic system
  - Two Types:
    - Hodgkins lymphoma: enlarged lymph nodes & biopsy shows distinctive large cell (Reed-Sternberg cells)
    - Non-Hodgkins lymphoma: more common form. Similar to Hodgkins, but without a Reed-Sternberg cell.
  - Hodgkins Lymphoma
    - Risk Factors
      - Probable viral cause such as Epstein Barr
      - 2- to 3-fold increase in Hodgkins in clients with history of mononucleosis
      - Genetic predisposition: Young adults 26-31yo; More frequent in Jewish; Siblings have 2 to 5x the risk.
  - Hodgkins: Clinical Manifestations
    - Painless lymphadenopathy, commonly in supraclavicular, cervical, mediastinal areas
    - Non productive cough
    - Mediastinal mass on CXR
    - Pericardial effusion
    - JVD based on changes in heart d/t tumor sitting there
    - Unexplained weight loss; night sweats & fevers of unknown origin
  - Hodgkins: Treatment
    - Chemotherapy combinations (can use lower doses of each drug)
      - MOPP (combo therapy)
      - ABVD – less side effects (this one used the most now)
      - BMT & stem cell transplantation
      - 70-80% survival rate with chemotherapy (yippee!)
  - Non Hodgkins Lymphoma
    - Increase in incidence 1973-91 attributed to increase in AIDS
    - 60 times more common in patients with AIDS
    - Men are affected more often than women
    - Higher in whites
    - Increased incidence in the 50s & 60s
    - Aggressive disease that needs high-dose therapy! Tougher to treat, and pt is likely to be immuno-deficient to begin with, so very tricky.
  - Non Hodgkins: Risk Factors
    - Immunodeficiency states
    - Auto immune disorders (such as SLE, RA)
    - Infectious agents
    - Viral cause is implicated: Herpes
    - H pylori infection (bacterial)
  - Non Hodgkins: Pathohysiology
    - Abnormal proliferation of neoplastic lymphocytes

- Cells fixed at 1 phase of development...they have arrested development and do not mature through the normal stages. As a result they are ineffective and they also proliferate and take over normal cells.
- Mechanical obstruction of enlarged lymph nodes
- Lymphocytic infiltration of abdomen or pharynx

- Non Hodgkins: Clinical Manifestations
  - Generalized lymphadenopathy: painless
  - Night sweats
  - Fever
  - Weight loss
  - Hepatomegaly / Splenomegaly
- Non Hodgkins: Management
  - Radiation Therapy (the use of high-energy ionizing radiation to treat a variety of cancers)
    - External beam radiation therapy is delivered froma source placed at some distance from the target site. The advantage is skin sparing effect b/c the maximum effect of radiation occurs at tumor depth and not on the skin surface.
    - Internal radiation therapy involves the placement of radioisotopes directly into or near the tumor, or into systemic circulation. Can be sealed source or unsealed (systemic)
    - Sealed source radiation therapy (also called "brachytherapy"). The radioactive substances are kept in place within the organ which is being treated.
    - Note: radiation destroys a cell's ability to reproduce, also induces apoptosis. Rapidly dividing cells are more vulnerable to radiation than slowly-dividing cells. Luckily, normal cells have greater ability to repair sublethal DNA damage from radiation.
  - Chemotherapy: CHOP: cyclophosphamide, hydroxydaunorubicin, vincristine & prednisone is considered first line therapy.
    - The goals of chemotherapy are to cure, control or palliate. Chemo is used when the disease is widespread, the risk of undetectable disease is high and the tumor cannot be resected and is resistant to XRT.

Nursing Management of Cancer Patients

- Nursing Care: Chemotherapy
  - Requires administration by specially trained RNs (the chemo drugs are highly toxic!)
  - Standards can be found in Oncology Nursing Society's Cancer Chemotherapy Guidelines.
  - Assessing complications is very important:
    - CBC, electrolytes
    - Watch for extravasation (watch IVs for patency)
    - Care is taken in vein selection (may not have good veins)
    - Neutropenia (highly susceptible to infection)
    - Care of venous access devices
  - Side Effects of Treatment
    - Altered oral mucous membranes
      - Inspect oral cavity daily
      - Instruct patient regarding proper oral care
      - Moistening gauze or toothettes instead of toothbrush (esp if plt count's <40,000)
      - Rinse with normal saline QID
      - Avoid commercial mouthwashes (don't want alcohol)
      - Cleanse mouth before and after meals
      - Provide a bland, soft diet to prevent trauma to the oral cavity and maintain oral hygiene.
    - Stomatitis: Instruct patient to report S/S:
      - Burning
      - Pain
      - Areas of redness
      - Open lesions on the lips
      - Pain with swallowing
      - Intolerance to temperature extremes

- Tx for stomatitis: Nursing treatment: normal saline rinses q 2 hours except while sleeping, use soft toothbrush or toothette, avoid use of dentures except during meals, moisten lips with a lubricant, avoid spicy foods or extreme temperature foods, also avoid foods that are difficult to chew, consider a topical anesthetic agent.
- Altered nutrition related to depressed appetite, nausea, and vomiting
  - Monitor accurate I and O
  - Nutritional assessment
  - Monitor nutritional labs: serum albumin, glucose, H/H, total protein & magnesium
  - Assess for s/s of malnutrition: Muscle wasting, edema, changes in hair and skin
  - Provide good oral care, give antiemetics and appetite stimulants
  - Encourage small, frequent meals that are high in calories and protein
  - Increase activity levels as tolerated
  - Provide environment suitable for eating...pain free, relaxed, clean, no unpleasant odors
- Potential for infection related to myelosuppresion (more stuff in notes r/t neutropenic precautions)
  - Infection control practices:
    - Monitor and record vital signs.
    - Assess for S/S of infection, notify MD immediately.
    - Obtain cultures prior to administering antibiotic therapy.
    - Administer antibiotics as prescribed.
    - Neutrapenic precautions if needed (usually instituted with WBC of < 0.5)
      - avoid contact with those who have known or recent infection or vaccination. Private room, avoid rectal or vaginal procedures (temperatures, examination, medications)
      - Administer stool softners to prevent straining
      - Meticulous oral hygiene
      - Avoid use of straight edge razor
      - Avoid raw mean or fish, fresh fruit and vegetables; No fresh flowers or plants.
      - Change solutions per protocol
      - Avoid IM injections
      - Strict aseptic technique when inserting medical devices
      - GOOD HANDWASHING
- Fatigue related to chemotherapy, anemia, hepatotoxicity, anorexia
  - Monitor ability to do ADLs.
  - Encourage frequent rest periods.
  - Assess nutritional intake.
  - Administer blood products per protocol.
  - Monitor I and O along with electrolytes.
  - Treat pain and discomfort.

- Body Image Disturbance related to alopecia, role changes, sexual function
  - Assess pt. feelings, coping abilities
  - Validate concerns
  - Advocate for participation in support groups and decision making
  - Facilitate a sense of control
  - Facilitate coping process
  - Prevent depersonalization ("Mr. Jones", not "leukemia pt in 38")
  - Instruct patient in self care – promote independence
- Potential for fluid volume deficit related to nausea, vomiting, diarrhea
  - Assess bowel pattern
  - Record frequency of vomiting & diarrhea
  - Establish and maintain IV access
  - Administer fluids per protocol & order
  - Record accurate I/O
  - Monitor serum electrolyte values
  - Monitor for skin breakdown (can be a huge issue for cancer pt)

- Administer anti-emetic and anti-diarrhea. agents per orders
- Potential for bleeding related to bone marrow suppression, hepatotoxicity
  - Monitor platelet counts.
  - Monitor LFT and coagulation studies
  - Assess for s/s of bleeding
  - Minimize venipunctures
  - Avoid rectal temperatures
  - Apply direct pressure to injection sites
  - Oral hygiene with soft toothbrush
  - Avoid commercial mouthwashes, straight edged razors, file nails, etc.
- Pain related to chemo, induced pancreatitis or neuropathy
  - Assess pain, using scale (1-10)
  - Assess discomfort characteristics to determine possible source of pain
  - Assess contributing factors: fear, anxiety, depression...
  - Patient to avoid irritants (housecleaning fumes and noise, provide rest periods, no perfume)
  - Humidify the air
  - Administer analgesics
  - Analgesics prior to procedures
  - Positioning, ice, heat, relaxing environment

Other Common Nursing Dx

Altered tissue perfusion
Decreased cardiac output
Potential for impaired gas exchange
Ineffective airway clearance
Impaired skin integrity
Ineffective coping
Knowledge deficit

Nursing. Care: Radiation Therapy

- Provide education.
- Minimize side effects (effects are felt/seen 10-14 days after treatment)
  - Skin reactions, alopecia
  - Mucositis, Xerostomia (dry mouth), Radiation caries (dental caries d/t radiation)
  - Esophagitis, Dysphagia
  - N/V, diarrhea, fatigue
  - Cystitis, urethritis
  - Bone marrow suppression. Areas of greatest risk are pelvic region, sacrum, skull, lumbar and thoracic spine, ribs, shoulder region and sternum
- Skin care within treatment field:
  - Keep the skin dry
  - Don't wash treatment area until permitted. Then wash gently, no hot water
  - Don't remove lines or ink marks on skin
  - Avoid lotions, powders, creams, alcohol and deodorants on treated skin
  - Avoid tape to treatment site
  - Electric razors only
  - Avoid direct sunlight (be aware of windows in their room)

NCLEX-RN Test Study Guide

TABLE OF CONTENTS

NCLEX Test Resources

Free NCLEX Practice Tests

http://www.testprepreview.com/nclex_practice.htm

Financial Aid Facts

http://www.finaidfacts.org

Scholarship Help

http://www.scholarshiphelp.org

Study Tips and Information

http://www.studyguidezone.com/resource_tips.htm

Introduction to this Guide

Your NCLEX score is one of the most critical elements to your qualification to become a nurse, so it is naturally much too important for you to take this test unprepared. The higher your NCLEX score, the better your chances of passing the boards.

Careful preparation, as described in this expert guide, along with hard work, will dramatically enhance your probability of success. In fact, it is wise to apply this philosophy not only to your board's exam, but to other elements of your life as well, to raise you above the competition. Your NCLEX score is one of the areas in the licensure process over which you have a substantial amount of control; this opportunity should not be taken lightly. Hence, a rational, prepared approach to your NCLEX test as well as the rest of the licensure process will contribute considerably to the likelihood of success.

Keep in mind, that although it is possible to take the NCLEX more than once, you should never take the test as an "experiment" just to see how well you do. It is of extreme importance that you always be prepared to do your best when taking the NCLEX. For one thing, it is extremely challenging to surmount a poor performance. If you are looking to take a "practice" run, look into review course, professionally developed mock NCLEX examinations, and, of course, this guide.

This guide provides you with the professional instruction you require for understanding the traditional NCLEX test. Covered are all aspects of the test and preparation procedures that you will require throughout the process. Upon completion of this guide, you'll have the confidence and knowledge you need for maximizing your performance on your NCLEX test.

Testing and Analysis

It won't take you long to discover that the NCLEX is unlike any test you've taken before, and it is probably unlike any test you will ever take again in your academic career. The typical high school or college test is a knowledge-based test. The NCLEX, however, is application-based.

What does this mean to you? It means that you'll have to prepare yourself in a completely different way! You won't simply be reciting memorized facts as they were phrased in some textbook, and you won't be applying any learned formulas to specific problems that will be laid out.

The NCLEX requires you to think in a thorough, quick and strategic manner...and still be accurate, logical and wise. This test is designed to judge your abilities in the ways that the licensure boards feel is vital to the success of first year nursing graduate.

To some extent, you have already gradually obtained these abilities over the length of your academic career. However, what you probably have not yet become familiar with is the capability to use these abilities for the purpose of maximizing performance within the complex and profound environment of a standardized, skills-based examination.

There are different strategies, mindsets and perspectives that you will be required to apply throughout the NCLEX. You'll need to be prepared to use your whole brain as far as thinking and assessment is concerned, and you'll need to do this in a timely manner. This is not something you can learn from taking a course or reading a book, but it is something you can develop through practice and concentration.

The following chapters in this guidebook will lay out the format and style of the NCLEX as well as give you sample questions and examples of the frame of mind you'll be expected to take. If there is one skill that you take with you from your preparation for the NCLEX, this should be it.

Introduction to the NCLEX

The purpose of the NCLEX is to establish a standard method of measurement for the skills that have been acquired by nursing school graduates. These skills are considered critical to the healthcare profession. The principle behind the NCLEX is similar to the SAT's that are required for application to American colleges. Although these tests are similar experiences in some respects, the NCLEX is a much more challenging and complex.

Fortunately, the NCLEX does not change very dramatically from year to year. What this means to you, is that it has become possible for quality practice tests to be produced, and if you should take enough of these tests, in addition to learning the correct strategies, you will be able to prepare for the test in an effective manner.

The NCLEX is not just a multiple-choice test. Fill in the blank questions and multiple right answer questions have been added to the test. Although these types of questions are not the majority of questions asked on the NCLEX. The main point is that the content has stayed the same. The nursing principles tested prior to these changes are still the same. The content has remained relatively the same. If you understand the content material of the exam, the type of testing question won't matter.

The NCLEX Scoring Scale

The minimum number of questions asked on the NCLEX-RN exam is 75. The maximum number of questions is 265. The exam is offered in CAT format which means the difficultly of the questions varies significantly. If you miss a question, the computer will give you an easier question. If you get it right, then you will get harder questions.

Many NCLEX test takers freak out if computer shuts off after 75 questions, or if they have to take the maximum number of questions. The main point is to be prepared to go the distance. Don't be sprinter and concentrate for 100 questions and then let your concentration begin to fade. Likewise, don't stress on how many questions you have to take. You won't know the outcome until you get your scores, so don't stress out.

Take some time for yourself and do something fun following the exam.

NCLEX Tips

1. Arrive early to the testing center.
2. Bring multiple forms of idea.
3. Wear layered clothing.
4. Get a good night's sleep before the test. (Don't cram)
5. Use a study partner when preparing for the exam.
6. Be familiar with the format of the exam.
7. Know your medical terminology.
8. Limit your distractions preparing for the exam.
9. Take time to unwind and reduce stress as you prepare.

10. Remember if you don't pass, you can retake the exam.

General Strategies

Strategy 1: Understanding the Intimidation

The test writers will generally choose some material on the exam that will be completely foreign to most test takers. You can't expect all of the medical topics to be a topic with which you have a fair amount of familiarity. If you do happen to come across a high number of topics/cases that you are extremely familiar with, consider yourself lucky, but don't plan on that happening.

Each case and scenario will be slightly different. Try and understand all of the material, while weeding out the distracter information. The cases will also frequently be drawn from real world experiences. Therefore, the passage that you will face on the test may almost seem out of context and as though it begins in the middle of a medical process. You won't have a nice title overhead explaining the general topic being covered but will immediately be thrown into the middle of a strange format that you don't recognize.

Getting hit by strange sounding medical topics that you don't recognize, of which you may only have a small exposure, is just normal on the NCLEX. Just remember that the questions themselves will contain all the information necessary to choose a correct answer.

Strategy 2: Finding your Optimal Pace

Everyone reads and tests at a different rate. It will take practice to determine what is the optimal rate at which you can read fast and yet absorb and comprehend the information. This is true for both the flyover that you should initially conduct and then the subsequent reading you will have to do as you go through and begin focusing on a specific question. However, on the flyover, you are looking for only a surface level knowledge and are not trying to comprehend the minutia of details that will be contained in the question. Basically, skim the question and then read the question slowly.

With practice, you will find the pace that you should maintain on the test while answering the questions. It should be a comfortable rate. This is not a speed-reading test. If you have a good pace, and don't spend too much time on any question, you should have a sufficient amount of time to read the questions at a comfortable rate. The two extremes you want to avoid are the dumbfounded mode, in which you are lip reading every word individually and mouthing each word as though in a stupor, and the overwhelmed mode, where you are panicked and are buzzing back and forth through the question in a frenzy and not comprehending anything.

You must find your own pace that is relaxed and focused, allowing you to have time for every question and give you optimal comprehension. Note that you are looking for optimal comprehension, not maximum comprehension. If you spent hours on each word and memorized the question, you would have maximum comprehension. That isn't the goal though, you want to optimize how much you comprehend with how much time you spend reading each question. Practice will allow you to determine that optimal rate.

Strategy 3: Don't be a Perfectionist

If you're a perfectionist, this may be one of the hardest strategies, and yet one of the most important. The test you are taking is timed, and you cannot afford to spend too much time on any one question.

If you are working on a question and you've got your answer split between two possible answer choices, and you're going back through the question and reading it over and over again in order to decide between the two answer choices, you can be in one of the most frustrating situations possible. You feel that if you just spent one more minute on the problem, that you would be able to figure the right answer out and decide between the two. Watch out! You can easily get so absorbed in that problem that you loose track of time, get off track and end up spending the rest of the test playing catch up because of all the wasted time, which may leave you rattled and cause you to miss even more questions that you would have otherwise.

Therefore, unless you will only be satisfied with a perfect score and your abilities are in the top .1% strata of test takers, you should not go into the test with the mindset that you've got to get every question right. It is far better to accept that you will have to guess on some questions and possibly get them wrong and still have time for every question, than to analyze every question until you're absolutely confident in your answer and then run out of time on the test.

Strategy 4: Factually Correct, but Actually Wrong

A favorite ploy of question writers is to write answer choices that are factually correct on their own, but fail to answer the question, and so are actually wrong.

When you are going through the answer choices and one jumps out for being factually correct, watch out. Before you mark it as your answer choice, first make sure that you go back to the question and confirm that the answer choice answers the question being asked.

Strategy 5: Extraneous Information

Some answer choices will seem to fit in and answer the question being asked. They might even be factually correct. Everything seems to check out, so what could possibly be wrong?

Does the answer choice actually match the question, or is it based on extraneous information contained in the question. Just because an answer choice seems right, don't assume that you overlooked information while reading the question. Your mind can easily play tricks on you and make you think that you read something or that you overlooked a phrase.

Unless you are behind on time, always go back to the question and make sure that the answer choice "checks out."

Strategy 6: Avoiding Definites

Answer choices that make definite statements with no "wiggle room" are often wrong. Try to choose answer choices that make less definite and more general statements that would likely be correct in a wider range of situations and aren't exclusive.

Example:

A. The nurse should follow universal contact precautions at all times in every case.

B. The nursing assistant completely demonstrated poor awareness of transfer safety.

C. Never allow new medications to be accessible on the unit.

D. Sometimes, the action taken by the aide was not well planned.

Without knowing anything about the question, answer choice D uses the term "sometimes," which has wiggle room, meaning there could have been a few strong points and weak points about the aide's performance. All of the other answer choices have a more definite sense about them, implying a more precise answer choice without wiggle room that is often wrong.

Strategy 7: Using Common Sense

The questions on the test are not intended to be trick questions. Therefore, most of the answer choices will have a sense of normalcy about them that may be fairly obvious and could be answered simply by using common sense.

While many of the topics will be ones that you are somewhat unfamiliar with, there will likely be numerous topics that you have some prior indirect knowledge about that will help you answer the questions.

Strategy 8: Instincts are Right

When in doubt, go with your first instinct. This is an old test-taking trick that still works today. Oftentimes if something feels right instinctively, it is right. Unfortunately, over analytical test takers will often convince themselves otherwise. Don't fall for that trap and try not to get too nitpicky about an answer choice. You shouldn't have to twist the facts and create hypothetical scenarios for an answer choice to be correct.

Strategy 9: No Fear

The depth and breadth of the NCLEX test can be a bit intimidating to a lot of people as it can deal with topics that have never been encountered before and are highly technical. Don't get bogged down by the information presented. Don't try to understand every facet of the nursing management process. You won't have to write an essay about the topics afterwards, so don't memorize all of the minute details. Don't get overwhelmed.

Strategy 10: Don't Get Thrown Off by New Information

Sometimes test writers will include completely new information in answer choices that are wrong. Test takers will get thrown off by the new information and if it seems like it might be related, they could choose that answer choice incorrectly. Make sure that you don't get distracted by answer choices containing new information that doesn't answer the question.

Example: Which conclusion is best supported?

A: Hyponatremia can cause the anxiety presented in this case.

Was anxiety even discussed in the question? If the answer is NO – then don't consider this answer choice, it is wrong.

Strategy 11: Narrowing the Search

Whenever two answer choices are direct opposites, the correct answer choice is usually one of the two. It is hard for test writers to resist making one of the wrong answer choices with the same wording, but changing one word to make it the direct opposite in meaning. This can usually cue a test taker in that one of the two choices is correct.

Example:

A. Calcium is the primary mineral linked to osteoporosis treatment.
B. Potassium is the primary mineral linked to osteoporosis treatment.

These answer choices are direct opposites, meaning one of them is likely correct. You can typically rule out the other two answer choices.

Strategy 12: You're not Expected to be Einstein

The questions will contain the information that you need to know in order to answer them. You aren't expected to be Einstein or to know all related knowledge to the topic being discussed. Remember, these questions may be about obscure topics that you've never heard of. If you would need to know a lot of outside knowledge about a topic in order to choose a certain answer choice – it's usually wrong.

Respiratory Conditions

Pulmonary Valve Stenosis

Causes:
Congenital
Endocarditis
Rheumatic Fever

Symptoms:
Fainting
SOB
Palpitations
Cyanosis
Poor weight gain

Tests:
Cardiac catheterization
ECG
Chest-Xray
Echocardiogram

Treatment:
Prostaglandins
Dieuretics
Anti-arrhythmics

Blood thinners

Valvuloplasty

ARDS- low oxygen levels caused by a build up of fluid in the lungs and inflammation of lung tissue.

Causes:

Trauma

Chemical inhalation

Pneumonia

Septic shock

Symptoms:

Low BP

Rapid breathing

SOB

Tests:

ABG

CBC

Cultures

Treatment:

Echocardiogram

Auscultation

Cyanosis

Chest X-ray

Mechanical Ventilation

Treat the underlying condition

Monitor the Patient for:

Pulmonary fibrosis

Multiple system organ failure

Ventilator associated pneumonia

Acidosis

Respiratory failure

Respiratory Acidosis- Build-up of Carbon Dioxide in the lungs that causes acid-base imbalances and the body becomes acidic.

Causes:

COPD

Airway obstruction

Hypoventilation syndrome

Severe scoliosis

Severe asthma

Symptoms:

Chronic cough

Wheezing

SOB

Confusion

Fatigue

Tests:

CAT Scan

ABG

Pulmonary Function Test.

Treatment:

Mechanical ventilation

Bronchodilators

Respiratory Alkalosis: CO2 levels are reduced and pH is high.

Causes:

Anxiety

Fever

Hyperventilation

Tests:

ABG

Chest X-ray

Pulmonary function tests

Symtpoms:

Dizziness

Numbness

Treatment:

Paper bag technique

Increase carbon dioxide levels

RSV (Respiratory synctial virus) - spread by contact, virus can survive for various time periods on different surfaces.

Symptoms:

Fever

SOB

Cyanosis

Wheezing

Nasal congestion

Croupy cough

Tests:

ABG

Chest X-ray

Treatment:

Ribvirin

Ventilator in severe cases

IV fluids

Bronchodilators

Monitor the patient for:

Pneumonia

Respiratory failure

Otitis Media

Hyperventilation

Causes:

COPD

Panic Attacks

Stress

Ketoacidosis

Aspirin overdose

Anxiety

Apnea: no spontaneous breathing.

Causes:

Obstructive sleep apnea

Seizures

Cardiac Arrhythmias

Brain injury

Nervous system dysfunction

Drug overdose

Prematurity

Bronchospasm

Encephalitis

Choking

Lung surgery

Causes:

Cancer

Lung abscesses

Atelectasis

Emphysema

Pneumothorax

Tumors

Bronchiectasis

Pneumonia: viruses the primary cause in young children, bacteria the primary cause in adults. Bacteria: Streptococcus pneumoniae, Mycoplasma pneumoniae

pneumoniae (pneumococcus).

Types of pneumonia:

Viral pneumonia

Walking pneumonia

Legionella pneumonia

CMV pneumonia

Aspiration pneumonia

Atypical pneumonia

Legionella pneumonia

Symptoms:

Fever

Headache

Ribvirin

SOB

Cough

Chest pain

Tests:

Chest X-ray

Pulmonary perfusion scan

CBC

Cultures of sputum

Presence of crackles

Treatment:

Antibiotics if caused by a bacterial infection

Respiratory treatments

Steroids

IV fluids

Vaccine treatments

Pulmonary actinomycosis –bacteria infection of the lungs caused by (propionibacteria or actinomyces)

Causes:

Microorganisms

Symptoms:

Pleural effusions

Facial lesions

Chest pain

Cough

Weight loss

Fever

Tests:

CBC

Lung biopsy

Thoracentesis

CT scan

Bronchoscopy

Monitor patient for:

Emphysema

Meningitis

Osteomyelitis

Alveolar proteinosis: A build-up of a phospholipid in the lungs were carbon dioxide and oxygen are transferred.

Causes:

May be associated with infection

Genetic disorder 30-50 yrs. Old

Symptoms:

Weight loss

Fatigue

Cough

Fever

SOB

Tests:

Chest X-ray

Presence of crackles

CT scan

Bronchoscopy

ABG- low O2 levels

Pulmonary Function tests

Treatment:

Lung transplantation

Special lavage of the lungs

Pulmonary hypertension: elevated BP in the lung arteries

Causes:

May be genetically linked

More predominant in women

Symptoms:

Fainting

Fatigue

Chest Pain

SOB with activity

LE edema

Weakness

Tests:

Pulmonary arteriogram

Chest X-ray

ECG

Pulmonary function tests

CT scan

Cardiac catheterization

Treatment:

Manage symptoms

Diuretics

Calcium channel blockers

Heart/Lung Transplant if necessary

Pulmonary arteriovenous fistulas: a congenital defect were lung arteries and veins form improperly, and a fistula is formed creating poor oxygenation of blood.

Symptoms:

SOB with activity

Presence of a murmur

Cyanosis

Clubbing

Paradoxical embolism

Tests:

CT Scan

Pulmonary arteriogram

Low O2 Saturation levels

Elevated RBC's

Treatment:

Surgery

Embolization

Pulmonary aspergilloma: fungal infection of the lung cavities causing abscesses.

Cause:

Fungus *Aspergillus*

Symptoms:

Wheezing

SOB

Chest pain

Fever

Cough

Tests:

CT scan

Sputum culture

Serum precipitans

Chest X-ray

Bronchoscopy

Treatment:

Surgery

Antifungal medications

Pulmonary edema: most commonly caused by Heart Failure, but may be due to lung disorders.

Symptoms:

Restless behavior

Anxiety

Wheezing

Poor speech

SOB

Sweating

Pale skin

Drowning sensation

Tests:

Murmurs may be present

Echocardiogram

Presence of crackles

Low O2 Saturation levels

Treatment:

Diuretics

Oxygen

Treat the underlying cause

Idiopathic pulmonary fibrosis: Thickening of lung tissue in the lower aspects of the lungs.

Causes:

Response to an inflammatory agent

Found in people ages 50-70.

Linked to smoking

Symptoms:

Cough

SOB

Chest pain

Cyanosis

Clubbing

Cyanosis

Tests:

Pulmonary function tests

Lung biopsy

Rule out other connective tissue diseases

CT scan

Chest X-ray

Treatment:

Lung transplantation

Corticosteroids

Anti-inflammatory drugs

Monitor the patient for:

Polycythemia

Pulmonary Htn.

Respiratory failure

Cor pulmonarle

Pulmonary emboli: Blood clot of the pulmonary vessels or blockage due to fat droplets, tumors or parasites.

Causes:

DVT- most common

Symptoms:

SOB (rapid onset)

Chest pain

Decreased BP

Skin color changes

LE and pelvic pain

Sweating

Dizziness

Anxiety

Tachycardia

Labored breathing

Cough

Tests:

Doppler US

Chest X-ray

Pulmonary angiogram

Monitor the patient for:

Shock

Pulmonary hypertension

Hemorrhage

Palpitations

Heart failure

Pulmonary perfusion test

Plethysmography

ABG

Check O2 saturation

Treatment:

Placement of an IVC filter

Administer Oxygen

Surgery

Thrombolytic Therapy if clot detected

Tuberculosis- infection caused by *Mycobaterium tuberculosis.*

Causes:

Due to airborne exposure

Symptoms:

Fever

Chest pain

SOB

Weight Loss

Fatigue

Wheezing

Phlegm production

Tests:

Thoracentesis

Sputum cultures

Presence of crackles

TB skin test

Chest X-ray

Bronchoscopy

Treatment:

Generally about 6 months

Rifampin

Pyrazinamide

Isoniazid

Cytomegalovirus – can cause lung infections and is a herpes-type virus.

Causes:

More common in immunocompromised patients

Often associated with organ transplantation

Symptoms:

Fever

SOB

Fatigue

Loss of appetite

Cough

Joint pain

Tests:

CMV serology tests

ABG

Blood cultures

Bronchoscopy

Treatment:

Antiviral medications

Oxygen therapy

Monitor the patient for:

Kidney dysfunction

Infection

Decreased WBC levels

Relapses

Viral pneumonia – inflammation of the lungs caused by viral infection.

Causes:

Rhinovirus

Herpes simplex virus

Influenza

Adenovirus

Hantavirus

CMV

RSV

Symptoms:

Fatigue

Sore Throats

Nausea

Joint pain

Headaches

Muscular pain

Cough

SOB

Tests:

Bronchoscopy

Open Lung biopsy

Sputum cultures

Viral blood tests

Treatment:

Antiviral medications

IV fluids

Monitor the patient for:

Liver failure

Heart failure

Respiratory failure

Pneumothorax: a build-up of a gas in the pleural cavities.

Types:

Traumatic pneumothorax

Tension pneumothorax

Spontaneous pneumothorax

Secondary spontaneous pneumothorax

Symptoms:

SOB

Tachycardia

Hypotension

Anxiety

Cyanosis

Chest pain-sharp

Fatigue

Tests:

ABG

Chest X-ray

Poor breath sounds

Treatment:

Chest tube insertion

Administration of oxygen

Circulatory System

Functions

The circulatory system serves:

(1) to conduct nutrients and oxygen to the tissues;

(2) to remove waste materials by transporting nitrogenous compounds to the kidneys and carbon dioxide to the lungs;

(3) to transport chemical messengers (hormones) to target organs and modulate and integrate the internal milieu of the body;

(4) to transport agents which serve the body in allergic, immune, and infectious responses;

(5) to initiate clotting and thereby prevent blood loss;

(6) to maintain body temperature;

(7) to produce, carry and contain blood;

(8) to transfer body reserves, specifically mineral salts, to areas of need.

General Components and Structure

The circulatory system consists of the heart, blood vessels, blood and lymphatics. It is a network of tubular structures through which blood travels to and from all the parts of the body. In vertebrates this is a completely closed circuit system, as William Harvey (1628) once demonstrated. The heart is a modified, specialized, powerful pumping blood vessel. Arteries, eventually becoming arterioles, conduct blood to capillaries (essentially endothelial tubes), and venules, eventually becoming veins, return blood from the capillary bed to the heart.

Course of Circulation

Systemic Route:

a. *Arterial system*. Blood is delivered by the pulmonary veins (two from each lung) to the left atrium, passes through the bicuspid (mitral) valve into the left ventricle and then is pumped into the ascending aorta; backflow here is prevented by the aortic semilunar valves. The aortic arch toward the right side gives rise to the brachiocephalic (innominate) artery which divides into the right subclavian and right common carotid arteries. Next, arising from the arch is the common carotid artery, then the left subclavian artery.

The subclavians supply the upper limbs. As the subclavian arteries leave the axilla (armpit) and enter the arm (brachium), they are called brachial arteries. Below the elbow these main trunk lines divide into ulnar and radial arteries, which supply the forearm and eventually form a set of arterial arches in the hand which give rise to common and proper digital arteries. The descending (dorsal) aorta continues along the posterior aspect of the thorax giving rise to the segmental intercostals arteries. After passage "through" (behind) the diaphragm it is called the abdominal aorta.

At the pelvic rim the abdominal aorta divides into the right and left common iliac arteries. These divide into the internal iliacs, which supply the pelvic organs, and the external iliacs, which supply the lower limb.

b. *Venous system*. Veins are frequently multiple and variations are common. They return blood originating in the capillaries of peripheral and distal body parts to the heart.

Hepatic Portal System: Blood draining the alimentary tract (intestines), pancreas, spleen and gall bladder does not return directly to the systemic circulation, but is relayed by the hepatic portal system of veins to and through the liver. In the liver, absorbed foodstuffs and wastes are processed. After processing, the liver returns the blood via hepatic veins to the inferior vena cava and from there to the heart.

Pulmonary Circuit: Blood is oxygenated and depleted of metabolic products such as carbon dioxide in the lungs.

Lymphatic Drainage: A network of lymphatic capillaries permeates the body tissues. Lymph is a fluid similar in composition to blood plasma, and tissue fluids not reabsorbed into blood capillaries are transported via the lymphatic system eventually to join the venous system at the junction of the left internal jugular and subclavian veins.

The Heart

The heart is a highly specialized blood vessel which pumps 72 times per minute and propels about 4,000 gallons (about 15,000 liters) of blood daily to the tissues. It is composed of:

Endocardium (lining coat; epithelium)

Myocardium (middle coat; cardiac muscle)
Epicardium (external coat or visceral layer of pericardium; epithelium and mostly connective tissue)
Impulse conducting system

Cardiac Nerves: Modification of the intrinsic rhythmicity of the heart muscle is produced by cardiac nerves of the sympathetic and parasympathetic nervous system. Stimulation of the sympathetic system increases the rate and force of the heartbeat and dilates the coronary arteries. Stimulation of the parasympathetic (vagus nerve) reduces the rate and force of the heartbeat and constricts the coronary circulation. Visceral afferent (sensory) fibers from the heart end almost wholly in the first four segments of the thoracic spinal cord.

Cardiac Cycle: Alternating contraction and relaxation is repeated about 75 times per minute; the duration of one cycle is about 0.8 second. Three phases succeed one another during the cycle:

a) atrial systole: 0.1 second,
b) ventricular systole: 0.3 second,
c) diastole: 0.4 second

The actual period of rest for each chamber is 0.7 second for the atria and 0.5 second for the ventricles, so in spite of its activity, the heart is at rest longer than at work.

Blood

Blood is composed of cells (corpuscles) and a liquid intercellular ground substance called plasma. The average blood volume is 5 or 6 liters (7% of body weight). Plasma constitutes about 55% of blood volume, cellular elements about 45%.

Plasma: Over 90% of plasma is water; the balance is made up of plasma proteins and dissolved electrolytes, hormones, antibodies, nutrients, and waste products. Plasma is isotonic (0.85% sodium chloride). Plasma plays a vital role in respiration, circulation, coagulation, temperature regulation, buffer activities and overall fluid balance.

Cardiovascular Conditions

Cardiogenic Shock: heart is unable to meet the demands of the body. This can be caused by conduction system failure or heart muscle dysfunction.

Symptoms of Shock:

Rapid breathing
Rapid pulse
Anxiety
Nervousness
Thready pulse
Mottled skin color
Profuse sweating
Poor capilary refill

Tests:

Nuclear Scans
Electrocardiogram
Echocardiogram
Electrocardiogram
ABG
Chem-7
Chem-20
Electrolytes
Cardiac Enzymes

Treatment:

Amrinone
Norepinephrine
Dobutamine
IV fluids
PTCA
Extreme cases-pacemaker, IABP

Aortic insufficiency: Heart valve disease that prevents the aortic valve from closing completely. Backflow of blood into the left ventricle.

Causes:

Rheumatic fever
Congenital abnormalities
Endocarditis
Marfan's syndrome
Ankylosing spondylitis

Reiter's syndrome

Symptoms:
Fainting
Weakness
Bounding pulse
Chest pain on occasion
SOB
Fatigue

Tests:
Palpation
Increased pulse pressure and diastolic pressure
Pulmonary edema present

Auscultation
Left heart cathereterization
Aortica angiography
Dopper US
Echocardiogram

Treatment:
Digoxin
Dieuretics
Surgical aorta valve repair

Monitor patient for:
PE
Left-sided heart failure
Endocarditis

Aortic aneurysm: Expansion of the blood vessel wall often identified in the thoracic region.

Causes:
Htn
Marfan's syndrome
Syphilis
Atherosclerosis (most common)
Trauma

Symptoms:
Possible back pain may be the only indicator

Tests:
Aortogram
Chest CT
X-ray

Treatment:

Varies depending on location

Stent

Circulatory arrest

Surgery

Monitor patient for:

Bleeding

Stroke

Graft infection

Irregular Heartbeats

Heart Attack

Hypovolemic shock: Poor blood volume prevents the heart from pumping enough blood to the body.

Causes:

Trauma

Diarrhea

Burns

GI Bleeding

Cardiogenic shock: Enough blood is available, however the heart is unable to move the blood in an effective manner.

Symptoms:

Anxiety

Weakness

Sweating

Rapid pulse

Confusion

Clammy skin

Tests:

CBC

Echocardiogram

CT scan

Endoscopy with GI bleeding

Swan-Ganz catheterization

Treatment:

Increase fluids via IV

Avoid Hypothermia

Epinephrine

Norepinephrine

Dobutamine

Myocarditis: inflammation of the heart muscle.

Causes:

Bacterial or Viral Infections

Polio, adenovirus, coxsackie virus

Symptoms:

Leg edema

SOB

Viral symptoms

Joint Pain

Syncope

Heart attack (Pain)

Fever

Unable to lie flat

Irregular heart beats

Tests:

Chest X-ray

Echocardiogram

ECG

WBC and RBC count

Blood cultures

Treatment:

Diuretics

Pacemaker

Antibiotics

Steroids

Monitor the patient for:

Pericarditis

Cardiomyopathy

Heart valve infection: endocarditis (inflammation), probable valvular heart disease. Can be caused by fungi or bacteria.

Symptoms:

Weakness

Fever

Murmur

SOB

Night sweats

Janeway lesions

Joint pain

Tests:

CBC

ESR

ECG
Blood cultures
Enlarged speen
Presence of splinter
hemorrhages

Treatment:
IV antibiotics

Surgery may be indicated

Monitor the patient for:
Jaundice
Arrhythmias
CHF
Glomerulonephritis
Emboli

Pericarditis: Inflammation of the pericardium.

Causes:
Viral- coxsackie, adenovirus, influenza, rubella viruses
Bacterial (various microorganisms)
Fungi
Often associated with TB, Kidney failure, AIDS, and autoimmune disorders.
Surgery

Symptoms:
Dry cough
Pleuritis
Fever
Anxiety
Crackles
Pleural effusion
LE swelling
Chest pain
Unable to lie down flat

Tests:
Auscultation
MRI scan
CT scan
Echocardiogram (key test)
ESR
Chest x-ray

Blood cultures

CBC

Treatment:

NSAIDS

Pericardiocentesis

Analgesics

Pericardiectomy

Monitor the patient for:

Constrictive pericarditis

A fib.

Supraventricular tachycardia (SVT)

Arrhythmias: Irregular heart beats and rhythms disorder

Types:

Bradycardia

Tachycardia

Ventricular fibrillation

Ectopic heart beat

Ventricular tachycardia

Wolff-Parkinson-white syndrome

Atrial fib.

Sick sinus syndrome

Sinus Tachycardia

Sinus Bradycardia

Symptoms:

SOB

Fainting

Palpitations

Dizziness

Chest pain

Irregular pulse

Tests:

Coronary angiography

ECG

Echocardiogram

Holter monitor

Treatment:

Defibrillation

Pacemaker

Medications

Monitor the patient for:

Heart failure

Stroke

Heart attack

Ischemia

Arteriosclerosis: hardening of the arteries.

Causes:
Smoking
Htn
Kidney disease
CAD
Stroke

Symptoms:
Claudication pain
Cold feet
Muscle acheness and pain in the legs
Hair loss on the legs
Numbness in the extremities
Weak distal pulse

Tests:
Doppler US
Angiography
IVSU
MRI test
Poor ABI (Ankle brachial index) reading

Treatment:
Analgesics
Vasodilation medications
Surgery if severe
Ballon surgery
Stent placement

Monitor the patient for:
Arterial emboli
Ulcers
Impotence
Gas gangreene
Infection of the lower extremities

Cardiomyopathy- poor hear pumping and weakness of the myocardium.

Causes:
Htn
Heart attacks
Viral infections

Types:

Alcoholic cardiomyopathy- due to alcohol consumption

Dilated cardiomyopathy-left ventricle enlargement

Hypertrophic cardiomyopathy-abnormal growth left ventricle

Ischemic cardiomyopathy- weakness of the myocardium due to heart attacks.

Peripartum cardiomyopathy- found in late pregnancy

Restrictive cardiomyopathy-limited filling of the heart due to inability to relax heart tissue.

Symptoms:

Chest pain

SOB

Fatigue

Ascites

LE swelling

Fainting

Poor Appetite

Htn

Palpitations

Tests:

ECG

CBC

Isoenzyme tests

Coronary Angigraphy

Chest X-ray

MRI

Auscultation

Treatment:

Ace inhibitors

Dieuretics

Blood thinners

LVAD – Left Ventricular Assist Device

Digoxin

Vasodilators

Congestive Heart Failure:

Class I describes a patient who is not limited with normal physical activity by symptoms.
Class II occurs when ordinary physical activity results in fatigue, dyspnea, or other symptoms.
Class III is characterized by a marked limitation in normal physical activity.
Class IV is defined by symptoms at rest or with any physical activity.

Causes:

CAD
Valvular heart disease
Cardiomyopathies
Endocarditis
Extracardiac infection
Pulmonary embolus

Symptoms:

Skin cold or cyanotic
Wheezing
Mitral valvular deficits
Lower extremity edema
Pulsus alternans
Hypertension
Tachypnea

Heart Sounds:

S1- tricuspid and mitral valve close

S2- pulmonary and aortic valve close

S3- ventricular filling complete

S4-elevated atrial pressure (atrial kick)

Wave Review

ST segment: ventricles depolarized

P wave: atrial depolarization

PR segment: AV node conduction

QRS complex: ventricular depolarization

U wave: hypokalemia creates a U wave

T wave: ventricular repolarization

Wave Review Indepth:

1. P WAVE - small upward wave; indicates atrial depolarization
2. QRS COMPLEX - initial downward deflection followed by large upright wave followed by small downward wave; represents ventricular depolarization; masks atrial repolarization; enlarged R portion - enlarged ventricles; enlarged Q portion - probable heart attack.
3. T WAVE - dome shaped wave; indicates ventricular repolarization; flat when insufficient oxygen; elevated with increased K levels
4. P - R INTERVAL - interval from beginning of P wave to R wave; represents conduction time from initial atrial excitation to initial ventricular excitation; good diagnostic tool; normally < 0.2sec.

5. S-T SEGMENT - time from end of S to beginning to T wave; represents time between end of spreading impulse through ventricles and ventricular repolarization; elevated with heart attack; depressed when insufficient oxygen.
6. Q-T INTERVAL - time for singular depolarization and repolarization of the ventricles. Conduction problems, myocardial damage or congenital heart defects can prolong this.

Arrhythmias Review

Supraventricular Tachyarrhythmias

Atrial fibrillation – Abnormal QRS rhythm and poor P wave appearance. (>300bpm.)

Sinus Tachycardia- Elevated ventricular rhythum/rate.

Paroxysmal atrial tachycardia- Abnormal P wave, Normal QRS complex

Atrial flutter- Irregular P Wave development. (250-350 bpm.)

Paroxysmal supraventricular tachycardia- Elevated bpm (160-250)

Multifocal atrial tachycardia- bpm (>105). Various P wave appearances.

Ventricular Tachyarrhythmias

Ventricular Tachycardia- Presence of 3 or greater PVC's (150-200bpm), possible abrupt onset. Possibly due to an ischemic ventricle. No P waves present.

(PVC)- Premature Ventricular Contraction- In many cases no P wave followed by a large QRS complex that is premature, followed by a compensatory pause.

Ventricular fibrillation- Completely abnormal ventricular rate and rhythum requiring emergency innervention. No effective cardiac output.

Bradyarrhythmias

AV block (primary, secondary (I,II) Tertiary
Primary- >.02 PR interval
Secondary (Mobitz I) – PR interval Increase
Secondary (Mobitz II) – PR interval (no change)
Tertiary- most severe, No signal between ventricles and atria noted on ECG. Probable use of Atrophine indicated. Pacemaker required.

Right Bundle Branch Block (RBBB)/Left Bundle Branch Block (LBBB)

Sinus Bradycardia- <60 bpm, with presence of a standard P wave.

Cardiac Failure Review

Right Sided Heart Failure

A. Right Upper Quadrant Pain
B. Right Ventricular heave
C. Tricuspid Murmur
D. Weight gain
E. Nausea
F. Elevated Right Atrial pressure
G. Elevated Central Venous pressure
H. Peripheral edema
I. Ascites
J. Anorexia
K. Hepatomegaly

Left Sided Heart Failure

A. Left Ventricular Heave
B. Confusion
C. Paroxysmal noturnal dyspnea
D. DOE
E. Fatigue
F. S_3 gallop
G. Crackles
H. Tachycardia
I. Cough
J. Mitral Murmur
K. Diaphoresis
L. Orthopnea

ECG Changes with MI

T Wave inversion

ST Segment Elevation

Abnormal Q waves

ECG Changes with Digitalis

Inverts T wave

QT segment shorter

Depresses ST segment

ECG Changes with Quinidine

Inverts T wave

QT segment longer

QRS segment longer

ECG Changes with Potassium

Hyperkalemia- Lowers P wave, Increases width of QRS complex

Hypokalemia- Lowers T wave, causes a U wave

ECG Changes with Calcium

Hypercalcemia-Makes a longer QRS segment

Hypocalcemia- Increases time of QT interval

Endocrine Review

Hypothyroidism: Poor production of thyroid hormone:

Primary- Thyroid cannot meet the demands of the pituitary gland.

Secondary- No stimulation of the thyroid by the pituitary gland.

Causes:

Surgical thyroid removal

Irradiation

Congenital defects

Hashimoto's thyroiditis (key)

Symptoms:

Constipation

Weight gain

Weakness

Fatigue

Poor taste

Hoarse vocal sounds

Joint pain

Muscle weakness

Poor speech

Color changes

Depression

Tests:

Decreased BP and HR

Chest X-ray

Elevated liver enzymes, prolactin, and cholesterol

Decreased T4 levels and serum sodium levels

Presence of anemia

Low temperature

Poor reflexes

Treatment:

Increase thyroid hormone levels

Levothyroxine

Monitor the patient for:

Hyperthyroidism symptoms following treatment

Heart disease

Miscarriage

Myxedema coma if untreated

Hyperthyroidism: excessive production of thyroid hormone.

Causes:
Iodine overdose
Thyroid hormone overdose
Graves' disease (key)
Tumors affecting the reproductive system

Symptoms:
Skin color changes
Weight loss
Anxiety
Possible goiter
Nausea
Exophthalmos
Diarrhea
Hair loss
Elevated BP
Fatigue
Sweating

Tests:
Elevated Systolic pressure noted
T3/T4 (free) levels increased
TSH levels reduced

Treatment:
Radioactive iodine
Surgery
Beta-blockers
Antithyroid drugs

Congenital adrenal hyperplasia: Excessive production of androgen and low levels of aldosterone and cortisol. (Geneticially inherited disorder). Different forms of this disorder that affect males and females differently.

Causes: Adrenal gland enzyme deficit causes cortisol and aldosterone to not be produced. Causing male sex characteristics to be expressed prematurely in boys and found in girls.

Symptoms:

Boys:

Small testes development

Enlarged penis development

Strong musculature appearance

Girls:

Abnormal hair growth

Low toned voice

Abnormal genitalia

Lack of menstruation

Tests:

Salt levels

Low levels of cotisol

Low levels of aldosterone

Increased 17-OH progesterone

Increased 17-ketosteroids in urine

Treatment:

Reconstructive surgery

Hydrocoristone

Dexamethasone

Primary/Secondary Hyperaldosteronism

Primary Hyperaldosteronism: problem within the adrenal gland causing excessive production of aldosterone.

Secondary Hyperaldosteronism: problem found elsewhere causing excessive production of aldosterone.

Causes:

Primary:

Tumor affecting the adrenal gland

Possibly due to HBP

Secondary:

Nephrotic syndrome

Heart failure

Cirrhosis

Htn

Symptoms:

Paralysis

Fatigue

Numbness sensations

Htn

Weakness

Tests:

Increased urinary aldosterone

Abnormal ECG readings
Decreased potassium levels
Decreased renin levels

Treatment:
Primary: Surgery
Secondary: Diet/Drugs

Cushing's syndrome: Abnormal production of ACTH which in turn causes elevated cortisol levels.

Causes:
Corticosteroids prolonged use
Tumors

Symptoms:
Muscle weakness
Central obesity distribution
Back pain
Thirst
Skin color changes
Bone and joint pain
Htn
Headaches
Frequent urination
Moon face
Weight gain
Acne

Tests:
Dexamethasone suppression test
Cortisol level check
MRI- check for tumors

Treatment:
Surgery to remove tumor
Monitor corticosteroid levels

Monitor the patient for:
Kidney stones
Htn
Bone fractures
DM
Infections

Diabetic ketoacidosis: increased levels of ketones due to a lack of glucose.

Causes: Insufficient insulin causing ketone production which end up in the urine. More common in type I vs. type 2 DM.

Symptoms:

Low BP

Abdominal pain

Headaches

Rapid breathing

Loss of appetite

Nausea

Fruit breath smell

Mental deficits

Tests:

Elevated glucose levels

Increased amylase and potassium levels

Ketones in urine

Check BP

Treatment:

Insulin

IV fluids

Monitor the patient for:

Renal failure

MI

Coma

T3/T4 Review

Both are stimulated by TSH release from the Pituitary gland

T4 control basal metabolic rate

T4 becomes T3 within cells. (T3) Active form.

T3 radioimmunoassay- Check T3 levels

Hyperthyroidism- T3 increased, T4 normal- (in many cases)

Medications that increase levels of T4:

Methadone

Oral contraceptives

Estrogen

Cloffibrate

Medications that decrease levels of T4:
Lithium
Propranolol
Interferon alpha
Anabolic steroids
Methiamazole

Lymphocytic thyroiditis: Hyperthyroidism leading to hypothyroidism and then normal levels.
Causes: Lymphocytes permeate the thyroid gland causing hyperthyroidism initially.

Symptoms:
Fatigue
Menstrual changes
Weight loss
Poor temperature tolerance
Muscle weakness
Hyperthyroidism symptoms

Tests:
T3/T4 increased
Increased HR
Lymphocyte concentration noted with biopsy

Treatment:
Varies depending on symptoms. (Beta blockers may be used.)

Monitor the patient for:
Autoimmune thyroditis
Hashimoto's thyroiditis
Goiter
Stuma lymphomatosoma

Graves' disease: most commonly linked to hyperthyroidism, and is an autoimmune disease. Exophthalmos may be noted (protruding eyeballs). Excessive production of thyroid hormones.

Symptoms:

Elevated appetite

Anxiety

Menstrual changes

Fatigue

Poor temperature tolerance

Diplopia

Exophthalmos

Tests:

Elevated HR

Increased T3/T4 levels

Serum TSH levels are decreased

Goiter

Treatment:

Beta-blockers

Surgery

Prednisone

Radioactive iodine

Monitor the patient for:

Fatigue

CHF

Depression

Hypothyroidism (over-correction)

Type I diabetes (Juvenile onset diabetes)

Causes: Poor insulin production from the beta cells of the pancreas. Excessive levels of glucose in the blood stream that cannot be used due to the lack of insulin. Moreover, the patient continues to experience hunger, due to the cells not getting the fuel that they need. After 7-10 years the beta cells are completely destroyed in many cases.

Symptoms:

Weight loss

Vomiting

Nausea

Abdominal pain

Frequent urination

Elevated thirst

Tests:

Fasting glucose test

Insulin test

Urine analysis

Treatment:

Insulin

Relieve the diabetic ketoacidosis symptoms

Foot ulcer prevention

Monitor for infection:

Monitor for hypoglycemia conditions if type I is over-corrected.

Glucagon may need to be administered if hypoglycemia conditions are severe.

Monitor the patient for ketone build-up if type I untreated.

Get the eyes checked- once a year

Type II diabetes

The body does not respond appropriately to the insulin that is present. Insulin resistance is present in Type II diabetes. Results in hyperglycemia.

Risk factors for Type II Diabetes:

Obesity

Limited exercise individuals

Race-Minorities have a higher distribution

Elevated Cholesterol levels

Htn

Symptoms:

Blurred vision

Fatigue

Elevated appetite

Frequent urination

Thirst

Note: A person may have Type II and be symptom free.

Tests:

Random blood glucose test.

Oral glucose tolerance test

Fasting glucose test.

Treatment:

Tlazamide

Glimepiride

Control diet

Increase exercise levels

Repaglidine/Nateglinide

Glycosylated hemoglobin

BUN/ECG

Frequent blood sugar testing

Acarbose

Diabetic Ulcer prevention

Monitor the patient for:

Neuropathy

CAD

Increased cholesterol

Retinopathy

PVD

Htn

Diabetes Risk Factors:

Bad diet

Htn

Weight distribution around the waist/overweight.

Certain minority groups

History of diabetes in your family

Poor exercise program

Elevated triglyceride levels

Microbiology Review

Characteristics of Bacteria Types

Rickettsias- gram-negative bacteria, small
Rickettsia rickettsii

Spirochetes- spiral shape, no flagella, slender
Lyme disease, Treponema pallidum-syphilis

Gram positive cocci- Hold color with Gram stain, ovoid or spherical shape
Staphlyococcus aureus, Streptococcus pneumoniae

Gram negative cocci- Loose color with Gram stain, spherical or oval shape
Neisseria meningidis (meningococcus*), Neisseria gonorrhoeae* (gonococcus)

Mycoplasmas- *Mycoplasma pneumoniae*

Acid-fast bacilli- Hold color with staining even when stained with acid in most cases. *Mycobacterium leprae, Mycobacterium tuberculosis*

Acitinomycetes- Stained positive with a gram stain, narrow filaments
Nocardia, Actinomyces israelii

Gram positive- Rod shaped, hold color with gram stain

Clostridium tetani, Bacillus anthracis

Gram negative- Do not hold color with gram stain, also rod shaped. *Pseudomonas aeruginosa, Escherichia coli, Klebsiella pneumoniae*

Diseases and Acid Fast Bacilli Review

Disease	Bacteria	Primary Medication
Tuberculosis, renal and meningeal infections	*Mycobacterium tuberculosis*	Isoniazid + rifampin + pyrazinamide
Leprosy	*Mycobacterium leprae*	Dapsone + rifampin

Diseases and Spirochetes Review

Disease	Bacteria	Primary Medication
Lyme Disease	*Borrelia burgdorferi*	Tetracycline
Meningitis	*Leptospira*	Penicillin G
Syphilis	*Treponema pallidum*	Penicillin G

Diseases and Actinomycetes Review

Disease	Bacteria	Primary Medication
Cervicofacial, and other lesions	*Actinomyces israelii*	Penicillin G

Diseases and Gram-Negative Bacilli Review

Disease	Bacteria	Primary Medication
Meningitis	*Flavobacterium meningosepticum*	Vancomycin
UTI's Bacteremia	*Escherichia coli*	Ampicillin+/- aminoglycoside
Gingivitis, Genital infections, ulcerative pharyngitis	*Fusobacterium nucleatum*	Penicillin G
Abscesses	*Bacteroides species*	Clindamycin/Penicillin G
Hospital acquired infections	*Acinetobacter*	Aminoglycoside
Abscesses, Endocarditis	*Bacteroides fragilis*	Clindamycin, metronidazole
Legionnaires' Disease	*Legionella pneumonphila*	Erythromycin
UTI's	*Proteus mirabilis*	Ampicillin/Amoxicillin
Pneumonia, UTI's, Bacteremia	*Pseudomonas aeruginosa*	Penicillin-Broad
Bacteremia, Endocarditis	*Streptobacillus moniliformis*	Penicillin G
Pneumonia, UTI	*Klebsiella pneumoniae*	Cephalosporin
Bacteremia, Wound infections	*Pasteurella multocida*	Penicillin G

Diseases and Gram-Positive Bacilli Review

Disease	Bacteria	Primary Medication
Gas Gangrene	*Clostridium*	Peniçillin G
Tetanus	*Clostridium tetani*	Penicillin G
Pharyngitis	*Corynebacterium diphtheriae*	Penicillin G
Meningitis, Bacteremia	*Listeria monocytogenes*	Ampicillin
Anthrax / pneumonia	*Bacillus anthracis*	Penicillin G
Endocarditis	*Corynebacterium species*	Penicillin G/Vancomycin

Diseases and Cocci Review

Disease	Bacteria	Primary Medication
Genital infections, arthritis-dermatitis syndrome	*Neisseria gonorrhoeae*	Ampicillin, Amoxicillin
Meningitis, Bacteremia	*Neisseria meningitidis*	Penicillin G
Endocarditis, Bacteremia	*Streptococcus (viridans group)*	Gentamicin
Bacteremia, brain and other absesses	*Streptococcus (anaerobic species)*	Penicillin G
Endocarditis, Bacteremia	*Streptococcus agalactiae*	Ampicillin
Pneumonia, Osteomyelitis,	*Staphyloccus aureus*	Penicillin G/Vancomycin

abscesses		
UTI's, Endocarditis	*Streptococcus faecalis*	Ampicillin, Penicillin G
Pneumonia, sinusitis, otitis, Arthritis	*Streptococcus pneumoniae*	Penicillin G or V
Cellulitis, Scarlet fever, bacteremia	*Streptococcus pyogenes*	Penicillin G or V
Bacteremia, endocarditis	*Streptococcus bovis*	Penicillin G

DNA Virus Review

DNA Virus	*Infection*
Adenovirus	Eye and Respiratory infections
Hepatitis B	Hepatitis B
Cytomegalovirus	Cytomegalic inclusion disease
Epstein-Barr	Infectious mononucleosis
Herpes Types 1 and 2	Local infections oral and genital
Varicella-zoster	Chickenpox, herpes zoster
Smallpox	Smallpox

RNA Virus Review

RNA Virus	*Infection*
Human respiratory virus	Respiratory tract infection
Hepatitis A virus	Hepatitis A
Influenza virus A-C	Influenza
Measles virus	Measles
Mumps virus	Mumps

Respiratory syncytial virus	Respiratory tract infection in children
Poliovirus	Poliomyelitis
Rhinovirus types 1-89	Cold
Human immunodeficiency virus	AIDS
Rabies virus	Rabies
Alphavirus	Encephalitis
Rubella virus	Rubella

Immunoglobulin isotypes

IgA– can be located in secretions and prevents viral and bacterial attachment to membranes.

IgD- can be located on B cells

IgE-main mediator of mast cells with allergen exposure.

IgG- primarily found in secondary responses. Does cross placenta and destroys viruses/bacteria.

IgM- primarily found in first response. Located on B cells

Cytokines Review

IL-1 Primarily stimulate of fever response. Helps activate B and T cells. Produced by macrophages.

IL-2 Aids in the development of Cytotoxic T cells and helper cells. Produced by helper T cells.

IL-3 Aids in the development of bone marrow stem cells. Produced by T-cells.

IL-4 Aids in the growth of B cells. Produced by helper T-cells. Aids in the production of IgG and IgE

IL-5 Promotes the growth of eosinophils. Produced by helper T-cells. Also promotes IgA production.

IL-8 Neutrophil factor

TNF-α Promotes the activation of neutrophils and is produced by macrophages.

TNF-β Produced by T lymphocytes and encourages the activation of neutrophils

γ-interferon (Activates macrophages and is produced by helper T cells.)

Controlled Substance Categories

Schedule I	Highest potential abuse, used mostly for research. (heroin, peyote, marijuana)
Schedule II	High potential abuse, but used for therapeutic purposes (opioids, amphetamines and barbiturates)
Schedule III	Mild to moderate physical dependence or strong psychological dependence on both. (opioids such as codeine, hydrocodone that are combined with other non-opoid drugs)
Schedule IV	Limited potential for abuse and physical and/or psychological dependence (benzodiazepines, and some low potency opioids)
Schedule V	Lowest abuse potential of controlled substances. Used in cough medications and anti-diarrheal preps.

Dose Response- the relationship between dose and the body's response is called a dose-response curve (DRC).

Potency- relates to the dosage required to produce a certain response. A more potent drug requires a lower dosage than does a less potent drug to produce a given effect.

Efficacy- usually refers to maximum efficacy. Maximum efficacy is plateau (or maximum response), but may not be achievable clinically due to undesirable side effects. In general, the steepness of the curve dictates the range of doses that are useful therapeutically.

LD_{50}/ED_{50} -- Quantal dose response curve is the relationship between the dose of the drug and the occurrence of a certain response.

Therapeutic index (TI)- the ratio of the median effective dose (ED_{50}) and the toxic dose (TD_{50}) is a predictor of the safety of a drug. This ratio is called the therapeutic index. Note: Acetominophin has TI of 27. Meperidine (DEMEROL) has a TI of 8.

Pharmacology

Drug Suffix	Example	Action
-azepam	Diazepam	Benzodiazepine
-azine	Chlorpromazine	Phenothiazine
-azole	Ketoconazole	Anti-fungal
-barbital	Secobarbital	Barbiturate
-cillin	Methicillin	Penicillin
-cycline	Tetracycline	Antibiotic
-ipramine	Amitriptyline	Tricyclic Anti-depressant
-navir	Saquinavir	Protease Inhibitor
-olol	Timolol	Beta Antagonist
-oxin	Digoxin	Cardiac glycoside
-phylline	Theophylline	Methylxanthine
-pril	Enalapril	ACE Inhibitor
-terol	Albuterol	Beta 2 Agonist
-tidine	Ranitidine	H_2 Antagonist
-trophin	Somatotrophin	Pituitary Hormone
-zosin	Doxazosin	Alpha 1 Antagonist

Cardiovascular Pharmacology

Antiarrhythmics- Na+ channel blockers (Class I)

Class IA	Class IB	Class IC
Procainamide	Mexiletine	Flecainide
Disopyramide	Lidocaine	Encainide
Amiodarone	Tocainide	Propafenone
Quinidine		

Antiarrhythmics (Beta blockers) (Class II)

Metroprolol

Atenolol

Propranolol

Timolol

Esmolol

Antiarrhythmics (K+Channel blockers) (ClassIII)

Sotaolol

Amiodarone

Bretylium

Ibutilide

Antiarrhythmics (Ca2+ channel blockers) (Class IV)

Diltiazem

Verapamil

Vasodilators: Verapamil

Minoxidil

Hydralazine

Calcium Channel Blockers:

Verapamil

Diltiazem

Nifedipine

Sympathoplegics:

Beta blockers

Clonidine

Reserpine

Guanethidine

Prazosin

ACE Inhibitors:

Lisinopril

Enalapril

Captopril

Cardiac glycosides:

Digoxin

Dieuretics:

Loop Dieuretics

Hydrocholorothiazide

K+ Sparing Dieuretics

Spironolactone

Triamterene

Amiloride

CNS Pharmacology

Sympathomimetics:

Dopamine

Dobutamine

Epinephrine

Norephinephrine

Isoproterenol

Cholinomimetics:

Carbachol

Neostigmine

Pyridostigmine

Echothiophate

Bethanechol

Cholinoreceptor blockers:

Hexamethonium-Nicotinic blocker

Atropine-Muscarinic blocker

Beta blockers:

Atenolol

Nadolol

Propranolol

Metoprolol

Pindolol

Labetalol

Tricyclic Antidepressants:

Doxepine

Imipramine

Amitriptyline

Nortriptyline

Amitriptyline

Parkinson's Treatment:

L-dopa

Amantadine

Bromocriptine

Benzodiazepindes:

Iorazepam

Triazolam

Oxazepam

Diazepam

Opiod Analgesics:

Heroin

Methadone

Morphine

Codeine

Dextromethorphan

Meperidine

MAO Inhibitors:

Tranylcypromine
Phenelzine

Seroton specific Re-uptake inhibitors:
Paroxetine
Sertraline
Fluoxetine
Citalopram

Epilepsy Treatment:
Valproic acid
Phenobarbital
Benzodiazepines
Gabapentin
Ethosuximide
Carbamazepine

Barbiturates:
Pentobarbital
Thiopental
Phenobarbital
Secobarbital

IV Anethestics:
Midazolam
Ketamine
Morphine
Fentanyl
Propofol
Thiopental

Local Anesthetics:
Tetracaine
Procaine
Lidocaine

Neuroleptics (Antipsychotic drugs)
Chlorpromazine
Thioridazine
Clozapine
Fluphenazine
Haloperidol

Alpha 1 Selective blockers:
Terazosin
Prazosin
Doxazosin
Alpha 2 Selective blockers:
Yohimbine

Glaucoma Treatment:
Prostaglandins
Dieuretics
Alpha agonists
Beta Blockers

Cholinomimetics

Cancer Treatment Drugs:

Etoposide
Nitrosoureas
Cisplatin
Doxorubicin
Incristine
Paclitaxel

Methotrexate
6 – mercaptopurine
Busulfan
5 – fluorouracil
Lomustine
Carmustine

Throbolytics:
Urokinase
Anistreplase
Streptokinase
Alteplase

Cox 2 Inhibitors:
Rofecoxib
Celecoxib

NSAID's:
Naproxen
Indomethacin
Ibuprofen

Diabetic Treatment:
Sulfonylureas:
Chlorpropamide

Tolbutamide
Glyburide

Insulin- Key

Metformin

Asthma Treatment:

Corticosteroids:
Prednisone
Beclomethasone

Antileukotrienes:
Zafirlukast
Zileuton

Beta 2 agonists:
Salmeterol
Albuterol

Glitazones:
Rosiglitazone
Troglitazone
Pioglitazone

Nonselective Beta agonists:
Isoproterenolol

Muscarinic agonists:
Ipratropium

H_2 blockers:
Famotidine
Nizatidine
Cimetidine
Ranitidine

Anti-Microbial Drugs

Tetracyclines:

Tetracycline

Doxycycline

Minocycline

Demeclocycline

Macrolides:

Carithormycin

Erythromycin

Azithromycin

Aminoglycosides:

Amikacin

Gentamicin

Neomycin

Tobramycin

Streptomycin

Protein Synthesis Inhibitors:

Chloramphenicol

Aminoglycosides

Tetracyclines

TB Medications:

Isoniazid

Rifampin

Ethambutol

Pyrazinamide

Ethambutol

Fluoroquinolones:

Ciprofloxacin

Sparfloxacin

Enaxacin

Nalidixic acid

Norfloxacin

Mortifloxacin

Sulfonamides:

Sulfadiazine

Sulfisoxazole

Sulfamethoxazole

Malaria Treatment:

Chlorquine

Quinine

Mefloquine

Additional Mentionable Anti-viral Drugs:

Acyclovir

Amatadine

Ribavirin

Zanamivir

Ganciclovir

HIV Treatment:

Zidovudine (AZT)

Nevirapine

Didanosine

Protease Inhibitors-(HIV)

Saquinavir

Retinonavir

Nelfinavir

Measurement Equivalents

Weights Conversion Table

.1 mg	1/600 grain
.2 mg	1/300 grain
.5 mg	1/120 grain
1 mg	1/60 grain
10 mg	1/6 grain
30 mg	½ grain
60 mg	1 grain
300 mg	5 grains
1 gm	15 grains
4 gm	60 grains
15 gm	4 drams
30 gm	1 ounce

Volume Conversion Table

Household	*Metric*	*Apothecary*
1 quart	1000 ml	1 quart
1 pint	500 ml	1 pint
2 tablespoons	30 ml	1 ounce
1 tablespoons	15 ml	4 fluid drams
1 teaspoon	5 ml	1 fluid dram
15 drops	1ml	15 minims

Common Conversions

1 meter	1000 (mm)
1 meter	100 (cm)
.001 milligram	1 (mcg)
1 gram	1000(mg)
1000 grams	1 (kg)
1 tablespoon (T)	15 (ml)
1 teaspoon (tsp)	5 (ml)
20 drops	1 (ml)
2.2 (lb)	1 (kg)
1 (lb)	453.6 (gm)
1 (oz)	30 (gm)
1 (ml)	1 (cc)
1 (dl)	100 (ml)

Solid Conversions

Apothecary	*Avoirdupois*
2.7 (lb)	2.2 (lb)
1.33 (lb)	1 (lb)
480 (gr)	1 (ounce)
15 (gr)	15.4 (gr)
1 (gr)	1 (gr)

Liquid Conversions

Household	*Metric*	*Apothecary*
1 drop	.06 (ml)	1 minim
¼ teaspoon	1 (ml)	15 or 16 minims

1 teaspoon	4 or 5 (ml)	1 fluid dram
1 tablespoon	15 (ml)	4 fluid dram
2 tablespoons	30 (ml)	1 fluid ounce
1 cup	250 (ml)	8 fluid ounces
1 pint	500 (ml)	16 fluid ounces
1 quart	1000 (ml)	32 fluid ounces

Metric - (Apothecaries')

1/100 grain	.6 (mg)
1/60 grain	1 (mg)
1/30 grain	2 (mg)
1/20 grain	3 (mg)
1/15 grain	4 (mg)
1/10 grain	6 (mg)
1/6 grain	10 (mg)
1/5 grain	12 (mg)
1/3 grain	20 (mg)
3/8 grain	25 (mg)
½ grain	30 (mg)
1 grain	60 (mg)
1 ½ grains	100 (mg)
5 grains	300 (mg)
10 grains	600 (mg)

Drug Distribution

Bioavailability dependant on several things:

1. Route of administration
2. The drug's ability to cross membranes
3. The drug's binding to plasma proteins and intracellular components

Membrane Review:

1. Membranes separate the body in components
2. The ability of membranes to act as barriers is related to its structure
3. Lipid Soluable compounds (many drugs) pass through by becoming dissolved in the lipid bylayer.
4. Glucose, H20, electrolytes can't pass on their own. They use pores.
5. In excitable tissues, the pores open and close.
6. Movement occurs by:
    a. passive diffusion
    b. active transport
    c. facilitated diffusion
    d. endocytosis

Passive Diffusion Review:

1. No energy expended.
2. Weak acids and bases need to be in non-ionized form (no net charge).

3. Drugs can also move between cell junctions. BBB is exception.
4. Must be lipid soluable to pass through pores.
5. Osmosis is a special case of diffusion
    a. A drug dissolved in H2O will move with the water by "bulk flow"
    b. Usually limited to movement through gap junctions because size too large for pores.

Active Transport Review:

1. Requires energy and requires a transport protein
2. Drugs must be similar to some endogenous substance.
3. Can carry substances against a gradient
4. Some drugs may exert their effect by increasing or decreasing transport proteins.

Facilitated Diffusion Review:

1. Requires transport protein
2. Does not require energy
3. Very few drugs move this way

Endocytosis:

1. Drug gets engulfed by cell via invagination
2. Very few drugs move this way and only in certain cells.

Regulation of distribution determined by:

1. Lipid permeability
2. Blood flow

3. Binding to plasma proteins
4. Binding to subcellular components

Volume of Distribution (V_d) - is a calculation of where the drug is distributed.

$$V_d = \frac{\text{amount of drug given (mg)}}{\text{concentration in plasma (mg/ml)}}$$

Calculate the V_d and compare to the total amount of body H20 in a person.

-if V_d = total amount of body (approx. 42) is uniformly distributed

-if V_d is less than 42 – retained in plasma and probably bound to plasma proteins

-if V_d is more than 42 – concentrated in tissues

This is not a "real value" but tells you where the drug is being distributed.

Placental Transfer of Drugs

1. Some drugs cause congenital anomalies
2. Cross placenta by simple diffusion
3. Must be polar or lipid-insoluable Not to Enter
4. Must assume the fetus is subjected to all drugs taken by the mother to some extent.

Biotransformation of Drugs

Biotransformation refers to chemically altering the original drug structure. "Metabolite" refers to the altered version.

Biotransformation metabolites are generally more polar than the original drug. The kidney will excrete polar compounds, but reabsorb non-polar compounds.

Enzymatic reactions are either Phase I or Phase II reactions:

Phase I include:

1. hydrolysis rxns – split the original compound into separate parts
2. reduction rxns – either remove O2 or add H
3. oxidation rxns- adds an O2 molecule and removes a H molecule. These are the most predominant reactions for biotransforming drugs

Phase I reactions are generally more polar and usually inactive-some exceptions.

Phase II reactions are called conjugation rxns.

1. Lead to the formation of a covalent bond between the drug and another compound such as glucaronic acid, amino acids or acetate.
2. Products are highly polar and generally inactive- morphine is exception.
3. Products are rapidly excreted in urine and feces because poorly reabsorbed by kidney and intestine.
4. There is also a phenomenon known as entrohepatic recirculation – can result in re-entry of the parent drug back

into the circulation and leads to delayed elimination and prolonged effect of the drug.

Most metabolism takes place in the liver- 1st pass significant. Kidney, skin, GI, and lugs have significant metabolic capacity. Phase I reactions take place mostly in endoplasmic reticulum (ER). Phase II reactions take place mostly in cytosol.

Cytochrome P450 mono-oxygenase enzymes are the major catalyst in Phase I. The Cyt 450 system is a series of enzymes that are heme containing proteins. The catalyze oxidation/reduction reactions- which make compounds more + or -. These metabolites are subjected to conjugation reactions and then excreted.

Biotransformation Factors:

1. Induction- certain drugs induce synthesis of addition Cyt 450 enzymes
2. Inhibition- certain drugs inhibit Cyt 450 enzymes
3. Genetic Polymorphism-slow vs. fast metabolizers
4. Disease- impaired liver function, decreased hepatic blood flow
5. Age/Gender-rate of phase I/II reactions slow in infants, females may have reduced ability to metabolize certain compounds?

Drug Elimination

1. Renal elimination

a. Drugs get filtered and if not reabsorbed, gets excreted in urine
b. Renal excretion involves: glomerular filtration, active tubular secretion, and passive tubular reabsorption.

2. Elimination by other routes.
   a. Lungs mostly volatile compounds
   b. Bile/fecal excretion
   c. Saliva, sweat, tears, breast milk
   d. Hair, skin

General Pharmacokinetics Review

Clinical Pharmacokinetics attempts to quantify the relationship between dose and effect. Primary parameters that dictate dosage include:

1. Clearance
2. Volume of Distribution
3. Bioavailability

Clearance-measure of the body's ability to eliminate a drug. Clearance is an expression of the volume of plasma which is cleared of the drug per unit time (ml/hr) not the concentration of the drug cleared.

Clearance = flow (ml/min) x <u>amount of drug removed from the blood (mg/ml)</u>

Amount of drug going in to kidney (mg/ml)

Or

Cl = flow x <u>[C]in – [C]out (amount removed)</u>

[C] in (amount in blood)

The systems of drug elimination are not usually saturated so drug elimination is dependent on the concentration of drug in the plasma. This means the higher the concentration of the drug, the faster the blood is cleared. When this is true this is called 1st order kinetics. In

1st order kinetics a constant faction of the drug is eliminated/unit time. The time required to remove half of the drug is called t ½. T1/2 is constant in 1st order kinetics.

In 1st order kinetics the:

Rate of elimination = concentration of drug in plasma (mg/ml) x Cl (ml/hr). When the systems for drug elimination become saturated, now have zero order elimination. Zero order elimination means that the elimination rate is constant over time, regardless of the concentration of drug in the system.

The aim is to maintain a steady-state concentration of a drug within a known therapeutic range. Steady state is achieved when the rate of elimination = rate of availability.

$$\text{Availability} = \frac{\text{amount of drug in plasma}}{\text{amount of drug given}}$$

Rate of Elimination = Cl x concentration in plasma

Time to reach steady state depends on dosing interval and elimination t ½ . If you want to achieve steady state more rapidly, a loading dose can be given followed by a maintenance dose.

Loading dose (mg) = target concentration (mg/ml) x V_d (ml)

Maintenance dose = amount given must equal amount eliminated within dosing time.

If given at intervals shorter than elimination time = toxicity.

If given at intervals longer than elimination time = ineffective dose.

Pharmacodynamic Terms

1. Agonist – has affinity and efficacy
2. Partial agonist – has affinity and partial efficacy
3. Antagonist – has affinity, no efficacy
4. Additive effects- !+1 = 2
5. Synergistic effects- 1+1 = 3
6. Affinity – attraction between drug and (X)
7. Specificity- attraction between drug and specific (X)
8. Potentiation- one drug enhances the effect of another drug
   Ex. Aspirin bumps T3/T4 off plasma proteins- more free T3/T4

Autonomic Nervous System Receptors

1. Cholinergic Receptors – Ach binds both – prefers Muscarinic

   a. Nicotinic-preferentially binds nicotine. Found at ganglion on post synaptic fiber. Found in both SNS and PNS. Drugs that bind to nicotinic receptors affect both systems.

b. Muscarinic- preferentially binds muscarine. Found on target tissue in PNS and located on sweat gland in SNS.

2. Adrenergic Receptors:

Alpha- found NE excited target tissue and also inhibited further release of NE from nerve. (constricted VSM)
Beta- found that NE and EPI equally potent in heart but EPI 50x more potent

Specific Pediatric Conditions

Wilm's tumor: kidney tumor found in children. Cause: unknown/possible genetic link. Tumor will spread to other regions. Sometimes children will be born with aniridia. Do not exert pressure over the abdomen.

Symptoms:
Fever
Vomiting
Fatigue
Irregular urine coloration
Abdominal pain
Constipation
Abdominal mass
Increased BP

Tests:
BUN
Creatinine
Analysis of the urine
X-ray
CT Scan
Family history of cancer
CBC

Treatment:
Surgery
Chemotherapy

Radiation

Neuroblastoma: tumor in children that starts from nervous tissue. Capable of spreading rapidly. Cause unknown.

Symptoms:
Abdominal mass
Skin color changes
Fatigue
Tachycardia
Motor paralysis
Anxiety
Diarrhea
Random eye movements
Bone and joint pain
Labored breathing

Tests:
Bone scan
CBC
MIBG scan
Catecholamines tests
X-ray
CT scan
MRI

Treatment:
Radiation
Chemotherapy
Surgery

Monitor the patient for:
Kidney failure
Metastasis
Various Organ system failures
Liver failure

Cerebral palsy: Cerebrum injury causing multiple nerve function deficits.

Types:
Spastic CP 50%
Dyskinetic CP 20%
Mixed CP

Ataxic CP

Symptoms:

Poor respiration status

Mental retardation

Spasticity

Speech and language deficits

Delayed motor and sensory development

Seizures

Joint contractions

Tests:

Sensory and Motor Skill testing

Check for spasticity

CT scan/MRI

EEG

Treatment:

PT/OT/ST

Surgery

Seizure medications

Spasticity reducing medication

Croup: trouble breathing in infants and children that can be caused by bacteria, viruses, allergies or foreign objects. Primarily, caused by viruses.

Symptoms:

Labored breathing

Symptoms increased at night.

Noisy cough

Stridor

Tests:

X-rays

Breaths sounds check

Treatment:

Acetaminophen

Steroid medications

Intubation

Nebulizers

Monitor the patient for:

Respiratory arrest

Atelectasis

Dehydration

Epiglottitis

Kawasaki disease: a disease that affects young children primarily. Unknown origin probable autoimmune disease. Attacks the heart, blood vessels, and lymph nodes.

Symptoms:

Fever

Joint pain

Swollen lymph nodes

Peripheral edema

Rashes

Papillae on the tongue

Chapped/Red lips

Tests:

CBC

Presence of pyuria

Chest X-ray

ECGH

ESR

Urine Analysis

Treatment:

Gamma globulin

Salicylate treatment

Monitor the patient for:

Coronary aneurysm

MI

Vasculitis

Pyloric stenosis: a narrowing of the opening between the intestine and stomach. Most common in infants. May have genetic factors

Symptoms:

Diarrhea

Abdominal pain

Belching

Vomiting

Weight loss

Tests:

Abdomen distended

Barium X-ray

US

Electrolyte imbalance

Treatment:

Surgery

IV fluids

Vaccinations

Attenuated – Varicella, MMR

Inactivated – Influenza

Toxoid – Tetanus/Diptheria

Biosynthetic – Hib conjugate vaccine

Tetralogy of Fallot- 4 heart defects that are congenital. Poorly oxygenated blood is pumped to the body's tissues.

4 factors:

Right ventricular hypertrophy

Ventricular septal defect

Aorta from both ventricles

Stenosis of the pulmonic outflow tract

Symptoms:

Poor weight gain

Cyanosis

Death

Limited infant feeding

Clubbing

SOB

Tests:

Chest X-ray

EKG

Echocardiogram

Heart Catheterization

CBC

Heart Murmur

Treatment:

Surgery

Small meals

Limit child's anxiety

Monitor the patient for:

Seizures

Poor overall development

Cyanois

Atrial septal defect- congenital opening between the atria.

Symptoms:

Dyspnea

Reoccurring infections (respiratory)

SOB

Palpitations

Tests:

Catheterization

Echocardiography

ECG

MRI

Irregular heart rhythm/sounds

Treatment:

Surgery

Antibiotics

Monitor the patient for:

Heart failure

A fib.

Pulmonary Htn.

Endocarditis

Ventricular septal defect- opening between the ventricles of the heart.

Symptoms:

Poor weight gain

Labored breathing

Profuse sweating

SOB

Poor color

Irregular heart beat

Respiratory infections reoccurring

Tests:

Ausculatation

Echocardiogram

ECG

Chest X-ray

Treatment:

Digoxin

Surgery

Digitalis

Monitor the patient for:

Endocarditis

Pulmonary Htn.

Aortic insufficiency

Limited growth and development

Arrhythmias

CHF

Patent ductus arteriosus: open blood vessel (ductus ateriosus) that does not close after birth.

Symptoms:

SOB

Limited feeding

Tests:

ECG

Echocardiogram

Heart murmur

Chest X-ray

Treatment:

Surgery

Indomethacin

Decrease fluid volumes

Monitor the patient for:

Surgical complications

Endocarditis

Heart failure

Aortic coarctation: aorta becomes narrow at some point due to a birth defect

Symptoms:

Headache

Hypertension with activity

Nose bleeding

Fainting

SOB

Tests:

Check BP

Doppler US

Chest CT

MRI

ECG

Chest X-ray

Cardiac catheterization

Treatment:

Surgery

Monitor the patient for:

Stroke

Heart failure

Aortic aneurysm

Htn

CAD

Endocarditis

Aortic dissection

Tumor Review

Primary Tumors

Neuromas-80-90% of brain tumors, named for what part of nerve cell affected.

Meningiomas - outside of arachnoidal tissue, usually benign and slow growing

Glioblastoma Multiform-50% of all primary tumors, linked to specific genetic mutations

Secondary Tumors

Metastatic carcinomas

Scale –degree of anaplasia: differentiation of mature (good) vs. immature cells (bad)

Grade I: up to 25% anaplasia

Grade II: 26-50% anaplasia

Grade III: 51-75% anaplasia

Grade IV: 76-100% anaplasia

Primary Tumor Effect:

1. Headaches
2. Vomiting
1. Seizures
2. Neurological problems
3. Dementia
4. Drowsiness

Secondary Tumor Effect:

1. Direct compression/necrosis

2. Herniation of brain tissue
3. Increase ICP

Noteworthy Tumor Markers

1. AFP
2. Alkaline phosphatase
3. β-hCG
4. CA-125
5. PSA

Define the following terms:

Basal cell carcinoma:

Chondrosarcoma:

Ewing's sarcoma:

Giant cell tumor:

Melaonoma:

Meningioma:

Oligodendroglioma:

Pituitary ademona:

Schwannoma:

Squamous cell carcinoma:

Leukemia Review

Know the following four types of leukemias.

ALL- acute lymphocytic leukemia

AML- acute myelocytic leukemia

CLL- chronic lymphocytic leukemia

CML- chronic myeloid leukemia

GI Review

Zollinger-Ellison syndrome: Tumors of the pancreas that cause upper GI inflammation. The tumors secrete gastrin causing high levels of stomach acid.

Symptoms:
Diarrhea
Vomiting
Abdominal pain

Tests:
Abdominal CT
+ Calcium Infusion Test
+ Secretin Stimulation Test

Elevated gastrin levels
Tumors in the pancreas

Treatment:
Ranitidine
Cimetidine
Lansoprazole
Omeprazole
Surgery

Wilson's disease: High levels of copper in various tissues throughout the body. (Genetically linked- Autosomal recessive).

Key organs affected are:
Eyes
Brain
Liver
Kidneys

Symptoms:
Gait disturbances
Jaundice
Tremors

Abdominal pain/distention
Dementia
Speech problems
Muscle weakness
Spenomegaly
Confusion
Dementia

Tests:
Various lab tests:

Bilirubin/PT/ SGOT increased

Albumin/Uric acid production decreased

MRI

Genetic testing

Low levels of serum copper

Copper is found in the tissues

Kayser-Fleisher Rings in the eye

Treatment:

Pyridoxine

Low copper diet

Corticosteroids

Penicillamine

Monitor the patient for:

Cirrhosis

Muscle weakness

Joint pain/stiffness

Anemia

Fever

Hepatitis

Pancreatitis: Inflammation of the pancreas

Symptoms:

Fever

Vomiting

Nausea

Chills

Anxiety

Jaundice

Sweating

Tests:

X-ray

CT scan

Various Lab tests

Pancreatic Cancer: cancer of the pancreas. Higher rates in men.

Symptoms:

Nausea

Jaundice

Depression

Back pain

Indigestion

Abdominal pain

Weight loss

Tests:

CT scan

Biopsy

Abdominal US

Liver function test

Treatment:

Surgery

Chemotherapy

Radiation

Whipple procedure

Hepatitis A: Viral infection that causes liver swelling.

Symptoms:

Fatigue

Nausea

Fever

Itching

Vomiting

Tests:

Increased liver enzymes

Presence of IgG and IgM antibodies

Enlarged liver

Treatment:

Rest

Proper diet low in fatty foods

Hepatitis B: Sexually transmitted disease, also transmitted with body fluids and some individual may be symptom free but still be carriers.

Symptoms:

Jaundice

Dark Urine

Malaise

Joint pain

Fever

Fatigue

Tests:

Decreased albumin levels

+ antibodies and antigen

Increased levels of transaminase

Treatment:

Monitor for changes in the liver.

Recombinant alpha interferon in some cases.

Transplant necessary if liver failure occurs.

Hepatitis C

Symptoms:

Fatigue

Vomiting

Urine color changes (dark)

Jaundice

Abdominal pain

Tests:

ELISA assay

Increased levels of liver enzymes

No Hep. A or B antibodies

Treatment:

Interferon alpha

Ribavirin

Gastritis: can be caused by various sources (bacteria, viruses, bile reflux or autoimmune diseases). Inflammation of the stomach lining.

Symptoms:

Loss of appetite

Hiccups

Nausea

Vomiting blood

Abdominal pain

Tests:

EGC

X-Ray

CT scan

Ulcers

Peptic Ulcers-ulcer in the duodenum or stomach

Gastric Ulcers- ulcer in the stomach

Duodenum Ulcer-ulcer in the duodenum

Bacteria: Helicobacter pylori- often associated with ulcer formation.

Symptoms:

Weight loss

Chest pain

Heartburn

Vomiting

Indigestion

Fatigue

Tests:

EGD

Stool guaiac

GI X-rays

Treatment:

Bismuth

Famotidine

Sucralfate

Cimetidine

Omeprazole

Antibiotics

Diverticulitis – abnormal pouch formation that becomes inflamed in the intestinal wall.

Symptoms:

Fever

Diarrhea

Nausea

Vomiting

Constipation

Tests:

Barium enema

WBC count

Colonoscopy

CT Scan

Sigmoidoscopy

Intestinal obstruction: Can a paralytic ileus/false obstruction (children) or a mechanical obstruction:

Types of mechanical obstruction:

Tumors

Volvulus

Impacted condition

Hernia

Symptoms:

Constipation

Vomiting

Diarrhea

Breath

Abdominal swelling

Abdominal pain

Tests:

Barium enema

CT scan

Upper/Lower GI series

Poor bowel sounds

Carcinoid Syndrome: symptoms caused by cardinoid tumors. Linked to increased secretion of Serotonin.

Symptoms:

Flush appearance

Wheezing

Diarrhea

Onset of niacin deficiency

Abdominal pain

Decreased BP

Tests:

5-HIAA test

Increased levels of Chromogranin A and Serotonin

CT scan

MRI

Treatment:

Surgery

Sandostatin

Chemotherapy

Multivitamins

Octreotide

Interferon

Monitor the patient for:

Low BP

Right Sided Heart Failure

Hiatal Hernia: Stomach sticks into the chest through the diaphragm. Can cause reflux symptoms.

Symptoms:

Chest pain

Heartburn

Poor swallow

Tests:

EGD

Barium Swallow X-ray.

Treatment:

Weight loss

Surgical repair

Medications for reflux

(GERD) -Gastroesophageal reflux disease

Symptoms:

Nausea

Vomiting

Frequent coughing

Hoarseness

Belching

Chest pain

Anatacid relief

Sore Throat

Tests:

Barium swallow

Bernstein test

Stool guaiac

Endoscopy

Treatment:

Weight loss

Antacids

Proton pump inhibitors

Limit fat and caffeine

Histamine H2 blockers

Monitor the patient for:

Chronic pulmonary disease

Barrett's esophagus

Esophagus inflammation

Bronchospasms

Ulcerative colitis: chronic inflammation of the rectum and large intestine.

Symptoms:

Weight loss

Jaundice

Diarrhea

Abdominal pain

Fever

Joint pain

GI bleeding

Tests:

Barium edema

ESR

CRP

Colonoscopy

Treatment:

Corticosteroids

Mesalamine

Surgery

Ostomy

Azathioprine

Monitor the patient for:

Ankylosing spondylitis

Liver disease

Carcinoma

Pyoderma gangrenosum

Hemorrhage

Perforated colon

Eye, Ear, and Mouth Review

Disorders of the Eye

Diabetic retinopathy:

Blood vessels in the retina are affected. Can lead to blindness if untreated. Two primary stages (Proliferative and Nonproliferative. Retina may experience bleeding in nonproliferative stage. During the proliferative stage damage begins moving towards the center of the eye and there is an increase in bleeding. Any damage caused is non-reversible. Only further damage can be prevented.

Strabismus:

Eyes are moving in different stages. The axes of the eyes are not parallel. Normally, treated with an eyepatch; however, eye drops are now used in many cases. Atropine drops are placed in the stronger eye for correction purposes. Surgery may be necessary in some cases. Suture surgery will reduce the pull of certain eye muscles.

Macular Degeneration:

Impaired central vision caused by destruction of the macula, which is the center part of the retina. Limited vision straight ahead. More common in people over 60. Can be characterized as dry or wet types. Wet type more common. Vitamin C, Zinc, and Vitamin E may help slow progression.

Esotropia:

Appearance of cross-eyed gaze or internal strabismus.

Exotropia:

External strabismus or divergent gaze.

Conjunctivitis:

Inflammation of the conjuctiva, that can be caused by viruses or bacteria. Also known as pink eye. If viral source can be highly contagious. Antibiotic eye drops and warm cloths to the eye helpful treatment. Conjunctivitis can also be caused by chemicals or allergic reactions. Re-occurring conjunctivitis can indicate a larger underlying disease process.

Glaucoma:

An increase in fluid pressure in the eye leading to possible optic nerve damage. More common in African-Americans. Minimal onset symptoms, often picked to late. Certain drugs may decrease the amount of fluid entering the eye. Two major types of glaucoma are open-angle glaucoma and \angle-closure glaucoma.

Disorders of the Mouth

Acute pharyngitis:

Often the cause of sore throats, inflammation of the pharynx.

Acute tonsillitis:

Viral or Bacterial infection that causes inflammation of the tonsils.

Aphthous ulcer:

Also known as a canker sore. A sensitive ulcer in the lining of the mouth. 1 in 5 people have these ulcers. Cause is unknown in many cases.

Acute Epiglottitis

Inflammation of the epiglotitis that may lead to blockage of the respiratory system and death if not treated. Often caused by numerous bacteria. Intubation may be required and speed is critical in treatment. IV antibiotics will help reverse this condition in most cases. Common symptoms are high fever and sore throat.

Oral candidiasis:

This is a yeast infection of the throat and mouth by Candida albicans.

Oral leukoplakia:

A patch or spot in the mouth that can become cancerous.

Parotitis:

A feature of mumps and inflammation of the parotid glands.

Disorders of the Ear

Otitis media:

Most common caused by the bacteria (H.flu) and Streptococcus pneumoniae in about 85% of cases. 15% of cases viral related. More common in bottlefeeding babies. Can be caused by upper respiratory infections. Ear drums can rupture in severe cases. A myringotomy may be performed in severe cases to relieve pus in the middle ear.

Barotitis:

Atmospheric pressures causing middle ear dysfunction. Any change in altitude causes problems.

Mastoiditis:

May be caused by an ear infection and is known as inflammation of the mastoid.

Meniere's disease:

Inner ear disorder. Causes unknown. Episodic rotational vertigo, Tinnitus, Hearing loss, and Ringing in the ears are key symptoms. Dazide is the primary medication for Meniere's disease. Low salt diet and surgery are also other treatment options. Diagnosis is a rule-out diagnosis.

Labyrinthitis:

Vertigo associated with nausea and malaise. Related to bacterial and viral infections. Inflammation of the labyrinth in the inner ear.

Otitis externa:

Usually caused by a bacterial infection. Swimmer's ear. Infection of the skin with the outer ear canal that progress to the ear drum. Itching, Drainage and Pain are the key symptoms. Suctioning of the ear canal may be necessary. Most common ear drops (Volsol, Cipro, Cortisporin).

Obstetrics/Gynecology

Amniocentesis: Removal of some fluid surrounding the fetus for analysis. Fetus location is identified by US prior to the procedure. Results may take a month.

Used to check for:
Spina bifida
Rh compatibility
Immature lungs
Down syndrome

Chorionic villus sampling: Removal of placental tissue for analysis from the uterus during early pregnancy. US helps guide the procedure. 1-2 weeks get the results. Can be performed earlier than amniocentesis.

Used to check for:
Tay-Sachs disease
Down syndrome
Other disorders

Monitor the patient for:
Infection
Miscarriage
Bleeding

Preeclampsia: presence of protein in the urine, and increased BP during pregnancy. Found in 8% of pregnancies.

Symptoms:

Abnormal Rapid Weight gain
Headaches
Peripheral edema
Nausea
Anxiety
Htn
Low urination frequency

Tests:

Proteinuria
BP check
Weight gain analysis
Thrombocytopenia
Evidence of edema

Treatment:

Deliver the baby
Bed rest
Medications

Induced labor may occur with the following criteria:

Eclampsia
HELLP syndrome
High serum creatinine levels
Prolonged elevated diastolic blood pressure >100mmHg
Thrombocytopenia
Abnormal fetal growth

Eclampsia: seizures occurring during pregnancy, symptoms of pre-eclampsia have worsened. Factors that cause eclampsia vs. pre-eclampsia relatively unknown.

Symptoms:

Weight gain sudden

Seizures

Trauma

Abdominal pain

Pre-eclampsia

Tests:

Check liver function tests

Check BP

Proteinuria presence

Apnea

Treatment:

Magnesium sulfate

Bedrest

BP medications

Induced labor may occur with the following criteria:

Eclampsia

HELLP syndrome

High serum creatinine levels

Prolonged elevated diastolic blood pressure >100mmHg

Thrombocytopenia

Abnormal fetal growth

Amniotic fluid- greatest at 34 weeks gestation.

Functions:

Allows normal lung development

Freedom for movement

Fetus temperature regulation

Trauma prevention

Oligohydramnios: Low levels of amniotic fluid that can cause: fetal abnormalities, ruptured membranes and fetus disorders.

Polyhydamnios: High levels of amniotic fluid that can cause: gestational diabetes and congenital defects.

Polyhydaminos Causes:

Beckwith-Wiedemann syndrome

Hydrops fetalis

Multiple fetus development

Anencephaly

Esophageal atresia

Gastroschisis

Sheehan's syndrome: hypopituitarism caused by uterine hemorrhage during childbirth. The pituitary gland is unable to function due to blood loss.

Symptoms:

Amenorrhea

Fatigue

Unable to breast-feed baby

Anxiety

Decreased BP

Hair loss

Tests:

CT scan of Pituitary gland

Check pituitary hormone levels

Treatment:

Hormone therapy

Breast infections/Mastitis: Infection or inflammation due to bacterial infections. (S. aureus).

Symptoms:

Fever

Nipple pain/discharge

Breast pain

Swelling of the breast

Tests:

Physical examination

Treatment:

Antibiotics

Moist heat

Breast pump

Atrophic vaginitis- low estrogen levels cause inflammation of the vagina. Most common after menopause.

Symptoms:

Pain with intercourse

Itching pain

Vaginal discharge

Vaginal irritation after intercourse

Tests:

Pelvic examination

Treatment:

Hormone therapy

Vaginal lubricant

Cervicitis: infection, foreign bodies,or chemicals that causes inflammation of the cervix.

Symptoms:

Pain with intercourse

Vaginal discharge

Pelvic pain

Vaginal pain

Tests:

Pelvic examination

STD tests

Pap smear

Treatment:

Laser therapy

Antibiotics/antifungals

Cryosurgery

Pelvic inflammatory disease: infection of the fallopian tubes, uterus or ovaries caused by STD's in the majority of cases.

Symptoms:

Vagina l discharge

Fever

Pain with intercourse

Fever

Nausea

Urination painful

LBP

No menstruation

Tests:

Pelvic exam

Laparoscopy

ESR

WBC count

Pregnancy test

Cultures for infection

Treatment:

Antibiotics

Surgery

Toxic shock syndrome: infection of (S. aureus) that causes organ disorders and shock.

Symptoms:

Seizures

Headaches

Hypotension

Fatigue

Multiple organ involvement

Fever

Nausea

Vomiting

Tests:

Check BP

Multiple organ involvement

Treatment:

Dialysis- if kidneys fail

BP medications

IV fluids

Antibiotics

Monitor the patient for:

Kidney failure

Liver failure

Heart failure

Extreme shock

Hirsutism: development of dark areas of hair in women that are uncommon.

Causes:

Cushing's syndrome

Congenital adrenal hyperplasia

Hyperthecosis

PCOS

High Androgen levels

Certain medications

Treatment:

Laser treatment

Birth control medications

Electrolysis

Bleaching

Dysmenorrhea: painful menses.

Symptoms:

Constipation

Nausea

Vomiting

Diarrhea

Tests:

Determine if normal dysmenorhea is occurring.

Pain relief

Anti-inflammatory medications

Endometriosis: abnormal tissue growth outside the uterus.

Symptoms:

Spotting

Infertility

LBP

Periods (painful)

Sexual intercourse painful

Tests:

Pelvic US

Laparoscopy

Pelvic exam.

Treatment:

Progesterone treatment

Pain management

Surgery

Hormone treatment

Synarel treatment

Stress Incontinence: A laugh, sneeze or activity that causes involuntary urination. Urethral sphincter dysfunction.

Tests:

Rectal exam

X-rays

Pad test

Urine analysis

PVR test

Cystoscopy

Pelvic exam

Treatment:

Surgery

Medications (pseudoephedrine/phenylpropanolamine)/Estrogen

Pelvic floor re-training

Fluid intake changes

Urge incontinence- urine loss caused by bladder contraction.

Symptoms:

Frequent urination

Abdominal pain/distention

Tests:

Pelvic exam

X-rays

Cystoscopy

EMG

Pad test

Urinary stress test

PVR test

Genital exam-men

Treatment:

Surgery

Medications-(tolterodine, propatheline, imipramine, tolterodine, terbutaline)

Biofeedback training

Kegel strengthening

Dermatology Review

Atopic Dermatitis:

Scaling, Itching, Redness and Excoriation. Possible lichenification in chronic cases. Most common in young children around the elbow and knees. Adults are more common in neck and knees. May be associated with an allergic disorder, hay fever, or asthma.

Contact Dermatitis:

Itchy, weepy reaction with a foreign substance (Poison Ivy) or lotions. Skin becomes red.

Diaper Rash:

Inflammatory reaction in the region covered by a diaper. This may include chemical allergies, sweat, yeast, or friction irritation.

Ermatitis stasis:

Decreased blood flow the lower legs resulting in a skin irritation, possible ulcer formation.

Onychomycosis:

Fungal infection related to the fingernails or toenails. Often caused by Trichophyton rubrum.

Lichen planus:

Treated with topical corticosteroids. The presence of pink or purple spots on the legs and arms. Lesions are itchy, flat and polygonal. May cause hair loss.

Pityriasis rosea:

A mild to moderate rash that starts as a single pink patch and then numerous patches begin to appear on the skin. This may lead to itching. Found primarily in ages 10-35 years old.

Psoriasis:

An autoimmune disease mediated by T lymphocytes that can lead to arthritis. Generally, treated with UV light, tar soap and topical steroid cream. A reddish rash that can be found in numerous locations.

Stevens-Johnson syndrome:

An allergic reaction that can include rashes, and involve the inside of the mouth. May be due to drug sensitivity. Can lead to uveitis and keratitis. Other factors related to SJS include: pneumonia, fever, myalgia and hepatitis. SJS can be extremely similar to varicella zoster and pemphigus vulgaris conditions. There may also be the presence of herpes virus or Mycoplasma pneumoniae.

Bullous pemphigoid:

Eruptions of the skin caused by the accumulation of antibodies in the basement membrane of the skin. Treated with cortisone creams or internally. Skin biopsy offers definitive diagnosis.

Acne vulgaris:

Oil glands become inflamed, plugged or red. May be treated in moderate to severe cases with anti-inflammatory medications or creams.

Rosacea:

A redness that covers the middle part of the face. Blood vessels in the face dilate. Most common in adults 30-50 years old. Unable to be cured, only treated. May cause long term skin damage is left untreated. Antibiotics are often prescribed.

Seborrheic keratosis:

The development of skin "tags" or the barnacles of old age. Usually found in people over 30 years old. Appear to be tabs growing in groups or individually on your skin. Can be treated with Scrapping, Freezing or Electrosurgery.

Actinic keratosis:

A site that can become cancerous, usually small and rough on the skin that has been exposed to the sun a lot. Usually treated with cryosurgery and photodynamic therapy.

Scabies:

Caused by the human itch mite: Sarcaptes scabies, and identified by presence of raised, red bumps that are itchy. Closer identification with a visual aid will show streaks in the skin created by the mite.

Molluscum contagiosum:

Considered a STD. Small downgrowths called molluscum bodies that include the presence of soft tumors in the skin caused by a virus. Contagious.

Herpes zoster:

Infection caused by the varicella-zoster virus. Can cause chickenpox and then shingles in later years. The virus infects the dosal root ganglia of nerves and can cause intense itching.

St. Anthony's Fire:

Claviceps purpurea (fungus) can cause intense pain in the extremities by causing blood vessels to constrict. Fungus produces ergotamines.

Impetigo:

A skin infection caused by Staph or Streptococcus that causes itchy, red skin and pustules. Treated with topical antibiotics and primarily affects children.

Acanthosis nigricans:

The presence of dark velvety patches of skin around the armpit, back, neck and groin. Can occur with multiple diseases. Has been linked to patients with insulin dysfunction.

Hidradenitis suppurativa:

The presence of numerous abscess in the groin and armpit region.

Melasma:

"Mask of Pregnancy" Changes in the pigmentation of women that are pregnant. Occurs in 50% of all pregnancies.

Urticaria:

Elevated itchy areas that are linked to allergic reactions. May be accompanied with edema and may blanch with touch. "Hives"

Vitiligo:

Loss of melanocytes resulting in skin turning white. Hair in regions affected will also turn white. Primarily identified in ages 10-30.

Several genetic factors involved. May be associated with other more severe autoimmune disorders.

Axial Skeleton

The axial skeleton consists of 80 bones forming the trunk (spine and thorax) and skull.

Vertebral Column: The main trunk of the body is supported by the spine, or vertebral column, which is composed of 26 bones, some of which are formed by the fusion of a few bones. The vertebral column from superior to inferior consists of 7 cervical (neck), 12 thoracic and 5 lumbar vertebrae, as well as a sacrum, formed by fusion of 5 sacral vertebrae, and a coccyx, formed by fusion of 4 coccygeal vertebrae.

Ribs and Sternum: The axial skeleton also contains 12 pairs of *ribs* attached posteriorly to the thoracic vertebrae and anteriorly either directly or via cartilage to the *sternum* (breastbone). The ribs and sternum form the *thoracic cage*, which protects the heart and lungs. Seven pairs of ribs articulate with the sternum (*fixed ribs*) directly, and three do so via cartilage; the two most inferior pairs do not attach anteriorly and are referred to as *floating ribs*.

Skull: The skull consists of 22 bones fused together to form a rigid structure which houses and protects organs such as the brain, auditory apparatus and eyes. The bones of the skull form the *face* and *cranium* (brain case) and consist of 6 single bones (*occipital, frontal, ethmoid, sphenoid, vomer* and *mandible*) and 8 paired bones (*parietal, temporal, maxillary, palatine, zygomatic, lacrimal, inferior concha* and *nasal*). The *lower jaw* or *mandible* is the only movable bone of the skull (head); it articulates with the temporal bones.

Other Parts: Other bones considered part of the axial skeleton are the *middle ear bones* (*ossicles*) and the small U-shaped *hyoid bone* that is suspended in a portion of the neck by muscles and ligaments.

Appendicular Skeleton

The *appendicular skeleton* forms the major internal support of the appendages—the *upper* and *lower extremities* (limbs).

Pectoral Girdle and Upper Extremities: The arms are attached to and suspended from the axial skeleton via the *shoulder* (*pectoral*) *girdle*. The latter is composed of two *clavicles* (*collarbones)* and two *scapulae* (*shoulder blades*). The clavicles articulate with the sternum; the two *sternoclavicular joints* are the only sites of articulation between the trunk and upper extremity.

Each upper limb from distal to proximal (closest to the body) consists

Each upper limb from distal to proximal (closest to the body) consists of hand, wrist, forearm and arm (upper arm). The *hand* consists of 5 *digits* (fingers) and 5 *metacarpal* bones. Each digit is composed of three bones called *phalanges*, except the thumb which has only two bones.

Pelvic Girdle and Lower Extremities: The lower *extremities*, or legs, are attached to the axial skeleton via the *pelvic* or *hip girdle*. Each of the two coxal, or *hip bones* comprising the pelvic girdle is formed by the fusion of three bones—*illium, pubis,* and *ischium*. The coxal bones attach the lower limbs to the trunk by articulating with the sacrum.

THE HUMAN SKELETAL SYSTEM	
Part of the Skeleton	**Number of Bones**
Axial Skeleton	**80**
Skull	22
Ossicles (malleus, incus and stapes)	6
Vertebral column	26
Ribs	24
Sternum	1
Hyoid	1
Appendicular Skeleton	**126**
Upper extremities	64
Lower extremities	62

Characteristics of Bone

Bone is a specialized type of connective tissue consisting of cells (*osteocytes*) embedded in a calcified matrix which gives bone its characteristic hard and rigid nature. Bones are encased by a *periosteum*, a connective tissue sheath. All bone has a central marrow cavity. *Bone marrow* fills the marrow cavity or smaller marrow spaces, depending on the type of bone.

Types of Bone: There are two types of bone in the skeleton: *compact bone* and *spongy* (cancellous) bone.

Compact Bone. Compact bone lies within the periosteum, forms the outer region of bones, and appears dense due to its compact organization. The living osteocytes and calcified matrix are arranged in layers, or *lamellae*. Lamellae may be circularly arranged surrounding a central canal, the *Haversian canal*, which contains small blood vessels.

Spongy Bone. Spongy bone consists of *bars, spicules* or *trabeculae*, which forms a lattice meshwork. Spongy bone is found at the ends of long bones and the inner layer of flat, irregular and short bones. The trabeculae consist of osteocytes embedded in calcified matrix, which in definitive bone has a lamellar nature. The spaces between the trabeculae contain bone marrow.

Bone Cells: The cells of bone are osteocytes, osteoblasts, and osteoclasts. *Osteocytes* are found singly in *lacunae* (spaces) within the calcified matrix and communicate with each other via small canals in the bone known as *canaliculi*. The latter contain osteocyte cell processes. The osteocytes in compact and spongy bone are similar in structure and function.

Osteoblasts are cells which form bone matrix, surrounding themselves with it, and thus are transformed into osteocytes. They arise from undifferentiated cells, such as mesenchymal cells. They are cuboidal cells which line the trabeculae of immature or developing spongy bone.

Osteoclasts are cells found during bone development and remodeling. They are multinucleated cells lying in cavities, *Howship's lacunae*, on the surface of the bone tissue being resorbed. Osteoclasts remove the existing calcified matrix releasing the inorganic or organic components.

Bone Matrix: *Matrix* of compact and spongy bone consists of collagenous fibers and ground substance which constitute the organic component of bone. Matrix also consists of inorganic material which is about 65% of the dry weight of bone. Approximately 85% of the inorganic component consists of calcium phosphate in a crystalline form (hydroxyapatite crystals). Glycoproteins are the main components of the ground substance.

MAJOR TYPES OF HUMAN BONES

Type of Bone	Characteristics	Examples
Long bones	Width less than length	Humerus, radius, ulna, femur, tibia
Short bones	Length and width close to equal in size	Carpal and tarsal bones
Flat bones	Thin flat shape	Scapulae, ribs, sternum, bones of cranium (occipital, frontal, parietal)
Irregular bones	Multifaceted shape	Vertebrae, sphenoid, ethmoid
Sesamoid	Small bones located in tendons of muscles	----------

Joints

The bones of the skeoeton articulate with each other at *joints*, which are variable in structure and function. Some joints are immovable, such as the *sutures* between the bones of the cranium. Others are *slightly movable joints*; examples are the *intervertebral joints* and the *pubic symphysis* (joint between the two pubic bones of the coxal bones).

TYPES OF JOINTS

Joint Type	Characteristic	Example
Ball and socket	Permits all types of movement (abduction, adduction, flexion, extension, circumduction); it is considered a universal joint.	Hips and shoulder joints
Hinge (ginglymus)	Permits motion in one plane only	Elbow and knee, interphalangeal joints
Rotating or pivot	Rotation is only motion permitted	Radius and ulna, atlas and axis (first and second cervical vertebrae)
Plane or gliding	Permits sliding motion	Between tarsal bones and carpal bones
Condylar (condyloid)		

	Permits motion in two planes which are at right angles to each other (rotation is not possible)	Metacarop-phalangeal joints, temporomandibular

Adjacent bones at a joint are connected by fibrous connective tissue bands known as *ligaments*. They are strong bands which support the joint and may also act to limit the degree of motion occurring at a joint.

Musculoskeletal Conditions

Legg-Calve-Perthes disease: poor blood supply to the superior aspect of the femur. Most common in boys ages 4-10. The femur ball flattens out and deteriorates. 4x higher incidence in boys + Bony cresent sign.

Symptoms:
Hip and Knee pain
Limited AROM and PROM
Pain with gait and unequal leg length.

Tests:
X-ray Hip
Test ROM of hip

Treatment:
Surgery
Physical therapy
Brace
Bedrest

Developmental dysplasia of the hip: abnormal development of the hip joint found that is congenital.

Symptoms:
Fat rolls asymmetrical
Abnormal leg length
AROM limited

Tests:
US
X-ray of hips
AROM testing of hips

Treatment:
Cast
Surgery
Physical Therapy

Slipped capital femoral epiphysis: 2x greater incidence in males, most common hip disorder in adolescents. The ball of the femur separates from the femur along the epiphysis.

Symptoms:

Hip pain

Gait dysfunction

Knee pain

Abnormal Hip AROM

Tests:

X-ray

Palpation of the hips

Treatment:

Surgery

Polymyalgia Rheumatica- hip or shoulder pain disorder in people greater than 50 years old.

Symptoms:

Shoulder pain

Hip pain

Fever

Anemia

Fatigue

Tests:

ESR increased

CPK

Hemoglobin low

Treatment:

Pain management

Corticosteroids

Systemic lupus serythemtosus: autoimmune disorder that affects joints, skin and various organ systems. Chronic and inflammatory. 9x more common in females.

Symptoms:
Butterfly rash
Weight loss
Fever
Hair loss
Abdominal pain
Mouth sores
Fatigue
Seizures
Arthritis
Nausea
Joint pain
Psychosis

Tests:
CBC
Chest X-ray
ANA test
Skin rash observation
Coombs' test
Urine analysis
Test for various antibodies

Treatment:
NSAIDS
Protective clothing
Cytotoxic drugs
Hydroxychloroquine

Monitor the patient for:
Seizures
Infection
Hemolytic anemia
Myocarditis
Infection
Renal failure

Scleroderma: connective tissue disease that is diffuse.

Symptoms:
Wheezing
Heartburn
Raynaud's phenomenon

Skin thickness changes

Weight loss

Joint pain

SOB

Hair loss

Bloating

Tests:

Monitor skin changes

Chest x-ray

Antinuclear antibody test

ESR increased

Monitor the patient for:

Renal failure

Heart failure

Pulmonary fibrosis

Rheumatoid Arthritis: inflammatory autoimmune disease that affects various tissues and joints.

Symptoms:

Fever

Fatigue

Joint pain and swelling

ROM decreased

Hand/Feet deformities

Numbness

Skin color changes

Tests:

Rheumatoid factor tests

C-reactive protein

Synovial fluid exam

X-rays of involved joints

ESR increased

Treatment:

Physical therapy

Moist heat

Anti-inflammatory drugs

Corticosteroids

Anti-malarial drugs

Cox-2 inhibitors

Splinting

Juvenile Rheumatoid Arthritis: inflammatory disease that occurs in children.

Types:
Pauciarticular JRA- 50%
Polyarticular JRA- 40%
Systemic JRA- 10%

Symptoms:
Painful joints
Eye inflammation
Fever
Rash
Temperature changes (joints)
Poor AROM

Tests:
ANA test
HLA antigen test
CBC
Physical exam of joints
X-rays of joints
Eye exam
RA factor test

Treatment:
Physical therapy
Corticosteroids
NSAIDS
Infliximab
Hydrochloroquine
Methotrexate

Paget's disease: abnormal bone development that follows bone destruction.

Symptoms:
Joint pain
Bow legged appearance
Hearing loss
Neck and back pain
Headaches
Sharp bone pain

Tests:
Increased alkaline phophatase levels

X-rays- abnormal bone development.

Bone scan

Treatment:

NSAIDS

Calcitonin

Plicamycin

Etidronate

Tiludronate

Surgery

Monitor the patient for:

Spinal deformities

Hear loss

Paraplegia

Heart failure

Fractures

Osteoarthritis: chronic condition affecting the joint cartilage that may result in bone spurs being formed in the joints.

Symptoms:

Join pain

Morning stiffness

Limited AROM

Weight bearing increases symptoms

Tests:

X-ray

Passive testing of joints

Treatment:

Physical therapy

Cox 2 inhibitors

NSAIDS

Joint injections

Aquatic exercises

Surgery

Gout: uric acid development in the joints causing arthritis.

Stages:

Asymptomatic

Acute

Intercritical

Chronic

Symptoms:

Joint edema

Fever

Lower extremity and/or upper extremity joint pain

Tests:

Uric acid in the urine

Synovial biopsy

Synovial analysis

Monitor the patient for:

Kidney stones

Kidney disorders

Fibromyalgia: joint, muscle and soft tissue pain in numerous locations. Presence of tender points and soft tissue pain.

Symptoms:

Fatigue

Body aches

Poor exercise capacity

Muscle/Joint pain

Tests:

Rule-out diagnosis.

Treatment:

Anti-depressants

Physical therapy

Stress Management

Massage

Support group

Duchenne muscular dystrophy: Genetically X-linked recessive type of muscular dystrophy that starts in the lower extremities. Dystrophin-protein dysfunction.

Symptoms:

Falls

Fatigue

Muscle weakness

Gait dysfunction

Scoliosis

Joint contractures

Tests:

CPK levels increased

Cardiac testing

EMG

Muscle biopsy testing

Treatment:

Physical therapy

Braces

Mobility assistance

Monitor the patient for:

Contractures

Pneumonia

Respiratory failure

CHF

Cardiomyopathy

Limited mobility

Ankylosing spondylitis: Vertebrae of the spine fuse.

Symptoms:

Limited AROM

Back and neck pain

Joint edema

Fever Weight loss

Tests:

X-ray spine

CBC

ESR test

NSAIDS

Surgery

HLA-B27 antigen test

Monitor the patient for:

Pulmonary fibrosis

Aortic valve stenosis

Uveitis

Compartment syndrome: impaired blood flow and nerve dysfunction caused by nerve and blood vessel compression.

Symptoms:

Severe pain

Weakness

Skin color changes

Tests:

Muscular length testing

Treatment:

Surgery

Physical Therapy

Osteosarcoma: bone tumor that is malignant and found in adolescents.

Symptoms:

Bone pain

Fractures

Swelling

Tests:

CT scan

X-ray

Biopsy

Bone scan

Treatment:

Chemotherapy

Surgery

Special Report- High Frequency Terms

The following terms were compiled as high frequency NCLEX test terms. I recommend printing out this list and identifying the terms you are unfamiliar with. Then, use a medical dictionary or the internet to look up the terms you have questions about. Take one section per day if you have the time to maximize recall.

A

Acquired immunodeficiency syndrome
Acromegaly
Acute lymphoblastic leukemia
Acute myelogenous leukemia
Acute nonlymphocytic leukemia
Adenocarcinoma
Adjuvant disease
Agoraphobia
Alopecia
Alzheimer's dementia
Amebiasis
Amenorrhea
Amyloidosis
Anastomoses
Aneurysm
Angina pectoris
Angiogenesis
Anklyosing spondylitis
Anxiety
Appendicitis
Arterial disease
Arteriosclerosis
Arthralgia
Arthritis bacterial
Arthritis (Crohn's disease)
Arthritis (gouty)
Arthritis (Reiter's syndrome)
Arthritis (Rheumatoid arthritis
Atypical angina
Avascular necrosis
AZT

B

Barrett's oesophagus
Back pain (Sciatica)
Back pain (tumor)
Barlow's syndrome
Basal cell carcinoma
Behçet's disease
Benign prostate hypertrophy
Biliary disease
Bilirubin
Biliverdin
Blood cultures
Boerhaave's syndrome
Bornholm disease
Bowen's disease
Bradycardia
Braxton-Hicks contractions
Bronchiectasis
Budd-Chiari syndrome
Buerger's disease
Bulimia
Burkitt Lymphoma

C

CAD
Cancer (basal cell)
Cancer (pancreatic)
Cancer (prostate)
Cancer (squamous cell)
Candidiasis
Cardiac disease
Cardiac valvular disease
Carpal tunnel syndrome
Catecholamines
Cauda equina syndrome

Gestatoin
Giant cell tumor
Gilbert's syndrome
Gliosis
Glucagon
Glucose tolerance test
Goodpasture's syndrome
Graves disease
Guillai-Barre' syndrome
Gynecomastia

H

Haemochromatosis
Hand-foot syndrome
Hashimoto's thyroiditis
Hartmann's solution
Heart failure
Heart rate
Helper T cells
Hemarthrosis
Hematuria
Hemophilia
Hemorrhage
Henoch-Schönlein syndrome
Heparin
Hepatic encephalopathy
Hepatitis (A-E)
Herpes zoster
Hiatal hernia
Hirschsprung's disease
HIV
Hodgkin's disease
Homans sign
Homocystinuria
Hormone replacement therapy
Huntington's chorea
Hurler's syndrome
Hunter's syndrome
Hyalinization
Hypercortisolism
Hyperglycemia
Hyperplasia
Hyperparathyroidism
Hypnotic preparations
Hypochromia
Hyponatremia
Hypothyroidism
Hypoxia
Hysterectomy

I

IBD Inflammatory bowel disease
IBS Irritable bowel syndrome
Immune serum globulin
Immunoglobulins (IgE, IgG, IgM)
Inderal
Induration
Infectious arthritis
Inflammatory bowel disease
Inhibitors
Interferon
Interleukin (I), (II)
Interstitial cystitis
Intramedullary tumors
Iridocyclitis
Ischemic Heart Disease
Isographs
Isotonic solution

J

Jaundice
Joint pain (gout)
Joint pain (psoriatic arthritis)
Joint sepsis
Jevenile rheumatoid arthritis

K

Kaposi's sarcoma
Kawasaki disease
Kehr's sign
Kernicterus
Ketoacidosis
Kidney failure
Kidney stones
Kleihauer test

Definition of Root Words

A

abdomin/o abdomen
acou/o hearing
aden/o gland
adenoid/o adenoids
adren/o adrenal gland
alveol/o alveolus
amni/o amnion
andro/o male
angi/o vessel
ankly/o stiff
anter/o frontal
an/o anus
aponeur/o aponeurosis
appendic/o appendix
arche/o beginning
arteri/o artery
atri/o atrium
aur/i ear
aur/o ear
aut/o self

B

bacteri/o bacteria
balan/o glans penis
bi/o life
blephar/o eyelid
bronch/i bronchus
bronch/o bronchus

C

calc/i calcium
cancer/o cancer
carcin/o cancer
cardi/o heart
carp/o carpals
caud/o tail
cec/o cecum
celi/o abdomen
cephal/o head
cerebell/o cerebellum
cerebr/o cerebrum
cervic/o cervix
cheil/o lip
cholangi/o bile duct

chol/e gall
chondro/o cartilage
chori/o chorion
chrom/o color
clavic/o clavicle
col/o colon
colp/o vagina
core/o pupil
corne/o cornea
coron/o heart
cortic/o cortex
cor/o pupil
cost/o rib
crani/o cranium
cry/o cold
cutane/o skin
cyes/i pregnancy
cyst/o bladder

D

dacry/o tear
dermat/o skin
diaphragmat/o diaphragm
dipl/o double
dips/o thirst
dist/o distal
diverticul/o diverticulum
dors/o back
duoden/o duodenum
dur/o dura

E

ech/o sound
electr/o electricity
embry/o embryo
encephal/o brain
endocrin/o endocrine
enter/o intestine
epididym/o epididymis
epiglott/o epiglottis
episi/o vulva
epitheli/o epithelium
erythr/o red
esophag/o esophagus
esthesi/o sensation

F

femor/o femur
fet/i fetus
fet/o fetus
fibr/o fibrous tissue
fibul/o fibula

G

ganglion/o ganglion
gastr/o stomach
gingiv/o gum
glomerul/o glomerulus
gloss/o tongue
glyc/o sugar
gnos/o knowledge
gravid/o pregnancy
gynec/o woman

H

hem/o blood
hepat/o liver
herni/o hernia
heter/o other
hidr/o sweat
hist/o tissue
humer/o humerus
hydr/o water
hymen/o hymen
hyster/o uterus

I

ile/o ileum
ili/o ilium
irid/o iris
iri/o iris
ischi/o ischium
ischo/o blockage

J

jejun/o jejunum

K

kal/i potassium
kary/o nucleus
kerat/o hard
kinesi/o motion
kyph/o hump

L

lacrim/o tear duct
lact/o milk
lamin/o lamina
lapar/o abdomen
later/o lateral
lei/o smooth
leuk/o white
lingu/o tongue
lip/o fat
lith/o stone
lob/o lob/o
lord/o flexed forward
lumb/o lumbar
lymph/o lymph

M

mamm/o breast
mandibul/o mandible
mast/o breast
mastoid/o mastoid
maxill/o maxilla
meat/o opening
melan/o black
mening/o meninges
menisc/o meniscus
men/o menstruation
ment/o mind
metr/i uterus
metr/o uterus
mon/o one
muc/o mucus
myc/o fungus
myel/o spinal cord
my/o muscle

N

nas/o nose
nat/o birth
necr/o death
nephr/o kidney
neur/o nerve
noct/i night

O

ocul/o eye
olig/o few
omphal/o navel
onc/o tumor
onych/o nail
oophor/o ovary
ophthalm/o eye
opt/o vision
orchid/o testicle
orch/o testicle
organ/o organ
or/o mouth
orth/o straight
oste/o bone
ot/o ear
ox/i oxygen

P

pachy/o	thick
palat/o	palate
pancreat/o	pancreas
par/o	labor
patell/o	patella
path/o	disease
pelv/i	pelvis
perine/o	peritoneum
petr/o	stone
phalang/o	pharynx
phas/o	speech
phleb/o	vein
phot/o	light
phren/o	mind
plasm/o	plasma
pleur/o	pleura
pneumon/o	lung
poli/o	gray matter
polyp/o	small growth
poster/o	posterior
prim/i	first
proct/o	rectum
proxim/o	proximal
pseud/o	fake
psych/o	mind
pub/o	pubis
puerper/o	childbirth
pulmon/o	lung
pupill/o	pupil
pyel/o	renal pelvis
pylor/o	pylorus
py/o	pus

Q

quadr/i	four

R

rachi/o	spinal
radic/o	nerve
radi/o	radius
rect/o	rectum
ren/o	kidney
retin/o	retina
rhabd/o	striated
rhytid/o	wrinkles
rhiz/o	nerve

S

sacr/o	sacrum
scapul/o	scapula
scler/o	sclera
scoli/o	curved
seb/o	sebum
sept/o	septum
sial/o	saliva
sinus/o	sinus
somat/o	body
son/o	sound
spermat/o	sperm
spir/o	breathe
splen/o	spleen
spondyl/o	vertebra
staped/o	stapes
staphyl/o	clusters
stern/o	sternum
steth/o	chest
stomat/o	mouth
strept/o	chain-like
super/o	superior
synovi/o	synovia

T

tars/o	tarsal
ten/o	tendon
test/o	testicle
therm/o	heat
thorac/o	thorax

thromb/o clot
thym/o thymus
thyroid/o thyroid gland
tibi/o tibia
tom/o pressure
tonsill/o tonsils
toxic/o poison
trachel/o trachea
trich/o hair
tympan/o eardrum

U

uln/o ulna
ungu/o nail
ureter/o ureter
urethr/o urethra
ur/o urine
uter/o uterus
uvul/o uvula

V

vagin/o vagina
valv/o valve
vas/o vessel
ven/o vein
ventricul/o ventricle
ventro/o frontal
vertebr/o vertebra
vesic/o bladder
vesicul/o seminal vesicle

Prefixes

an- without
ante- before
bi- two
brady- slow
dia- through
dys- difficult
endo- within
epi- over
eu- normal
exo- outward
hemi- half
hyper- excessive
hypo- deficient
inter- between
intra- within
meta- change

multi-	numerous
nulli-	none
pan-	total
para-	beyond
per-	through
peri-	surrounding
post-	after
pre-	before
pro-	before
sub-	below
supra-	superior
sym-	join
syn-	join
tachy-	rapid
tetra-	four
trans-	through

Suffixes

-al	pertaining to
-algia	pain
-apheresis	removal
-ary	pertaining to
-asthenia	weakness
-capnia	carbon dioxide
-cele	hernia
-clasia	break
-clasis	break
-crit	separate
-cyte	cell
-desis	fusion
-drome	run
-eal	pertaining to
-ectasis	expansion
-ectomy	removal
-esis	condition
-genesis	cause
-genic	pertaining to
-gram	record
-graph	recording device
-ial	pertaining to
-iasis	condition
-iatrist	physician
-iatry	specialty
-ic	pertaining to
-ician	one that
-ictal	attack
-ior	pertaining to
-ism	condition of
-itis	inflammation
-lysis	separating
-malacia	softening
-meter	measure
-odynia	pain
-oid	resembling
-ology	study
-oma	tumor
-opia	vision
-opsy	view of
-orrhaphy	repairing
-orrhea	flow
-osis	condition
-otomy	cut into
-oxia	oxygen
-paresis	partial paralysis
-pathy	disease
-pepsia	digestion
-pexy	suspension
-phagia	swallowing, eating
-phobia	excessive fear of
-phonia	sound, voice
-physis	growth
-plasia	development
-plasm	a growth
-plegia	paralysis
-pnea	breathing
-poiesis	formation
-ptosis	sagging
-salpinx	fallopian tube
-sacoma	malignant tumor
-schisis	crack
-sclerosis	hardening
-stasis	standing
-stenosis	narrowing
-thorax	chest
-tocia	labor, birth
-tome	cutting device
-trophy	develop
-uria	urine